INTERNATIONAL DIETETICS AND NUTRITION TERMINOLOGY (IDNT) REFERENCE MANUAL:

Standardized Language for the Nutrition Care Process

First Edition

INTERNATIONAL DIETETICS AND NUTRITION TERMINOLOGY (IDNT)
REFERENCE MANUAL: Standardized Language for the Nutrition Care Process
First Edition

ISBN: 978-0-88091-417-8

10 9 8 7 6 5 4 3

INTERNATIONAL DIETETICS AND NUTRITION TERMINOLOGY (IDNT) REFERENCE MANUAL:
Standardized Language for the Nutrition Care Process
First Edition

Table of Contents

Please check the ADA Web site (http://www.eatright.org/cps/rde/xchg/ada/hs.xsl/career_9706_ENU_HTML.htm).
Sign in as a member and select Practice from the sidebar and then Nutrition Care Process and Model Resources.

Edition: 2008

Publication Highlights

PUBLICATIONS RELATED TO THE NUTRITION CARE PROCESS

Since the Nutrition Care Process and Model development, the American Dietetic Association (ADA) has printed several publications related to the Nutrition Care Process. Two *Journal of the American Dietetic Association* articles and three publications have been issued regarding the Nutrition Care Process and Model since 2002. The original article published in the 2003 *Journal* described the complete nutrition care process (1). Another 2005 *Journal* article described the implementation of Nutrition Diagnosis, Step 2 in the nutrition care process (2).

The first publication, entitled *Nutrition Diagnosis: A Critical Step in the Nutrition Care Process,* examined only Nutrition Diagnosis (3). In a follow-up publication, *Nutrition Diagnosis and Intervention: Standardized Language for the Nutrition Care Process,* the standardized languages for two of the four steps, nutrition diagnosis and nutrition intervention, were defined and a nutrition assessment matrix was created from the nutrition diagnoses reference sheets (4). This publication contains all four steps in the nutrition care process, with standardized taxonomies for nutrition diagnosis, nutrition intervention, and nutrition monitoring and evaluation. It represents the first revision to the nutrition diagnoses, comprehensive information and reference sheets about nutrition counseling in the nutrition intervention section, and a standardized language for monitoring and evaluation. Various tools (e.g., reference sheets, patient/client examples, camera-ready pocket guides) are included for practitioners to implement the process in their practice.

NEW IN THIS PUBLICATION

The **Nutrition Assessment** section is **REVISED** and reflects the changes to the assessment data matrix associated with the revisions to the nutrition diagnoses. The Standardized Language Committee will articulate and publish a nutrition assessment taxonomy in a future edition of this publication.

The **Nutrition Diagnosis** section is **REVISED** and represents the first substantive changes to the nutrition diagnoses based upon research findings and member recommendations.

They include:
- Deletion of two previously published nutrition diagnoses
- Deletion of individual Etiologies or Signs/Symptoms
- Addition of individual Etiologies or Signs/Symptoms
- Revision of individual Definitions, Etiologies, or Signs/Symptoms

Refer to the section on nutrition diagnoses for additional information.

The **Nutrition Intervention** section is **ENHANCED** with detailed information in the introduction and reference sheets for the nutrition counseling section of nutrition intervention. Education on skill development was added to nutrition education section of nutrition intervention. This additional information was developed in response to member requests, and is filled with practice and research potential.

The **Nutrition Monitoring and Evaluation** section is **NEW**. The ADA has developed a language and methodology to aid in standardizing the practitioner's approach to the nutrition monitoring and evaluation step of the nutrition care process. Within nutrition monitoring and evaluation, practitioners monitor progress and measure and evaluate the nutrition care outcomes achieved by the patient/client.

Monitor progress
- Check patient/client's understanding and compliance with nutrition intervention
- Determine if the intervention is being implemented as prescribed
- Provide evidence that the nutrition intervention is or is not changing the patient/client's behavior or status
- Identify other positive or negative outcomes
- Gather information indicating reasons for lack of progress
- Support conclusions with evidence

Measure outcomes
- Select the nutrition care outcome indicator(s) (markers) to measure the desired outcome(s)
- Use standardized nutrition care outcome indicator(s) to increase the validity and reliability of the measurements of change

Evaluate outcomes
- Compare monitoring data with the nutrition prescription/goals or reference standards to assess progress and determine future action

The nutrition monitoring and evaluation reference sheets, in this publication, identify nutrition care outcomes and specific indicators are based on scientific literature. They provide guidance to practitioners for measuring and evaluating nutrition outcomes.

ALSO NEW IN THIS PUBLICATION

Each step in the process has a **NEW** *SNAPshot* document. These were developed to see, at-a-glance, a quick summary of the key concepts within the steps.

The ***Bibliography*** is a **NEW** document in the publication that lists the publications, *Journal* articles, and web resources related to the nutrition care process and standardized language.

NOT INCLUDED IN THIS PUBLICATION

Details and the rational for changes to the Nutrition Diagnoses are available in the Nutrition Care Process and Model Resource section of the ADA website, www.eatright.org, in the either the Research or Practice sections. Each nutrition diagnosis reference sheet that was modified includes a notation on the last page indicating the publication year in which it was updated, e.g., Updated: 2008 Edition. Editorial changes, not affecting the content, were not included in the document.

Case Studies A and B, published previously, have been **REVISED** to include the nutrition monitoring and evaluation. Case Study A has **EXPANDED** nutrition counseling information utilizing the new nutrition intervention reference sheet terminology. Case Study C is a **NEW** case example of how nutrition monitoring and evaluation is utilized for performance improvement. All three of the Case Studies are available in the Nutrition Care Process and Model Resource section of the ADA Web site, www.eatright.org, in the either the Research or Practice sections.

The *Scope of Dietetics Practice Framework, Standards of Practice in Nutrition Care and Updated Standards of Professional Performance*, and the *Standards of Practice in Nutrition Care Appendix* have been **REMOVED** from the publication and are available on the ADA Web site, www.eatright.org, in the either the Research or Practice Sections.

REFERENCES

1. Lacey K, Pritchett E. Nutrition care process and model: ADA adopts road map to quality care and outcomes management. *J Am Diet Assoc.* 2003;103:1061-1072.
2. Mathieu J, Foust M, Ouellette P. Implementing nutrition diagnosis, step two in the nutrition care process and model: Challenges and lesions learned in two health care facilities. *J Am Diet Assoc.* 2005;105:1636-1640.
3. American Dietetic Association. *Nutrition Diagnosis: A Critical Step in the Nutrition Care Process.* Chicago, IL: American Dietetic Association; 2006.
4. American Dietetic Association. *Nutrition Diagnosis and Intervention: Standardized Language for the Nutrition Care Process.* Chicago, IL: American Dietetic Association; 2007.

Nutrition Care Process Summary

INTRODUCTION

Continually emerging from the American Dietetic Association's (ADA) strategic plan are priority actions that guide work groups and taskforces in creating tools to advance the dietetics profession. In 2002, to achieve the Association's strategic goals of promoting demand for dietetics practitioners and help them be more competitive in the marketplace, the ADA Quality Management Committee appointed the Nutrition Care Model Workgroup. This Workgroup developed the Nutrition Care Process and Model, a systematic process describing how dietetics practitioners provide care with patients/clients (1).

The nutrition care process is designed to improve the consistency and quality of individualized patient/client care and the predictability of the patient/client outcomes. It is not intended to standardize nutrition care for each patient/client but to establish a standardized process for providing care.

> **Special Note.** The terms **patient/client** are used in association with the NCP; however, the process is also intended for use with groups. In addition, family members or caregivers are an essential asset to the patient/client and dietetic practitioner in the NCP. Therefore, **groups, families, and caregivers** of patients/clients are implied each time a reference is made to patient/client.

There are four steps in the process—Nutrition Assessment, Nutrition Diagnosis, Nutrition Intervention, and Nutrition Monitoring and Evaluation. Three of the nutrition care process steps are very familiar to dietetics practitioners and nutrition textbooks skillfully cover their content—nutrition assessment, nutrition intervention, and nutrition monitoring and evaluation. However, the Workgroup identified a less well-defined aspect of nutrition care: nutrition diagnosis. Further, it recognized that a standard taxonomy for the second step in the process would greatly enhance the profession's ability to document, communicate, and research its impact.

As a result, the ADA's Standardized Language Task Force was formed to create a taxonomy for the profession's unique nutrition diagnosis language. The language was described during presentations at the 2005 Food and Nutrition Conference and Exhibition and made available in a publication at that meeting (2). The follow-up publication, *Nutrition Diagnosis and Intervention: Standardized Language for the Nutrition Care Process*, was published in 2007 (3). The nutrition diagnosis language is undergoing study in a number of research projects. This publication incorporates the first substantive changes to the nutrition diagnosis terminology. Future modifications will be made based on the results of the additional research.

The Standardized Language Task Force has examined in depth three of the four steps and developed and published standardized languages for: nutrition diagnosis, nutrition intervention, and now nutrition monitoring and evaluation. Through the committee's exploration of nutrition monitoring and evaluation, it is clear that there is substantial overlap between nutrition assessment and nutrition monitoring and evaluation. Many data points may be the same or related; however, the data purpose and use are distinct in these two steps. We anticipate needing to add terms for Nutrition Assessment that are necessary to diagnose a nutrition problem, but would not be used for evaluating the impact of the nutrition intervention in the nutrition monitoring and evaluation step. Therefore, this publication illustrates a nearly complete language for describing the nutrition care process for nutrition practitioners and provides tools for practitioners to implement the process into their practice.

NUTRITION CARE PROCESS STEPS

Step 1. Nutrition Assessment

Nutrition assessment is the first step in the process and is a method for obtaining, verifying, and interpreting data that is needed to identify a nutrition-related problem. From the nutrition assessment data, the dietetic practitioner is able to determine whether a nutrition diagnosis/problem exists. This step, while well known to dietetics practitioners, would be greatly enhanced by use of standardized nutrition assessment language for communicating about patients/clients with similar disorders.

More effective comparison of nutrition assessment findings would be achieved with a standardized language. Thus, the Standardized Language Task Force will focus its efforts to describe the differences between nutrition assessment and nutrition monitoring and evaluation, which will be published in the future. Many opportunities for research exist in nutrition assessment, which will result in improved determinations of the most appropriate nutrition assessment data to use for individuals and populations and practice settings.

Step 2: Nutrition Diagnosis

Nutrition diagnosis is a critical step between nutrition assessment and nutrition intervention. The purpose of a standardized nutrition diagnosis language is to describe consistently nutrition problems so that they are clear within and outside the profession. The standard language will enhance communication and documentation of nutrition care, and it will provide a minimum data set and common data elements for future research.

In simple terms, a nutrition practitioner identifies and labels a specific nutrition diagnosis (problem) that, in general, he or she is responsible for treating independently (e.g., excessive carbohydrate intake). With nutrition intervention, the nutrition diagnosis ideally resolves, **or at least the signs and symptoms improve.** In contrast, a medical diagnosis describes a disease or pathology of organs or body systems (e.g., diabetes). In some instances, such as the nutrition diagnosis Swallowing Difficulty NC-1.1, nutrition practitioners are labeling or diagnosing the functional problem that has a nutritional consequence. Nutrition practitioners do not identify medical diagnoses; they diagnose phenomena in the nutrition domain.

ADA's Standardized Language Task Force developed a framework that outlines three domains—Clinical, Intake, and Behavioral-Environmental—within which the nutrition diagnoses/problems fall. With the changes incorporated from the research studies and recommendations accepted by the Task Force, sixty nutrition diagnoses/problems have been identified. A reference was developed and it describes each nutrition diagnosis and incorporates expert input (2).

It is this step in the nutrition care process that results in the documentation of the nutrition diagnosis statement or PES statement. This statement is composed of three distinct components: the problem (P), the etiology (E) and the signs and symptoms (S). The PES statement is derived from the synthesis of information from the nutrition assessment data.

Step 3: Nutrition Intervention

Nutrition intervention is the third step in the nutrition care process. Nutrition interventions are specific actions used to remedy a nutrition diagnosis/problem, and can be used with individuals, a group, or the community at large. These nutrition interventions are intended to change a nutrition-related behavior, environmental condition, or aspect of nutritional health. A dietetics practitioner collaborates, whenever possible, with the patient/client(s) and other health care providers during the nutrition intervention.

Nutrition intervention consists of two interrelated components—planning and implementation. Planning involves prioritizing the nutrition diagnoses; conferring with the patient, others, and practice guides and policies; jointly establishing goals; and defining the nutrition prescription and identifying specific nutrition intervention(s). Implementing the nutrition intervention is the action phase, which includes carrying out and communicating the plan of care, continuing the data collection, and revising the nutrition intervention, as warranted, based on the patient/client response. This step cannot be completed unless both components are in place to support the nutrition intervention.

The nutrition intervention is, almost always, aimed at the etiology (E) of the nutrition diagnosis/problem identified in the PES statement. In very specific instances, the nutrition intervention is directed at reducing the effects of the signs and symptoms (S) to reduce the signs and symptoms. Generally, the signs and symptoms form the basis for the next step in the nutrition care process: nutrition monitoring and evaluation (Step 4).

Four domains of nutrition intervention have been identified—Food and/or Nutrient Delivery, Nutrition Education, Nutrition Counseling, and Coordination of Care. The terminology is defined and reference sheets for each specific nutrition intervention are available for use by the profession. It is believed that the information necessary for medical record documentation, billing, and the description of the nutrition interventions for research are included in the terminology.

A dietetics practitioner will note that while some interventions are closely related (e.g., education and counseling), the terms are intentionally separated to distinguish between them. Additionally, specific descriptors of a nutrition intervention encounter (i.e., interactions, visits, contacts, sessions) are provided to assist a dietetics practitioner with the details of his/her encounters with patient/client(s). Examples of descriptors include encounters with individuals or groups, face to face or electronically, and the degree to which the dietetics practitioner is responsible for the patient/client care, to name a few.

Step 4: Nutrition Monitoring and Evaluation

The purpose of nutrition monitoring and evaluation is to determine the amount of progress made by the patient/client and if goals are being met. Nutrition monitoring and evaluation tracks patient/client outcomes relevant to the nutrition diagnosis and intervention plans and goals. Nutrition care outcomes—the desired results of nutrition care—have been defined, and specific indicators that can be measured and compared to established criteria have been identified.

Selecting the appropriate nutrition care indicators is determined by the nutrition diagnosis and its etiology and signs or symptoms and the nutrition intervention used. The medical diagnosis and health care outcome goals, and quality management goals for nutrition also influence which nutrition care outcome indicators are chosen. Other factors, such as practice setting, patient/client population, and disease state and/or severity also affect the indicator selection.

The nutrition monitoring and evaluation outcomes are organized in four domains: Nutrition-Related Behavioral and Environmental Outcomes, Food and Nutrient Intake Outcomes, Nutrition-Related Physical Sign and Symptom Outcomes, and Nutrition-Related Patient/Client-Centered Outcomes.

During this step, dietetics practitioners monitor the patient/client progress by determining whether the nutrition intervention is being implemented and by providing evidence that the nutrition intervention is or is not *changing* the patient/client behavior or nutrition/health status. Dietetics practitioners measure the outcomes by selecting the appropriate nutrition care outcome indicator(s) and comparing the findings with previous status, nutrition intervention goals, and/or reference standards. The use of standardized indicators and criteria increases the validity and reliability of the outcome data and their collection facilitates electronic charting, coding, and outcomes measurement.

NUTRITION CARE PROCESS AND MEDICAL NUTRITION THERAPY

The nutrition care process and medical nutrition therapy (MNT) are not synonymous terms. MNT is one type of nutrition care, whereas the nutrition care process describes the approach to a spectrum of nutrition care. The nutrition care process defines specific steps a dietetics practitioner uses when providing MNT. Other activities, such as referral to a community program, are not MNT, but use the same nutrition care process.

Edition: 2008

IMPLEMENTATION OF THE NUTRITION CARE PROCESS AND FUTURE DIRECTIONS

Publications and Resources

This publication represents the third major publication related to the nutrition care process in three years. Several exciting research projects are ongoing, including pilot tests of individual steps as well as multiple steps in the nutrition care process, which will influence future publications of this reference manual.

Dietetics practitioners across the country are implementing the nutrition care process. This reference manual provides extensive detail and explanation about the standardized language for dietetics. For a portable resource with essential excerpts from the reference manual, the ADA has created a companion publication—*Pocket Guide for the International Dietetics and Nutrition Terminology Reference Manual, First Edition.*

At this time, three *Toolkits* are available from ADA for the on-line Evidence-Based Nutrition Practice Guidelines, based upon evidence analyses (4-6). They contain sample forms and examples incorporating the terms in the nutrition care process steps. These are available for purchase from ADA for dietetic practitioners to use at the "Store" tab at www.adaevidencelibrary.com. Dietetics practitioners may find useful the extensive resources provided on the ADA Web site, www.eatright.org, in the either the Research or Practice sections.

Members have completed numerous presentations and newsletter articles for national, state, and Dietetic Practice Group audiences, with nearly 8,000 individuals reached through presentations thus far. ADA also facilitates a peer network of dietetics practitioners who are leading the way in implementing the nutrition care process in their facilities and communities.

ADA is moving ahead in a variety of ways to implement the standardized language of the nutrition care process. In addition to numerous association activities, there are applications in the broader dietetics and medical communities.

International Information Sharing and Standardized Medical Languages

In 2005, the ADA Foundation funded an ADA hosted meeting to expand the dialogue with other international dietetic associations about ADA's standardized nutrition diagnosis language and similar efforts other associations have made. The meeting also initiated a dialogue between the foremost medical informatics organizations and the international nutrition and dietetics community. As a result of this dialogue:

- A presentation regarding the nutrition care process has been accepted at the XV International Congress of Dietetics, September 8 - 11, 2008 in Yokohama, Japan.
- The Dietitians Association of Australia has initiated a research study evaluating the face validity of the Nutrition Diagnoses.
- The Dutch Association of Dietitians (Nederlandse Vereniging van Diëtisten) has requested permission to use the Nutrition Diagnoses in their health care databases.

Indeed, as the world moves fully into electronic health care records, health informatics, and common databases, the international community of nutrition and dietetics practitioners have the opportunity to work in partnership with the medical informatics organizations to ensure that data elements critical to capturing nutrition care are included in databases and collected in a consistent way.

ADA is working toward including the concepts from the nutrition care process and the specific terms in standards for electronic health records and incorporation into standardized informatics languages, such as the Systematized Nomenclature of Medicine International (SNOMED), Logical Observation Identifiers Names and Codes (LOINC), and United Medical Language System (UMLS). ADA has already begun the dialogue with these groups to let them know the direction that the Association is headed and to keep them appraised of progress. Thus far, the feedback from the database and informatics groups has been quite positive, and they have expressed a need for documenting the unique nature of nutrition services.

SUMMARY

This publication contains all four steps in the nutrition care process, with a standardized taxonomy for nutrition diagnosis, nutrition intervention, and nutrition monitoring and evaluation. It represents the first revision to the nutrition diagnoses, enhanced information about nutrition counseling in the nutrition intervention section, and a new nutrition language for monitoring and evaluation. Various tools (e.g., reference sheets, patient/client examples, camera-ready pocket guides) are included for dietetics practitioners to implement the process in their practice. Future publications will provide a new taxonomy for nutrition assessment and revisions to the other steps based upon research findings.

From conception of the nutrition care process in 2002 through its implementation now, the Standardized Language Task Force continues to update ADA's House of Delegates, the Board of Directors, and members through reports, articles, presentations, publications, and the ADA Web site.

However, to see the strategic goals of an increased demand for dietetics practitioners who are more competitive in the marketplace come to fruition, practitioners need to take a historic step by implementing the nutrition care process today.

REFERENCES

1. Lacey K, Pritchett E. Nutrition care process and model: ADA adopts road map to quality care and outcomes management. *J Am Diet Assoc.* 2003;103:1061-1072.
2. American Dietetic Association. *Nutrition Diagnosis: A Critical Step in the Nutrition Care Process.* Chicago, IL: American Dietetic Association; 2006.
3. American Dietetic Association. *Nutrition Diagnosis and Intervention: Standardized Language for the Nutrition Care Process.* Chicago, IL: American Dietetic Association; 2007.
4. American Dietetic Association. Critical illness evidence-based nutrition guideline, 2006. Available at: http://www.adaevidencelibrary.com/topic.cfm?cat=2809. Accessed November 1, 2006.
5. American Dietetic Association. Disorders of Lipid Metabolism Toolkit. Available at: https://www.adaevidencelibrary.com/store.cfm. Accessed April 10, 2007.
6. American Dietetic Association. Adult Weight Management Evidence-Based Nutrition Practice Guideline, 2006. Available at: http://www.adaevidencelibrary.com/topic.cfm?cat=2798. Accessed April 10, 2007.

Edition: 2008

SNAPshot
NCP Step 1. Nutrition Assessment

What is the purpose of Nutrition Assessment? The purpose is to collect and interpret relevant patient/client* information to identify nutrition-related problems and their causes. This contrasts with nutrition monitoring and evaluation data where dietetics practitioners use similar, or even the same, data to determine changes in patient/client behavior or nutrition status and the efficacy of nutrition intervention.

How does a dietetics practitioner determine where to obtain Nutrition Assessment data? It depends on the practice setting. For individuals, data can come directly from the patient/client through interview, observation and measurements, in addition to information from the referring health care provider or agency, medical record and laboratory tests. For population groups, data from surveys, administrative data sets, and epidemiological or research studies are used. A nutrition assessment matrix that links nutrition assessment parameters with nutrition diagnoses was developed to assist practitioners in identifying nutrition diagnoses.

How are Nutrition Assessment data organized? In five categories.

Food/Nutrition History	Biochemical Data, Medical Tests, and Procedures	Anthropometric Measurements	Physical Examination Findings	Client History
Food and nutrient intake, nutrition related knowledge and practices, physical activity, and food availability	*Laboratory data (e.g., electrolytes, glucose, lipid panel) and tests (e.g., gastric emptying time, resting metabolic rate)*	*Height, weight, body mass index, growth rate, and rate of weight change*	*Oral health, physical appearance, muscle and subcutaneous fat, wasting, and mental status*	*Medication and supplement use, medical/health history, and social, personal/family history*

What is done with the Nutrition Assessment data? Nutrition assessment data are compared to relevant norms and standards for interpretation and decision-making. These may be national, institutional, or regulatory norms and standards. Nutrition assessment findings are documented and are used in nutrition diagnosis statements and nutrition intervention goal setting.

Critical thinking during this step...
- Determining appropriate data to collect and selecting valid and reliable tools
- Distinguishing relevant from irrelevant data.
- Selecting appropriate norms and standards for comparing the data
- Organizing and categorizing the data in a meaningful way that relates to nutrition problems

---

Is there a standardized language or taxonomy for Nutrition Assessment? Not at this time. Nutrition assessment has been well-described in the nutrition textbooks and literature. Use of standardized nutrition assessment procedures for patient/clients with similar disorders allows for effective comparison of nutrition assessment findings and outcome measurements resulting from nutrition intervention; therefore, the Nutrition Care Process Standardized Language Committee will articulate a nutrition assessment taxonomy to be published in a future edition.

Are dietetics practitioners limited to the Nutrition Assessment data included in the Nutrition Assessment Matrix and used in the Nutrition Diagnoses? Nutrition assessment data listed in the nutrition diagnoses reference sheets are undergoing study and research to confirm (validate) which data are most relevant to specific nutrition diagnoses. However, based on their patient/client population, practice setting and purpose, dietetics practitioners may utilize additional nutrition assessment parameters.

Detailed information about this step can be found in the International Dietetics and Nutrition Terminology (IDNT) Reference Manual: Standardized Language for the Nutrition Care Process, First Edition, American Dietetic Association.

*Patient/client refers to individuals, groups, family members, and/or caregivers.

Nutrition Care Process Step 1. Nutrition Assessment

INTRODUCTION

Nutrition Assessment is the first of four steps in the Nutrition Care Process (1). At its simplest, it is a method of identifying and evaluating data needed to make decisions about a nutrition-related problem/diagnosis. While the types of data collected in nutrition assessments may vary among nutrition settings, the process and intention are the same. When possible, the assessment data is compared to reliable norms and standards for evaluation. Further, nutrition assessment initiates the data collection process that is continued throughout the nutrition care process and forms the foundation for reassessment and reanalysis of the data in nutrition monitoring and evaluation.

WHAT IS NEW IN THIS EDITION RELATED TO NUTRITION ASSESSMENT?

At this time, a standardized language for nutrition assessment has not been developed. This section contains a matrix of the five categories of nutrition assessment—food/nutrition history; biochemical data, medical tests, and procedures; anthropometric measurements; physical examination findings; and client history—and the nutrition diagnoses associated each individual sign/symptom.

In this publication, all five categories of the nutrition assessment matrix have been modified. A notation is on the last page of each nutrition assessment category indicating the publication year in which it was updated, e.g., Updated: 2008 Edition. There are two overall reasons for changes to the nutrition assessment and diagnosis matrix—a) changes to clarify the matrix and b) changes due to modifications to the nutrition diagnosis reference sheets.

Changes made to clarify the nutrition assessment and diagnosis matrix:
- **Addition of nutrition diagnosis codes that were unintentionally omitted** from the 2007 publication for a particular assessment data point (2). Specifically, the signs/symptoms were on the nutrition diagnosis sheets; however, they were inadvertently omitted in the compilation of the nutrition assessment data.
- **Revision of the nutrition assessment data language for clarity.** Some nutrition diagnoses listed individual signs/symptoms (e.g., nausea), while others listed multiple signs/symptoms (e.g., nausea, vomiting, diarrhea, and abdominal pain). These were originally listed both ways in the matrix, now all of the signs/symptoms are listed individually.
- **Revisions of the nutrition assessment data language for consistency.** Some nutrition diagnoses use terms such as "sight impairment (e.g., Impaired ability to prepare foods/meals NB-2.4) whereas other nutrition diagnoses use terms such as "vision problems" (Intake of unsafe food NB-3.1). Since there were no discernable differences between the two terms, one nutrition assessment term entitled "vision problems" was used with both diagnoses listed.

Changes due to modifications to the nutrition diagnosis reference sheets:
- Revision of the nutrition assessment matrix reflecting the additions or deletions to the nutrition diagnosis reference sheets. Based upon research findings or member recommendations, the signs/symptoms listed in the nutrition diagnosis were modified in this publication. If a sign/symptom was added to a nutrition diagnosis, the alphanumeric code (e.g. NB 2.3) was added to the nutrition assessment matrix for that data point. Likewise, if a sign/symptom was deleted from a nutrition diagnosis, the alphanumeric code was removed from the nutrition assessment matrix. Revisions or wording changes to the nutrition diagnosis signs/symptoms were only reflected in the matrix if the change altered the meaning or interpretation of the data.

Further information regarding the changes to the nutrition diagnoses can be found in the section for Step 2.

With the identification of inconsistency in language used in the nutrition assessment matrix and development of standardized languages for the other three steps in the nutrition care process, it has become clear that a standard taxonomy for nutrition assessment would support a consistent approach to nutrition assessment and the nutrition care process as well as enhance communication and research.

In fact, the process of defining a nutrition monitoring and evaluation taxonomy made it clear that there is substantial overlap in concepts/terms between nutrition monitoring and evaluation and nutrition assessment. However, the data purpose and use are distinct in these two steps. Therefore, it will be necessary to define nutrition assessment terminology in a future edition of the International Dietetics and Nutrition Terminology (IDNT) Reference Manual. There may be additional terms added that are specific to nutrition assessment that are necessary to diagnose the nutrition problem, but would not be valid indicators to use in the nutrition monitoring and evaluation step to determine if the problem was being resolved.

NUTRITION CARE PROCESS AND NUTRITION ASSESSMENT

Step 1, Nutrition Assessment, of the nutrition care process forms the foundation for progressing through the other three steps in the process. Of initial significance, this systematic method for obtaining, verifying, and interpreting data is needed to make decisions about the significance and cause of a nutrition-related problem.

Several data sources can contribute to a nutrition assessment, such as information gained from the referring health care provider or agency, patient/client interview, medical record, patient/client rounds, community-based surveys, administrative data, and epidemiological studies. Data sources may vary among nutrition settings. Each patient/client presents unique aspects that may influence the approach for the nutrition assessment, and critical thinking skills are especially important at this step. The nature of the individual or group and the practice setting/ environment lead to the appropriate tools to use in the assessment collection to ensure valid and reliable data. Critical thinking skills also help a dietetics practitioner distinguish relevant from irrelevant data and appropriate comparative norms and standards.

> **Special Note.** The terms **patient/client** are used in association with the NCP; however, the process is also intended for use with groups. In addition, family members or caregivers are an essential asset to the patient/client and dietetics practitioner in the NCP. Therefore, **groups and families and caregivers** of patients/clients are implied each time a reference is made to patient/client.

Based on the nutrition assessment, the dietetics practitioner is able to determine whether a nutrition diagnosis/ problem exists. It also leads to the appropriate determination for the continuation of care, such as progression through the nutrition care process or the need for additional information/testing prior to continuing in the process. The data collection procedure persists throughout the nutrition care process and forms the foundation for reassessment and reanalysis of the data.

CATEGORIES OF NUTRITION ASSESSMENT DATA

In the development of the standardized nutrition diagnosis language, the following five categories of nutrition assessment data were identified—food/nutrition history; biochemical data, medical tests, and procedures; anthropometric measurements; physical examination findings; and client history. Because the nutrition assessment forms the basis for identifying a nutrition diagnosis, these terms are reflected on each nutrition diagnosis reference sheet (see pages 49-170) and the signs/symptoms are grouped by the categories of nutrition assessment data.

Following are some examples of data collected within each assessment category; however, these examples are not all-inclusive:

Food/Nutrition History consists of four areas: food intake, nutrition and health awareness and management, physical activity and exercise, and food availability.

> Food intake may include factors such as composition and adequacy of food and nutrient intake, meal and snack patterns, environmental cues to eating, food and nutrient tolerance, and current diets and/or food modifications.

> Nutrition and health awareness and management include, for example, knowledge and beliefs about nutrition recommendations, self-monitoring/management practices, and past nutrition counseling and education.

> Physical activity and exercise consists of functional status, activity patterns, amount of sedentary time (e.g., TV, phone, computer), and exercise intensity, frequency, and duration.

> Food availability encompasses factors such as food planning, purchasing, preparation abilities and limitations, food safety practices, food/nutrition program utilization, and food insecurity.

Biochemical Data, Medical Tests, and Procedures include laboratory data (e.g., electrolytes, glucose, lipid panel, and gastric emptying time).

Anthropometric Measurements include height, weight, body mass index (BMI), growth rate, and rate of weight change.

Physical Examination Findings include oral health, general physical appearance, muscle and subcutaneous fat wasting, and affect.

Client History consists of four areas: medication and supplement history, social history, medical/health history, and personal history.

> Social history may include items such as socioeconomic status, social and medical support, cultural and religious beliefs, housing situation, and social isolation/connection.

> Personal history consists of factors including age, occupation, role in family, and education level.

> Medical/health history includes chief nutrition complaint, present/past illness, surgical history, chronic disease or complication risk, family medical history, mental/emotional health, and cognitive abilities.

> Medication and supplement history includes, for instance, prescription and over-the-counter drugs, herbal and dietary supplements, and illegal drugs.

Definitions for the nutrition assessment terms described have been published in comprehensive resources on the topic and are beyond the scope of this publication. One resource for nutrition assessment includes *ADA Pocket Guide to Nutrition Assessment* (3). A companion resource, *ADA Pocket Guide to Pediatric Nutrition Assessment*, will be published by ADA related to nutrition assessment for pediatrics in 2008 (4).

In regard to the Biochemical, Medical Tests, and Procedures category of nutrition assessment, the nutrition diagnoses contain normal test levels and ranges only for guidance.

Special Note. Laboratory parameters within the nutrition diagnosis reference sheets are provided only for guidance.
- Laboratory values may be different depending on the laboratory performing the test.
- Scientific consensus concerning selection of biochemical tests, laboratory methods, reference standards or interpretation of data does not always exist.
- Laboratory findings may be evaluated for their significance or lack of significance depending on the patient/client population, disease severity, and/or treatment goals.
- Current national, institutional, and regulatory guidelines that affect practice should be applied as appropriate to individual patient/clients.

Edition: 2008

Nutrition interventions should be individualized based on many factors, and laboratory values alone are not diagnostic. A nutrition diagnosis is assigned based on the clinical judgment of an appropriately educated, experienced individual.

NUTRITION ASSESSMENT AND DIAGNOSIS MATRIX

The matrix identifies the pertinent nutrition assessment data for each nutrition diagnosis. This tool is intended to assist in identifying a list of possible diagnoses based on data collected. The matrix enables the dietetics practitioner to identify possible nutrition diagnoses by reading down the list of data to find the identified parameter (e.g., increased BMI), then reading across the matrix to identify possible diagnoses (e.g., NI 1.5, NC 3.3, NB 1.5). This process may be repeated with additional data (e.g., excess energy intake from energy-dense foods: NI 1.5, NI 2.2, NI 2.4, NI 2.5, and NC 3.3), until a list of possible diagnoses is developed. The nutrition diagnostic language reference sheets provide additional detail.

Numerous changes have been made to update and clarify the nutrition assessment and diagnosis matrix in this publication. It is likely that as more research emerges, there will be changes in the matrix in future versions of this publication.

SUMMARY

Nutrition assessment is the first step in the nutrition care process, but it is used throughout each cycle of the nutrition care process and is not an isolated event. Dietetics practitioners recognize that nutrition assessment is a dynamic process that develops throughout the nutrition care process. For example, a dietetics practitioner may be in the middle of the nutrition education intervention when the client provides a new piece of information that may cause a modification of the nutrition diagnosis, PES statement, or even the nutrition intervention.

Future research will continue to shed light on the appropriate data to collect and its application in nutrition assessment with a patient/client or group. Moreover, as the profession utilizes nutrition assessment within the other steps of the nutrition care process, the most valid and reliable assessment data to use in nutrition diagnosis, nutrition intervention, and nutrition monitoring and evaluation will also become evident.

REFERENCES

1. Lacey K, Pritchett E. Nutrition care process and model: ADA adopts road map to quality care and outcomes management. *J Am Diet Assoc.* 2003;103:1061-1072.
2. American Dietetic Association. *Nutrition Diagnosis and Intervention: Standardized Language for the Nutrition Care Process.* Chicago, IL: American Dietetic Association; 2007.
3. American Dietetic Association. Pamela Charney, Ainsley Malone, eds. *ADA Pocket Guide to Nutrition Assessment.* Chicago, IL: American Dietetic Association; 2004.
4. Leonberg, BL. *ADA Pocket Guide to Pediatric Nutrition Assessment.* Chicago, IL: American Dietetic Association; 2008.

Nutrition Assessment Matrix
Food and Nutrition History Data and Related Nutrition Diagnostic Terminology

Parameter (not all-inclusive)	Nutrition Diagnostic Terminology		
Excess intake of			
Alcohol and/or binge drinking	NI 4.3	NC 3.4	
Amino acids (specify)	NI 5.7.3		
Bioactive substances	NI 4.2		
Convenience foods, pre-prepared meals, and foods prepared away from home	NI 2.2	NB 2.4	
Energy from energy dense or high fat foods/beverages,	NI 1.5	NI 2.2	NI 2.4
PN or EN	NC 3.3		
Fat, foods prepared with added fat	NI 5.4	NI 5.6.2	NC 2.2
Fat from high-risk lipids (saturated fat, trans fat, cholesterol)	NI 5.6.2	NI 5.6.3	
Fiber	NI 5.4	NI 5.8.6	NC 2.2
Fluid	NI 3.2		
Foods without available vitamins	NI 5.9.1		
Fortified foods and supplements containing vitamins	NI 5.9.2		
Food in a defined time period	NB 1.5		
Iron	NI 5.5		
Manganese	NI 5.5		
Mercury	NB 3.1		
Minerals	NI 5.10.2		
Parenteral or enteral nutrition	NI 1.5		
Phosphorus	NI 5.4	NC 2.2	
Plant foods containing soluble fiber, β-glucan, or plant sterol and stanol esters	NI 4.2		
Protein	NI 4.2 NC 2.2	NI 5.4	NI 5.7.2
Sodium	NI 3.2 NC 2.2	NI 5.4	
Substances which interfere with digestion or absorption	NI 4.2		
Associated factors			
Binge eating patterns	NI 2.2		
Change in way clothes fit	NC 3.2		
Highly variable calorie intake	NI 2.2		
Lipid or dextrose infusions, peritoneal dialysis or other medical treatments that provide significant calories	NI 2.4		

Edition: 2008

Nutrition Assessment Matrix
Food and Nutrition History Data and Related Nutrition Diagnostic Terminology

Parameter (not all-inclusive)	Nutrition Diagnostic Terminology		
Insufficient intake of			
Carbohydrate	NI 5.8.1		
Energy	NI 1.4	NI 2.1	NI 5.2
Fiber, soy protein, β-glucan, or plant sterol and stanol esters	NI 4.1	NI 5.8.5	
Fluid	NI 3.1		
Fat, essential fatty acids	NI 5.6.1		
Fat, monounsaturated, polyunsaturated, or omega-3 fatty acids	NI 5.6.3		
Food/supplements and nutrients	NI 5.1	NI 5.3	NI 5.9.1
	NI 5.10.1	NC 1.2	NB 2.4
	NB 3.2		
Food or food from specific foods/groups due to GI symptoms	NC 1.4	NC 2.1	
Minerals	NI 5.10.1	NC 2.2	
Vitamins	NI 5.9.1	NC 2.2	
Parenteral or enteral nutrition	NI 1.4	NI 2.3	
Protein	NI 2.1	NI 5.2	NI 5.7.1
Vitamin D intake/sunlight exposure	NI 5.9.1	NI 5.10.1	
Associated factors			
Anorexia	NI 2.1	NI 5.10.2	NC 2.2
Changes in appetite or taste	NI 2.1	NC 2.3	
Changes in recent food intake	NC 1.2	NC 3.2	NC 3.4
Failure to recognize foods	NB 2.6		
Forgets to eat	NB 2.6		
Hunger	NC 3.1	NB 3.2	
Infant coughing, crying, latching on and off, pounding on breasts	NC 1.3		
Infant lethargy	NC 1.3		
Infant with decreased feeding frequency/duration, early cessation of feeding, and/or feeding resistance	NC 1.3		
Infant with fewer than six wet diapers in 24 hours	NC 1.3		
Infant with hunger, lack of satiety after feeding	NC 1.3		
Lack of interest in food	NI 1.4	NI 5.2	NI 5.9.1
	NI 5.10.1		
Lack of strength or stamina for eating	NB 2.6		
Mealtime resistance	NC 1.1		
Mother doesn't hear infant swallowing	NC 1.3		
Mother with lack of confidence in ability to breastfeed	NC 1.3		
Mother with small amount of milk when pumping	NC 1.3		
Nausea	NI 2.1	NC 2.2	
Recent food avoidance and or/lack of interest in food	NI 5.3		
Refusal to eat; chew	NC 3.1	NB 2.6	
Satiety, early	NC 3.2		
Spitting food out or prolonged feeding time	NC 1.2		
Swallowing, difficulty	NI 3.1		
Thirst	NI 3.1		

Nutrition Assessment Matrix
Food and Nutrition History Data and Related Nutrition Diagnostic Terminology

Parameter (not all-inclusive)	Nutrition Diagnostic Terminology		
Intake different from recommended			
Carbohydrate	NI 5.8.2	NI 5.8.3	NI 5.8.4
Carbohydrate, protein and/or fat intake from enteral and/or parenteral nutrients	NI 2.5		
Food, inappropriate use of	NB 2.6		
Food choices, inappropriate	NI 5.8.1		
Food group/nutrient imbalance	NB 1.2		
Food intake includes raw eggs, unpasturized milk products, soft cheeses, undercooked meats, wild plants, berries and mushrooms	NB 3.1		
Food variety, limited	NB 3.2		
Intake that does not support replacement or mitigation of OTC, prescribed drugs, herbals, botanicals, or dietary supplements	NC 2.3		
Medication (over the counter or prescribed), herbal, botanical, or dietary supplement intake that is problematic or inconsistent with recommended foods	NC 2.3		
Protein or other supplementation	NI 5.7.2	NI 5.7.3	
US Dietary Guidelines, any nutrient	NI 5.9.2	NB 1.7	
Food and nutrient intolerance			
Allergic reactions to certain carbohydrate foods or food groups	NI 5.8.3		
Coughing and choking with eating	NC 1.1		
Decreased intake or avoidance of food difficult to form into a bolus	NC 1.2		
Diminished joint mobility or wrist, hand or digits that impair ability to independently consume food	NI 1.4	NI 5.8.1	
Diarrhea in response to high refined carbohydrate intake	NI 5.8.3		
Dropping cups, utensils	NB 2.6		
Dropping food from utensil on repeated attempts to feed	NB 2.6		
Feeling of food "getting stuck" in throat	NC 1.1		
Foods provided not conducive to self feeding	NB 2.6		
Nausea, vomiting, diarrhea, high gastric residual volume	NI 2.5		
Pain on swallowing	NC 1.1		
Poor lip closure, drooling	NC 1.1	NB 2.6	
Pouching food	NC 1.1		
Prolonged chewing, feeding time	NC 1.1		
Utensil biting	NB 2.6		

Edition: 2008

Nutrition Assessment Matrix
Food and Nutrition History Data and Related Nutrition Diagnostic
Terminology

Parameter (not all-inclusive)	Nutrition Diagnostic Terminology		
Nutrition and health awareness			
Avoidance of food or calorie containing beverages	NB 1.5	NC 1.1	
Avoidance of foods of age-appropriate texture	NC 1.2		
Avoidance of foods/food groups	NB 1.2		
Belief that aging can be slowed by dietary limitations	NB 3.2		
Chronic dieting behavior	NI 5.10.1	NB 1.5	
Cultural or religious practices that limit intake	NI 5.7.1		
Cultural or religious practices that limit modification of dietary carbohydrate intake	NI 5.8.2		
Defensiveness, hostility, or resistance to change	NB 1.3		
Denial of hunger	NB 1.5		
Denial of need for food- and nutrition-related changes	NB 1.3		
Eating alone, feeling embarrassed by the amount of food eaten	NB 1.5		
Eating much more rapidly than normal, eating until feeling uncomfortably full, consuming large amounts of food when not feeling hungry	NB 1.5		
Embarrassment or anger at need for self-monitoring	NB 1.4	NB 2.3	
Emotional distress, anxiety, or frustration surrounding mealtimes	NB 2.6		
Excessive reliance on nutrition terming and preoccupation with nutrient content of food	NB 1.5		
Expected food/nutrition related outcomes are not achieved	NB 1.6		
Failure to complete any agreed homework	NB 1.6		
Failure to keep appointments/schedule or engage in counseling	NB 1.3	NB 1.6	
Fear of foods or dysfunctional thoughts regarding food or food experiences	NB 1.5		
Feeling disgusted with oneself, depressed, or guilty after overeating	NB 1.5		
Food faddism, pica	NC 3.1	NB 1.2	NB 3.2
Food preoccupation	NB 1.5		
Frustration or dissatisfaction with MNT recommendations	NB 2.5		
Frustration over lack of control	NB 2.5		
Harmful beliefs and attitudes of parent/caregiver	NB 3.2		
Incomplete self-monitoring records	NB 1.4		
Inflexibility with food selection	NB 1.5		
Irrational thoughts about food's effect on the body	NB 1.5		
Knowledge about current fad diets	NB 1.5		
Lack of appreciation of the importance of making recommended nutrition-related changes	NB 1.6		
Negative body language (note: varies by culture)	NB 1:3		
Previous failures to effectively change target behavior	NB 1.3		
Prolonged use of substances known to increase vitamin requirements or reduce vitamin absorption	NI 5.9.1		
Sense of lack of control of overeating during the episode	NB 1.5		
Unwillingness or disinterest in applying nutrition related recommendations	NC 3.3		
Verbalizes unwillingness/disinterest in learning	NB 1.1		
Weight preoccupation	NB 1.5		

Nutrition Assessment Matrix
Food and Nutrition History Data and Related Nutrition Diagnostic Terminology

Parameter (not all-inclusive)	Nutrition Diagnostic Terminology		
Food and nutrient knowledge and skill			
Food and nutrition-related knowledge deficit	NI 5.1	NC 2.2	
Inability to apply food- and nutrition-related information	NC 3.3	NB 1.1	
Inability to apply guideline information	NB 1.7		
Inability to change food- or activity-related behavior	NB 2.5		
Inability to interpret data or self management tools	NB 2.3		
Inability to maintain weight or regain of weight	NC 3.3		
Inability to recall agreed upon changes	NB 1.6		
Inability or unwillingness to select, or disinterest in selecting food consistent with guidelines	NB 1.7		
Inaccurate or incomplete understanding of information related to guidelines or needed changes	NB 1.1	NB 1.7	
Lack of ability to prepare meals	NI 5.3		
Lack of compliance or inconsistent compliance with plan	NB 1.6		
Lack of efficacy to make changes or to overcome barriers to change	NB 1.3		
Limited knowledge of carbohydrate composition of foods or of carbohydrate metabolism	NI 5.8.3		
Mother has insufficient knowledge of breastfeeding or infant hunger/satiety signals	NC 1.3		
Mother is concerned about breastfeeding/lack of support	NC 1.3		
No prior knowledge of need for food and nutrition-related recommendations	NB 1.1		
Provides inaccurate or incomplete written response to questionnaire/written tool, or is unable to read written tool	NB 1.1		
Relates concerns about previous attempts to learn information	NB 1.1	NB 2.5	
Uncertainty as to how to consistently apply food/nutrition information	NB 1.6		
Uncertainty of how to complete monitoring records	NB 1.4		
Uncertainty regarding appropriate foods to prepare based upon nutrition prescription	NB 2.4		
Uncertainty regarding changes that could/should be made in response to data in self-monitoring records	NB 1.4	NB 2.3	
Uncertainty regarding nutrition-related recommendations	NC 3.3		
Physical activity			
Decreased or sedentary activity level (due to barriers or other reasons)	NC 3.3		
Increased physical activity	NI 1.2	NC 3.1	NB 2.2
Excessive physical activity (ignoring family, job; exercising without rest/rehabilitation days, or while injured or sick)	NB 1.5	NB 2.2	
Low level of NEAT (non-exercise activity thermogenesis)	NB 2.1		
Overtraining	NB 2.2		

Edition: 2008

Nutrition Assessment Matrix
Food and Nutrition History Data and Related Nutrition Diagnostic Terminology

Parameter (not all-inclusive)	Nutrition Diagnostic Terminology		
Food availability			
Economic constraints that limit availability of appropriate foods	NI 2.1 NI 5.8.4	NI 5.8.2	NI 5.8.3
Food insecurity/unwillingness to use available resources	NB 2.5		
Inability to purchase and transport foods to one's home	NB 2.4		
Intake consistent with estimated or measured energy needs	NC 3.4		
Lack of facilities or accommodations for breastfeeding in community or at work	NC 1.3		
Ready access to available foods/products with bioactive substance	NI 4.2		
Unfavorable QOL or other quality of life rating	NB 2.5		
Other			
Ethnic and cultural related issues	NB 2.5		
Extreme hunger with or without palpitations, tremor, sweating	NC 3.4		
Lack of social and familial support	NB 2.5		
Intake consistent with estimated or measured energy needs	NC 3.4		
No self-management equipment	NB 1.4		
Normal intake in the face of illness	NC 3.2		
Use of narcotics	NC 3.4		

Updated: 2008 Edition

Nutrition Assessment Matrix
Anthropomorphic Data and Related Nutrition Diagnostic Terminology

Parameter (not all-inclusive)	Findings	Nutrition Diagnostic Terminology		
Anthropometric Data				
Body Mass Index (BMI)	decreased	NI 2.3	NI 5.1	NI 5.2
		NC 3.1	NB 1.5	NB 3.2
BMI	increased	NI 1.5	NC 3.3	NB 1.5
		NB 2.1		
Body fat distribution	changed	NC 3.4		
Body fat percentage	increased	NI 1.5		
Growth	delayed	NI 1.2	NI 2.1	NI 2.3
		NI 5.1	NI 5.2	NI 5.3
		NI 5.5	NI 5.7.2	NI 5.9.2
		NC 2.1	NB 1.4	NB 2.2
		NB 3.2		
Height	loss	NI 5.10.1		
Muscle circumference, mid-arm	decreased	NI 5.1	NC 3.1	
Muscle mass	increased	NI 1.2		
Skinfold thickness	increased	NC 3.3		
Skinfold thickness	decreased	NI 5.1	NC 3.1	
Waist circumference	increased	NC 3.3		
Wasting		NI-5.2		
Weight	change, rapid	NC 2.2	NB 1.5	
Weight	loss	NI 1.4	NI 2.1	NI 2.3
		NI 2.5	NI 3.1	NI 4.2
		NI 5.2	NI 5.3	NI 5.6.1
		NC 1.3	NC 2.1	NC 3.2
		NB 2.2	NB 2.6	
	unintentional	NI 1.2	NI 5.1	NI 5.2
		NI 2.3		
Weight	decreased	NC 3.1	NB 2.2	
Weight	gain	NI 1.4	NI 1.5	NI 2.2
		NI 3.2	NC 2.3	NC 3.3
		NC 3.4		
	in excess of lean tissue accretion	NI 2.4	NI 2.5	
	interdialytic	NI 5.4		
Weight	failure to gain as planned	NI 2.3	NI 5.2	NI 5.3
		NC 1.3	NB 1.6	NB 2.2

Updated: 2008 Edition

Nutrition Assessment Matrix
Biochemical Data, Medical Tests, and Procedures and Related Nutrition Diagnostic Terminology

Parameter (not all-inclusive)	Findings	Nutrition Diagnostic Terminology		
Biochemical data				
3-methyl histidine, urine	increased	NI 5.7.3		
Albumin, serum	decreased	NI 5.1	NI 5.2	NC 3.4
Alcohol, blood	increased	NI 4.3		
Alpha tocopherol, plasma	decreased	NI 5.9.1		
Amino acids (specific levels)	increased	NI 5.7.3	NC 2.1	
Ammonia, serum	increased	NI 5.7.3	NC 2.2	
Amylase, serum	increased	NI 5.6.2	NI 5.6.3	
AST, aspartate aminotransferase	increased	NI 4.3	NC 2.2	NB 2.2
ALT, alanine aminotransferase	increased	NC 2.2		
Bilirubin, total serum	increased	NI 5.6.2	NI 5.6.3	NC 2.2
BUN	increased	NI 3.1	NI 5.4	NI 5.7.2
BUN:creatinine ratio	increased	NI 5.7.3 NB 1.5	NI 2.4	NC 2.2
Calcium, serum	decreased	NI 2.3		
Calcium, serum ionized	decreased	NI 5.9.1		
Calcium, serum ionized	increased	NI 5.9.2		
Calcium, urine	decreased	NI 5.10.1		
Chloride, serum	decreased	NB 1.5		
Cholesterol, HDL	decreased	NI 5.4 NI 5.10.2	NI 5.6.2	NI 5.6.3
Cholesterol, LDL	increased	NI 5.4	NI 5.6.2	NI 5.6.3
Cholesterol, serum	decreased	NI 4.2	NI 5.1	
Cholesterol, serum	increased	NI 5.4 NB 1.5	NI 5.6.2	NI 5.6.3
Copper	decreased	NI 2.3	NI 5.10.1	
Cortisol levels	increased	NB 2.2		
C-reactive protein	elevated	NI 5.1	NI 5.6.3	
Creatinine	elevated	NI 5.4	NC 2.2	
Digestive enzymes	altered	NC 1.4	NC 2.1	
D-xylose	abnormal	NC 1.4	NC 2.1	
Fat, fecal	increased	NI 5.6.2	NC 1.4	NC 2.1
Ferritin, serum	decreased	NB 2.2		
Ferritin, serum	increased	NI 5.10.2		
Folic acid, serum	decreased	NI 5.9.1		
Folic acid, erythrocyte		NI 5.9.2		
GFR, glomerular filtration rate	decreased	NI 5.4 NC 2.2	NI 5.7.2	NI 5.7.3
GGT, gamma-glutamyl transferase	elevated	NI 4.3		
Glucose, blood	increased	NI 2.4 NI 5.8.4	NI 5.8.2 NC 2.2	NI 5.8.3 NC 3.4

Nutrition Assessment Matrix
Biochemical Data, Medical Tests, and Procedures and Related Nutrition Diagnostic Terminology

Parameter (not all-inclusive)	Findings	Nutrition Diagnostic Terminology		
Biochemical data				
Glucose, blood	decreased	NI 5.8.3 NB 1.5	NI 5.8.4	NC 2.2
Glucose, blood	inadequate control	NC 2.2		
Glutathione reductase, erythrocyte	increased	NI 5.9.1		
GTT (glucose tolerance test)	abnormal	NI 5.8.2		
Hematocrit	increased	NB 2.2		
Hemoglobin	decreased	NI 5.10.1		
Hemoglobin A1c	increased	NI 5.8.2	NC 2.2	
Hormone levels	fluctuating	NC 3.4		
Homocysteine	increased	NI 5.9.1		
Hydrogen breath test	abnormal	NC 1.4	NC 2.1	
IGF binding protein	abnormal	NB 2.2		
Immune function	suppressed	NB 2.2		
Iodine, urinary	decreased	NI 5.10.1		
Iron	decreased	NI 2.3		
Iron binding capacity	decreased	NI 2.3		
Ketones, urine	present	NB 1.5		
Leucopenia	present	NB 1.5		
Lipase	increased	NI 5.6.2	NI 5.6.3	
Lipid profile, serum	abnormal	NC 2.2 NB 1.7	NC 3.4	NB 1.5
Liver enzymes	elevated	NI 1.5 NI 4.2 NI 5.6.3	NI 2.4 NI 5.4 NC 2.2	NI 2.5 NI 5.6.2 NB 2.2
Magnesium, serum	decreased	NI 5.1	NI 5.5	NI 5.10.1
Magnesium, serum	increased	NI 5.10.2		
Mean corpuscular volume	increased	NI 4.3		
N'methyl-nicotanimide	decreased	NI 5.9.1		
N'methyl-nicotanimide	increased	NI 5.9.2		
Osmolality, serum	increased	NI 3.1		
Osmolality, serum	decreased	NI 3.2		
Parathyroid hormone	increased	NI 5.9.1	NI 5.9.2	
pCO_2	abnormal	NI 2.4	NC 2.2	
Phosphorus, serum	decreased	NI 5.1 NI 5.10.1	NI 5.5	NI 5.9.1
Phosphorus, serum	increased	NI 2.5	NI 5.4	NI 5.10.2
pO_2	abnormal	NC 2.2		
Potassium, serum	decreased	NI 2.5 NC 2.2	NI 5.1 NB 1.5	NI 5.5
Potassium, serum	increased	NI 5.1	NI 5.4	NC 2.2
Prealbumin	decreased	NI 5.1		
Pyrodoxal 5'phosphate, plasma	decreased	NI 5.9.1		
Pyrodoxal 5'phosphate, plasma	increased	NI 5.9.2		

Nutrition Assessment Matrix
Biochemical Data, Medical Tests, and Procedures and Related Nutrition Diagnostic Terminology

Parameter (not all-inclusive)	Findings	Nutrition Diagnostic Terminology		
Biochemical data				
Retinol, serum	decreased	NI 5.9.1		
Retinol, serum	increased	NI 5.9.2		
Sodium, serum	decreased	NI 3.2	NC 3.4	NB 1.5
Sodium, serum	increased	NI 3.1		
Stool culture	positive	NC 1.4	NB 3.1	
Thyroid function tests (TSH, T4, T3)	abnormal	NI 5.10.2	NB 1.5	
Toxicology reports	positive	NB 3.2		
Transketolase activity, erythrocyte	increased	NI 5.9.1		
Transferrin	increased	NI 4.3		
Triene:tetraene ratio	increased	NI 5.6.1		
Triglycerides	increased	NI 5.4	NI 5.6.2	NI 5.6.3
Vitamin B12	decreased	NI 5.9.1		
Vitamin C, plasma	decreased	NI 5.9.1		
Vitamin K (PT, PTT, INR)	abnormal	NI 2.3	NI 5.9.1	NI 5.9.2
Zinc, serum	decreased	NI 2.3	NB 2.2	
Medical tests and procedures				
Gastric emptying study	abnormal	NC 1.4		
Mineral density, bone	decreased	NI 5.10.1		
Respiratory quotient	abnormal	NI 1.5	NI 2.3	
Metabolic rate, resting	increased	NI 1.2		
Small bowel transit time	abnormal	NC 1.4		

Updated: 2008 Edition

Nutrition Assessment Matrix
Physical Examination Data and Related Nutrition Diagnostic Terminology

Parameter (not all-inclusive)	Findings	Nutrition Diagnostic Terminology		
Head and neck				
Eyes:				
Bitot's spots	present	NI 5.9.1		
Dryness	present	NI 5.9.2		
Night blindness	present	NI 5.9.1		
Vision	decreased	NC 3.2		
Xeropthalmia	present	NI 5.9.1		
Tongue:				
Bright red	present	NI 5.9.1		
Glossitis	present	NI 5.9.1	NC 2.1	
Extrusion	present	NB 2.6		
Impaired tongue movement	present	NC 1.2		
Frenulum abnormality (infants)	present	NC 1.3		
Magenta	present	NI 5.9.1		
Taste, sense	decreased	NC 3.2		
Mouth and throat:				
Cheilosis	present	NI 5.9.1	NC 2.1	
Dry mucous membranes, hoarse or wet voice, tongue extrusion	present	NI 2.3 NC 1.1 NB 3.1	NI 3.1 NC 1.2	NI 5.9.2 NB 2.6
Gums, inflamed or bleeding	present	NI 2.3	NI 5.1	NI 5.9.1
Ketone smell on breath	present	NI 5.8.1		
Lesions, oral	present	NC 1.2	NC 2.1	
Lips	dry or cracked	NI 5.9.2		
Mucosa (mouth and pharynx)	edema	NI 5.9.1		
Parotid glands	enlarged	NB 1.5		
Stomatitis	present	NI 5.9.1		
Teeth	missing, caries, damaged enamel, poorly fitting dentures	NI 1.4 NB 1.5	NI 5.8.2	NC 1.2
Head:				
Cranial nerve function (V, VII, IX, X, XII)	altered	NC 1.1	NC 1.2	
Fontanelle, bulging (in infants)	present	NI 5.9.2		
Hair, changes, brittle and lifeless	present	NI 5.10.2	NB 1.5	
Hairs, coiled	present	NI 5.9.1		
Hair loss	present	NI 2.3 NI 5.9.2	NI 5.1	NI 5.2
Headache	present	NI 5.9.2		
Lanugo hair formation on face and trunk	present	NB 1.5		
Mucosa, nasal	dryness	NI 5.9.2		
Occipital wasting	present	NI 5.2		
Smell, sense	decreased	NC 3.2		

Edition: 2008

Nutrition Assessment Matrix
Physical Examination Data and Related Nutrition Diagnostic Terminology

Parameter (not all-inclusive)	Findings	Nutrition Diagnostic Terminology		
Gastrointestinal system				
Ascites	present	NI 3.2	NC 2.2	
Bowel sounds	abnormal	NC 1.4	NC 2.1	
Constipation	present	NI 4.2	NI 5.5	NC 1.4
Distention, abdominal	present	NC 1.4	NC 2.1	
Diarrhea	present	NI 2.3	NI 4.2	NI 5.5
Diarrhea in response to carbohydrate feeding	present	NI 5.8.2		
Nausea	present	NI 2.3	NI 5.9.2	
Vomiting	present	NI 2.3	NI 5.9.2	
Neurologic system				
Confusion	present	NI 5.9.1		
Concentration	impaired	NB 1.5		
Motor and gait disturbances	present	NI 5.9.1		
Neurological changes	present	NI 4.2	NI 5.7.3	
Vibratory and position sense	decreased	NI 5.9.1		
Cardiovascular-pulmonary system				
Cardiovascular changes	arrythmias	NI 4.2	NB 1.5	
Edema, pulmonary	crackles or rales	NI 3.2		
Extremities and musculoskeletal system				
Arthralgia; joint effusions	present	NI 5.9.1		
Bone alterations	fragility	NI 5.9.2		
Bones	obvious prominence	NI 5.2		
Bones, long	widening at ends	NI 5.9.1		
Fat, body	decreased	NC 3.2 NB 2.2	NC 3.3	NB 1.5
Fat, body	increased	NC 3.3	NB 3.2	
Hands and feet	cyanosis	NB 1.5		
Hands and feet	tingling and numbness	NI 5.9.1		
Injuries	frequent and prolonged	NB 2.2		
Muscle mass	decreased	NI 2.3 NB 1.5	NI 2.5 NB 2.1	NI 5.1
Muscle soreness	chronic	NB 2.2		
Nail beds	blue, clubbing	NC 2.2		
Nail beds	pale	NI 2.3	NI 5.1	
Nail changes	present	NI 5.10.2		
Russell's sign	present	NB 1.5		

Nutrition Assessment Matrix
Physical Examination Data and Related Nutrition Diagnostic Terminology

Parameter (not all-inclusive)	Findings	Nutrition Diagnostic Terminology		
Skin				
Calcification of soft tissues (calcinosis)	present	NI 5.9.2		
Changes consistent with nutrient deficiency/excess	present	NI 5.6.1	NB 1.7	NB 3.2
Dermatitis	present	NI 5.6.1	NI 5.6.3	
Edema, peripheral	present	NI 2.4	NI 2.5	NI 5.2
		NC 2.2	NB 1.5	
Erythema, scaling and peeling of the skin	present	NI 5.9.2		
Ecchymosis	present	NI 5.9.1		
Follicular hyperkeratosis	present	NI 5.9.1		
Jaundice and itching	present	NC 2.2		
Skin	dry, scaly	NI 2.1	NI 3.1	NI 5.2
		NI 5.6.1	NB 1.5	
Skin integrity	decreased	NI 2.3	NI 5.1	
Skin lesions	present	NI 5.9.1		
Skin turgor	decreased	NI 3.1	NC 1.1	
Skin turgor	increased	NI 2.3	NI 3.2	NI 5.4
Seborrheic dermatitis	present	NI 5.9.1		
Perifolicular hemorrhages	present	NI 5.9.1		
Petechiae	present	NI 5.9.1		
Pressure ulcers (stage II-IV)	present	NI 2.3	NI 5.1	
Wound healing	decreased	NI 5.1	NI 5.2	NI 5.3
		NI 5.9.1		
Xanthomas	present	NI 5.6.2	NI 5.6.3	
Vital signs				
Blood pressure	decreased	NI 5.2	NB 1.5	
Blood pressure	increased	NI 4.2		
Heart rate	decreased	NB 1.5		
Heart rate	increased	NC 3.2		
Respiratory rate	increased	NI 1.5	NC 3.2	
Temperature	decreased	NB 1.5		
Temperature	increased	NI 1.2	NC 3.2	
Urine output	decreased	NI 3.1		
Miscellaneous				
Body language (note: varies by culture)	negative	NB 1.3	NB 1.6	

Updated: 2008 Edition

Nutrition Assessment Matrix
Client History Data and Related Diagnostic Terminology

Parameter (not all-inclusive)	Nutrition Diagnostic Terminology		
Social history			
Abuse, physical, sexual or emotional	NC 3.3		
Alcohol intake during pregnancy despite knowledge of risk	NI 4.3		
Alcohol intake, excessive	NI 4.3	NC 1.2	
Avoidance of social events where food is served	NB 1.5		
Change in living environment/independence	NI 5.10.1		
Chronic non-compliance	NB 1.3		
Substance abuse	NI 1.4	NC 3.2	NB 1.5
Environmental conditions, e.g., infants exclusively fed breast milk with limited exposure to sunlight (vitamin D)	NI 5.9.1		
Geographic latitude and history of UVB exposure/sunscreen use	NI 5.10.1		
Geographic location and socioeconomic status associated with altered nutrient intake of indigenous phenomenon	NI 5.2		
Giving birth to an infant with fetal alcohol syndrome	NI 4.3		
Hunger in the face of inadequate access to food supply	NI 5.3		
Illness or physical disability	NC 3.1	NB 3.2	
Lack of ability to prepare meals	NI 5.3		
Lack of developmental readiness	NC 1.2		
Lack of funds for purchase of appropriate foods	NI 5.3		
Lack of suitable support system to access food	NB 3.2		
Lifestyle changes, recent	NB 2.5		
Low cardiorespiratory fitness and/or low muscle strength	NB 2.1		
New medical diagnosis or change in existing	NI 4.3	NB 1.1	NB 1.4
diagnosis or condition	NB 2.3	NB 2.5	
Occupation of athlete, dancer, gymnast	NC 3.1		
Physical activity, easy fatigue with increased activity; unable to achieve desired levels	NI 2.3		
Physical disability or limitation	NC 3.3	NB 2.6	
Unrealistic expectations of weight gain or ideal weight	NI 2.4		
Personal/Family history			
Of childhood obesity	NC 3.3		
Of eating disorders, depression, obsessive compulsive disorders, anxiety disorders	NB 1.5		
Of familial obesity	NC 3.3		
Of hyperlipidemia, atherosclerosis or pancreatitis	NI 5.6.2	NI 5.6.3	
Of inability to lose weight through conventional weight loss intervention	NC 3.3		

Nutrition Assessment Matrix
Client History Data and Related Diagnostic Terminology

Parameter (not all-inclusive)	Nutrition Diagnostic Terminology		
Medical/Health history			
AIDS/HIV	NI 2.1	NI 2.3	NI 5.1
	NI 5.6.1	NC 3.2	
Alcoholism	NI 1.4	NC 2.2	
Alzheimer's disease	NI 1.2	NI 3.1	NC 1.2
	NB 2.6		
Anemia	NI 5.6.1	NI 5.9.1	NI 5.10.1
	NB 1.5		
Anxiety disorder	NI 2.2	NB 2.1	
Arthritis	NB 2.1		
Asthma	NC 3.4		
Atherosclerosis	NI 5.6.2		
Biliary disease	NI 5.6.2	NI 5.6.3	
Binge eating	NB 2.2		
Breast surgery	NC 1.3		
Bulimia nervosa	NB 2.2		
Burns	NI 2.3	NI 5.1	NC 3.2
Cadidiasis	NC 1.3		
Cancer, head, neck or pharyngeal	NC 1.2		
Cancer (other)	NI 5.9.2	NC 3.2	NB 1.2
Cardiac, neurologic, respiratory changes	NB 3.1		
Cardiovascular disease	NI 3.2	NI 4.1	NI 4.2
	NI 5.3	NI 5.4	NI 5.6.3
	NI 5.9.2	NC 2.2	NB 1.2
	NB 2.3		
Celiac disease	NI 5.8.1	NI 5.9.1	NI 5.10.1
	NC 1.4	NC 2.1	
Cerebral palsy	NI 1.2	NC 1.2	NB 2.4
Chronic fatigue syndrome	NB 2.1		
Chronic obstructive pulmonary disease	NI 1.2	NC 3.2	
Chronic or acute disease or trauma, geographic location and socioeconomic status associated with nutrient intake of indigenous phenomenon	NI 5.2		
Cleft lip/palate	NC 1.2	NC 1.3	
Cognitive or emotional impairment	NB 2.3	NB 2.4	
Constipation	NI 5.8.5	NI 5.8.6	
Crohn's disease	NI 2.3	NI 5.1	
	NC 1.4	NC 2.1	
Cushing's syndrome	NC 3.4		
Cystic fibrosis	NI 1.2	NI 5.6.2	
Dementia	NI 1.2	NI 1.4	NI 3.1
	NB 2.6	NB 3.2	
Depression	NI 2.1	NI 4.3	NC 3.2
	NC 3.3	NB 1.5	NB 2.1

Edition: 2008

Nutrition Assessment Matrix
Client History Data and Related Diagnostic Terminology

Parameter (not all-inclusive)	Nutrition Diagnostic Terminology		
Medical/Health history, continued			
Developmental delay	NB 2.6		
Diabetes mellitus	NI 5.6.3	NI 5.8.2	NI 5.8.3
	NI 5.8.4	NC 2.2	NB 1.2
	NB 1.4	NB 2.3	
Diverticulitis	NI 5.8.6	NC 1.4	
Dysphasia	NC 1.1		
Eating disorder	NI 1.4	NI 5.8.6	
Encephalopathy, hepatic	NI 5.4		
Fatigue	NC 3.4		
Fluorosis	NI 5.10.2		
Foodborne illness, e.g., bacterial, viral, and parasitic infection	NB 3.1		
Fractures, stress	NB 2.2		
Gastrointestinal stricture	NI 5.8.6		
Headache	NB 3.1		
Hyperemia	NI 5.9.1		
Hyperlipidemia	NI 5.6.2		
Hypertension	NI 4.2	NI 4.3	NI 5.4
Hyperthyroidism (pre- or untreated)	NC 3.2		
Hypertriglyceridemia, severe	NI 4.3		
Hypoglycemia	NI 5.8.3	NI 5.8.4	
Hypothyroidism	NC 3.3	NC 3.4	
Illness, recent	NI 5.3		
Inborn errors of metabolism	NI 5.7.3		
Infection	NI 5.8.2		
Inflammatory bowel disease	NI 5.8.5	NI 5.10.1	
Irritable bowel syndrome	NI 5.4	NI 5.8.6	NC 1.4
Kidney stones	NI 5.10.1		
Lactase deficiency	NI 5.8.2		
Liver disease	NI 3.2	NI 5.2	NI 5.4
	NI 5.6.3	NI 5.8.1	NI 5.9.2
	NI 5.10.2	NB 2.3	
Malabsorption, protein and/or nutrient	NI 2.1	NI 5.7.1	NI 5.7.2
Maldigestion	NC 1.4		
Malnutrition	NI 5.2	NI 5.3	NC 3.1
Mastitis	NC 1.3		
Mental illness	NI 1.4	NI 5.8.6	NC 3.1
	NB 1.1	NB 1.2	NB 1.7
	NB 3.1	NB 3.2	
Metabolic syndrome	NI 2.2	NI 5.8.3	NI 5.8.4
Multiple sclerosis	NB 2.6		
Nephrotic syndrome	NI 3.2		

Nutrition Assessment Matrix
Client History Data and Related Diagnostic Terminology

Parameter (not all-inclusive)	Nutrition Diagnostic Terminology		
Medical/Health history, continued			
Neurological disorders	NB 2.6		
Obesity, morbid	NB 2.1		
Obesity/overweight	NI 2.2	NI 5.6.3	NI 5.8.3
	NI 5.8.4	NB 1.4	
Oral soft issue infection, e.g., candidiasis, leukoplakia	NC 1.2		
Osteomalacia	NI 5.9.1		
Pancreatic disease	NI 4.3	NI 5.8.1	
Paralysis	NB 2.6		
Paraplegia	NB 2.4		
Parkinson's disease	NI 1.2		
Pellegra	NI 5.9.1		
Personality disorder	NB 1.5		
Phytobezoar	NI 5.8.6		
Poisoning by drugs, medicinals or biological substances	NB 3.1		
Poisoning from food stuffs or poisonous plants	NB 3.1		
Polycystic ovary disease	NI 5.10.1		
Polyps, colon	NI 5.10.1		
Postmenopause without estrogen supplementation	NI 5.10.1		
Premature birth	NC 1.3		
Premenstrual syndrome	NI 5.10.1		
Prolapsing hemorrhoids	NI 5.8.6		
Psychiatric illness	NC 3.4		
Pulmonary failure	NI 5.3		
Rachitic rosary in children	NI 5.9.1		
Renal disease, end stage	NI 3.2	NI 5.4	NB 2.3
Rickets	NI 5.9.1		
Rheumatic conditions	NC 3.4		
Seizure disorder	NI 5.8.1		
Sepsis or severe infection	NI 5.6.1	NI 5.8.2	NI 5.8.5
Short bowel syndrome	NI 5.8.6	NI 5.9.1	NI 5.10.1
SIADH	NI 3.2		
Stroke	NB 2.6		
Tardive dyskinesia	NB 2.6		
Thrush	NC 1.3		
Trauma	NC 3.2		
Tremors	NB 2.6		
Tuberculosis	NI 2.1	NI 5.6.1	
Ulcer disease	NI 5.8.5	NI 5.8.6	
Upper respiratory infections or pneumonia	NC 1.1		
Vagotomy	NC 1.4		
Vision problems	NB 2.4	NB 3.1	
Weight loss	NB 2.6		
Wired jaw	NC 1.2		

Edition: 2008

Nutrition Assessment Matrix
Client History Data and Related Diagnostic Terminology

Parameter (not all-inclusive)	Nutrition Diagnostic Terminology		
Mental status			
Evidence of addictive, obsessive, or compulsive tendencies	NB 2.2		
Signs and symptoms			
Abdominal cramping	NI 5.8.6		
Abdominal pain	NC 2.1	NC 1.4	
Achalasia	NC 1.1		
Acute or chronic pain	NI 1.4	NI 2.1	
Amenorrhea	NB 2.2		
Angina	NI 5.6.2		
Anorexia	NC 1.4		
Bloating	NB 3.1		
Chills	NB 3.1		
Cholesterol, serum	NI 4.1	NI 4.2	
Constipation	NC 1.4		
Contributes to the development of anemia	NI 5.5		
Cramping	NB 3.1		
Diarrhea	NI 5.5	NI 5.6.2	NI 5.6.3
	NI 5.8.6	NC 2.1	NB 3.1
	NC 1.4		
Discomfort or pain associated with intake of foods rich in bioactive substances	NI 4.2		
Dizziness	NB 3.1		
Dysphagia	NC 3.2		
Engorgement	NC 1.3		
Enteral or parenteral nutrition intolerance	NI 2.5		
Epigastric pain	NI 5.5	NI 5.6.2	NI 5.6.3
Falls, unexplained	NI 4.3		
Feeding tube or venous access in the wrong position or removed	NI 2.3		
Fever	NB 3.1		
Flatulence, excessive	NI 5.8.6		
Gastrointestinal disturbances	NI 5.10.2		
High stool volume or frequency that causes discomfort to the individual	NI 5.8.6		
Hunger, use of alcohol or drugs that reduce hunger	NI 1.4	NI 2.1	NI 5.2
Muscle weakness	NC 3.4		
Muscle weakness, fatigue, cardiac arrhythmia, dehydration, and electrolyte imbalance	NB 1.5		
Nausea	NI 5.5	NI 5.8.6	NB 3.1
	NC 1.4		
Oral manifestations of systemic disease	NC 1.2		
Report of always feeling cold	NB 1.5		
Self-induced vomiting, diarrhea, bloating, constipation, flatulence	NB 1.5		
Shortness of breath, dyspnea on exertion/rest	NI 3.2	NB 2.6	

Nutrition Assessment Matrix
Client History Data and Related Diagnostic Terminology

Parameter (not all-inclusive)	Nutrition Diagnostic Terminology		
Signs and symptoms, continued			
Steatorrhea	NI 5.6.2	NC 1.4	
Stool volume, low	NI 5.8.5		
Vomiting	NI 5.5	NI 5.8.6	NB 3.1
	NC 1.4		
Treatments			
Bowel resection	NC 1.4	NC 2.1	
Chemotherapy with oral side effects	NC 1.2		
Enteral or parenteral nutrition therapy	NI 5.7.3		
Esophagostomy or esophageal dilatation	NC 1.4		
Gastrectomy	NC 1.4		
Gastric bypass	NC 1.4	NC 2.1	
Intestinal resection	NI 2.3		
Knee surgery	NB 2.1		
Oral surgery, recent major	NC 1.2		
Ostomy, new	NB 1.4		
Radiation therapy	NC 1.2	NC 2.1	
Rigorous therapy regimen	NB 2.4		
Surgery	NI 5.3	NC 3.2	NB 2.4
Surgery requiring recumbent position	NB 2.6		
Medications and supplements			
Insulin or insulin secretagogues	NI 5.8.4		
Medications that cause somnolence and decreased cognition	NB 2.1		
Medication associated with weight loss	NC 3.2		
Medication, lipid lowering	NI 5.6.2		
Medications administered in large amounts of fluid	NI 3.2		
Medications affecting absorption or metabolism	NI 5.1		
Medications associated with increased appetite	NC 3.4		
Medications that affect appetite	NI 1.4	NC 3.1	
Medications that cause altered glucose levels	NI 5.8.2	NI 5.8.3	NI 5.8.4
Medications that cause anorexia	NI 2.1		
Medications that impact RMR	NC 3.3		
Medications that impair fluid excretion	NI 3.2		
Medications that increase energy expenditure	NI 1.2		
Medications that reduce requirements or impair metabolism of energy, protein, fat or fluid	NI 2.4		
Medications that reduce thirst	NI 3.1		
Medications that require nutrient supplementation that cannot be accomplished with food intake	NC 2.3		
Medications with known food-medication interactions	NC 2.3		
Misuse of laxatives, enemas, diuretics, stimulants, and/or metabolic enhancers	NB 1.5		

Updated: 2008 Edition

SNAPshot
NCP Step 2. Nutrition Diagnosis

What is the purpose of a Nutrition Diagnosis? The purpose is to identify and describe a specific nutrition problem that can be resolved or improved through treatment/nutrition intervention by a dietetic practitioner. A nutrition diagnosis (e.g., inconsistent carbohydrate intake) is different from a medical diagnosis (e.g., diabetes).

How does a dietetics practitioner determine a Nutrition Diagnosis? Dietetics practitioners use the data collected in the nutrition assessment to identify and label the patient/client's* nutrition diagnosis using standard nutrition diagnostic terminology. Each nutrition diagnosis has a reference sheet that includes its definition, possible etiology/causes and common signs or symptoms identified in the nutrition assessment step.

How are the Nutrition Diagnoses organized? In three categories.

Intake	Clinical	Behavioral-Environmental
Too much or too little of a food or nutrient compared to actual or estimated needs	*Nutrition problems that relate to medical or physical conditions*	*Knowledge, attitudes, beliefs, physical environment, access to food, or food safety*

How is the Nutrition Diagnosis documented? Dietetics practitioners write a PES statement to describe the problem, its root cause, and the assessment data that provide evidence for the nutrition diagnosis. The format for the PES statement is "Nutrition problem label related to _____ as evidenced by _____".

(P) Problem or Nutrition Diagnosis Label	(E) Etiology	(S) Signs/Symptoms
Describes alterations in the patient/client's nutrition status.	Cause/Contributing Risk Factors Linked to the nutrition diagnosis label by the words "related to."	Data used to determine that the patient/client has the nutrition diagnosis specified. Linked to the etiology by the words "as evidenced by."

What are the guidelines for selecting the diagnoses and writing a clear PES statement? The most important and urgent problem to be addressed is selected. When specifying the nutrition diagnosis and writing the PES statement; dietetics practitioners ask themselves a series of questions that help clarify the nutrition diagnosis. (See the critical thinking box).

Critical thinking during this step…

Evaluate your PES statement by using the following

P- Can the nutrition professional resolve or improve the nutrition diagnosis for this individual, group or population? When all things are equal and there is a choice between stating the PES statement using two nutrition diagnoses from different domains, consider the Intake nutrition diagnosis as the one more specific to the role of the RD.

E - Evaluate what you have used as your etiology to determine if it is the "root cause or the most specific root cause that the RD can address with a nutrition intervention. If as an RD you can not resolve the problem by addressing the etiology, can the RD intervention at least lessen the signs and symptoms?

S - Will measuring the signs and symptoms indicate if the problem is resolved or improved? Are the signs and symptoms specific enough that you can monitor (measure/evaluate changes) and document resolution or improvement of the nutrition diagnosis?

PES Overall - Does the nutrition assessment data support a particular nutrition diagnosis with a typical etiology and signs and symptoms?

Are dietetics practitioners limited to the Nutrition Diagnoses terms? Nutrition diagnosis terms and definitions were developed with extensive input and should fit most situations; however, food and dietetics practitioners can submit proposals for additions or revisions using the Procedure for Nutrition Controlled Vocabulary/Terminology Maintenance/Review available from ADA.

Detailed information about this step can be found in the International Dietetics and Nutrition Terminology (IDNT) Reference Manual: Standardized Language for the Nutrition Care Process, First Edition, American Dietetic Association.

Patient/client refers to individuals, groups, family members, and/or caregivers.

Nutrition Care Process Step 2. Nutrition Diagnosis

INTRODUCTION

The ADA has identified and defined nutrition diagnoses/problems used in the profession of dietetics. Nutrition diagnosis is identifying and labeling an actual occurrence, risk of, or potential for developing a nutritional problem that a dietetics practitioner is responsible for treating independently. The standardized language of nutrition diagnoses/problems is an integral component in the Nutrition Care Process. In fact, several other professions, including medicine, nursing, physical therapy, and occupational therapy, utilize care processes with defined terms for making nutrition diagnoses specific to their professional scope of practice.

ADA's Standardized Language Task Force developed a conceptual framework for the standardized nutrition language and identified the nutrition diagnoses/problems. The framework outlines the domains within which the nutrition diagnoses/problems fall and the flow of the nutrition care process in relation to the continuum of health, disease, and disability.

The methodology for developing sets of terms such as these included systematically collecting data from multiple sources simultaneously. Data were collected from a select group of ADA recognized leaders and award winners prior to starting the project. A 12-member task force developed the terms with input from groups of community, ambulatory, acute care, and long-term care practitioners and obtained feedback from experts concerning the research supporting the terms and definitions.

The methodology for continued development and refinement of these terms has been identified. As with the ongoing updating of the American Medical Association Current Procedural Terminology (CPT) codes, these will also be published on an annual basis. The terms are being studied in a number of research projects to assess their validity. Based upon the results of two content validation studies, this edition of the publication reflects changes to the nutrition diagnoses that are discussed in greater detail in this chapter (1 and E.B. Enrione personal communication, December 2006). Further changes are anticipated as results of additional studies become available. The nutrition diagnostic terms are being incorporated into several research studies that explore use in ambulatory or inpatient settings or by specific types of practice, e.g., nutrition support and oncology.

As each of the research studies is completed, findings will be incorporated into future versions of these terms. Future iterations and changes to the nutrition diagnoses/problems and the reference sheet are expected as this standard language and the dietetics profession evolve. In addition, practitioners can submit suggested changes. The process for practitioners to submit suggested revisions to the nutrition diagnoses is included in this book on page 365.

ADA is working toward including the concepts from the Nutrition Care Process and these specific terms in standards for electronic health records and incorporation into standardized informatics languages, such as the Systematized Nomenclature of Medicine International (SNOMED), Logical Observation Identifiers Names and Codes (LOINC) and United Medical Language System (UMLS). ADA has already begun the dialogue with these groups to let them know the direction that the Association is headed and to keep them appraised of progress. Thus far, the feedback from the database and informatics groups has been quite positive, and they have expressed a need for documenting the unique nature of nutrition services.

WHAT IS NEW IN THIS EDITION RELATED TO NUTRITION DIAGNOSIS?

As mentioned, research studies evaluating the validity of the nutrition diagnoses are ongoing. Two content validation studies are complete and the nutrition diagnoses have been modified in this edition based upon these results and submissions by ADA members (1 and E.B. Enrione personal communication, December 2006). In total, 16 members submitted recommendations suggesting modifications or additions to the 2007 Edition of the nutrition diagnoses (2) using the Procedure for Nutrition Controlled Vocabulary/Terminology Maintenance/ Review available in this resource.

The changes include:

- **Deletion of two previously published nutrition diagnoses,** Hypermetabolism NI-1.1 and Hypometabolism NI-1.3. It was determined that these are not nutrition diagnoses that practitioners can treat. With these deletions, there are now 60 nutrition diagnoses with which to describe nutrition practice.
- **Deletion of individual Etiologies or Signs/Symptoms** determined not to be causes/contributing factors or defining characteristics, respectively.
- **Addition of individual Etiologies or Signs/Symptoms** determined to be causes/contributing factors or defining characteristics, respectively.
- **Revision of individual Definitions, Etiologies, or Signs/Symptoms** for clarity or expansion. For example in the 2007 Edition, Excessive Energy Intake NI-1.5 includes the sign/symptom of *Body mass index (BMI) > 25*. This sign/symptom was revised to *BMI > 25 (adults), BMI > 95th percentile (pediatrics)* to include a parameter for pediatrics.

Further:

- Each nutrition diagnosis reference sheet that has been modified includes a notation on the last page indicating the publication year in which it was updated, e.g., Updated: 2008 Edition.
- The Nutrition Assessment Matrix (Step 1) reflects all of the changes to the nutrition diagnoses.
- A document detailing all of the specific changes to the nutrition diagnoses, along with the rationale, is available in the Nutrition Care Process and Model Resource section of the ADA Web site, www. eatright.org, in the either the Research or Practice sections. Editorial changes not affecting the content were not included in this document.

NUTRITION CARE PROCESS AND NUTRITION DIAGNOSIS

Nutrition diagnosis is a critical step between nutrition assessment and nutrition intervention. The nutrition diagnosis is the identification and labeling of the specific nutrition problem that dietetics practitioners are responsible for treating independently.

Naming the nutrition diagnosis, identifying the etiology and signs and symptoms, provides a way to document the link between nutrition assessment and nutrition intervention and set realistic and measurable expected outcomes for each patient/client. Identifying the nutrition diagnosis also assists practitioners in establishing priorities when planning an individual patient/client's nutrition intervention.

> **Special Note.** The terms **patient/client** are used in association with the NCP; however, the process is also intended for use with groups. In addition, family members or caregivers are an essential asset to the patient/client and dietetics practitioner in the NCP. Therefore, **groups, families, and caregivers** of patients/clients are implied each time a reference is made to patient/client.

In simple terms, a nutrition practitioner identifies and labels a specific nutrition diagnosis (problem) that, in general, he or she is responsible for treating independently (e.g., excessive carbohydrate intake). With nutrition intervention, the nutrition diagnosis ideally resolves. In contrast, a medical diagnosis describes a disease or pathology of organs or body systems (e.g., diabetes). In some instances, such as the nutrition diagnosis Swallowing Difficulty NC-1.1, nutrition practitioners are labeling or diagnosing the functional problem that has a nutritional consequence. Nutrition practitioners do not identify medical diagnoses; they diagnose phenomena in the nutrition domain.

Categories of Nutrition Diagnostic Terminology

The 60 nutrition diagnoses/problems have been given labels that are clustered into three domains: intake, clinical, and behavioral-environmental. Each domain represents unique characteristics that contribute to nutritional health. Within each domain are classes and, in some cases, subclasses of nutrition diagnoses.

A definition of each follows:

The **Intake** domain lists actual problems related to intake of energy, nutrients, fluids, or bioactive substances through oral diet, or nutrition support (enteral or parenteral nutrition).

Class: Energy Balance (1)—Actual or estimated changes in energy (kcal).

Class: Oral or Nutrition Support Intake (2)—Actual or estimated food and beverage intake from oral diet or nutrition support compared with patient/client's goal.

Class: Fluid Intake (3)—Actual or estimated fluid intake compared with patient/client's goal.

Class: Bioactive Substances Intake (4)—Actual or observed intake of bioactive substances, including single or multiple functional food components, ingredients, dietary supplements, and alcohol.

Class: Nutrient Intake (5)—Actual or estimated intake of specific nutrient groups or single nutrients as compared with desired levels.

> Subclass: Fat and Cholesterol (5.6)
> Subclass: Protein (5.7)
> Subclass: Carbohydrate and Fiber (5.8)
> Subclass: Vitamin (5.9)
> Subclass: Mineral (5.10)

The **Clinical** domain is nutritional findings/problems identified as related to medical or physical conditions.

Class: Functional (1)—Change in physical or mechanical functioning that interferes with or prevents desired nutritional consequences.

Class: Biochemical (2)—Change in the capacity to metabolize nutrients as a result of medications, surgery, or as indicated by altered lab values.

Class: Weight (3)—Chronic weight or changed weight status when compared with usual or desired body weight.

The **Behavioral-Environmental** domain includes nutritional findings/problems identified that relate to knowledge, attitudes/beliefs, physical environment, access to food, and food safety.

Class: Knowledge and Beliefs (1)—Actual knowledge and beliefs as reported, observed, or documented.

Class: Physical Activity and Function (2)—Actual physical activity, self-care, and quality of life problems as reported, observed, or documented.

Class: Food Safety and Access (3)—Actual problems with food access or food safety.

Examples of nutrition diagnoses and their definitions include:

INTAKE DOMAIN • Energy Balance

Inadequate energy intake NI-1.4	Energy intake that is less than energy expenditure, established reference standards, or recommendations based on physiological needs. Exception: when the goal is weight loss or during end-of-life care.

CLINICAL DOMAIN • Functional

Swallowing difficulty NC-1.1	Impaired or difficult movement of food and liquid within the oral cavity to the stomach

BEHAVIORAL-ENVIRONMENTAL DOMAIN • Knowledge and Beliefs

Not ready for diet/lifestyle change NB-1.3	Lack of perceived value of nutrition-related behavior change compared to costs (consequences or effort required to make changes); conflict with personal value system; antecedent to behavior change.

Edition: 2008

NUTRITION DIAGNOSIS STATEMENTS (OR PES)

The nutrition diagnosis is summarized into a structured sentence named the *nutrition diagnosis statement*. This statement, also called a *PES statement*, is composed of three distinct components: the problem (P), the etiology (E), and the signs and symptoms (S). The practitioner obtains the etiology and the signs and symptoms during the nutrition assessment phase of the nutrition care process. The nutrition diagnosis is derived from the synthesis of nutrition assessment data, and the wording is obtained from the nutrition diagnoses reference sheets (see pages 49-170).

The generic format for the nutrition diagnosis statement is:

Problem (P) *related to* etiology (E) *as evidenced by* signs and symptoms (S).

Where:

The **Problem or Nutrition Diagnosis Label** describes alterations in the patient/client's nutrition status that dietetics practitioners are responsible for treating independently. A nutrition diagnosis allows the dietetics practitioner to identify realistic and measurable outcomes, formulate nutrition interventions, and monitor and evaluate change. (Select from terms on Page 39.)	The **Etiology** (Cause/Contributing Risk Factors) are those factors contributing to the existence, or maintenance of pathophysiological, psychosocial, situational, developmental, cultural, and/or environmental problems. It is linked to the nutrition diagnosis label by the words "related to." Identifying the etiology will lead to the selection of a nutrition intervention aimed at resolving the underlying cause of the nutrition problem whenever possible. Usually free text, but can also use some terms from Page 39.	The **Signs/Symptoms** (Defining Characteristics) consist of objective (signs) and/or subjective (symptoms) data used to determine whether the patient/client has the nutrition diagnosis specified. It is linked to the etiology by the words "as evidenced by." The clear identification of quantifiable data in the signs and symptoms will serve as the basis for monitoring and evaluating nutrition outcomes Usually free text, but can also use some terms from Page 39 as long as they are quantified.

A well-written nutrition diagnosis (PES) statement is:

- Simple, clear, and concise
- Specific to the patient/client or group
- Related to a single patient/client nutrition-related problem
- Accurately related to an etiology
- Based on reliable and accurate nutrition assessment data

Specific questions dietetics practitioners should use in evaluating the PES they have developed are:

P- Can the nutrition professional resolve or improve the nutrition diagnosis for this individual, group or population? When all things are equal and there is a choice between stating the PES statement using two nutrition diagnoses from different domains, consider the Intake nutrition diagnosis as the one more specific to the role of the RD.

E - Evaluate what you have used as your etiology to determine if it is the "root cause or the most specific root cause that the RD can address with a nutrition intervention. If as an RD you can not resolve the problem by addressing the etiology, can the RD intervention at least lessen the signs and symptoms?

S - Will measuring the signs and symptoms indicate if the problem is resolved or improved? Are the signs and symptoms specific enough that you can monitor (measure/evaluate changes) and document resolution or improvement of the nutrition diagnosis?

PES Overall - Does the nutrition assessment data support a particular nutrition diagnosis with a typical etiology and signs and symptoms?

Examples of nutrition diagnosis (PES) statements are:

Diagnosis or Problem		Etiology		Signs and/or Symptoms
Excessive fat intake	*Related to*	frequent consumption of fast-food meals	*As evidenced by*	serum cholesterol level of 230 mg/dL and 10 meals per week of hamburgers/sandwich and fries
Excessive energy intake	*Related to*	unchanged dietary intake and restricted mobility while fracture healing	*As evidenced by*	5# weight gain during last 3 weeks due to consumption of 500 kcal/day more than estimated needs
Disordered eating pattern	*Related to*	harmful belief about food and nutrition	*As evidenced by*	reported use of laxatives after meals and statements that calories are not absorbed when laxatives are used
Swallowing Difficulty	*Related to*	post stroke complications	*As evidenced by*	results of swallowing tests and reports of choking during mealtime

NUTRITION DIAGNOSIS REFERENCE SHEET

A reference sheet is available for each nutrition diagnosis. Reference sheets contain four distinct components: nutrition diagnosis label, definition of nutrition diagnosis label, examples of common etiologies, and signs/symptoms. Following is a description of the four components of the reference sheet.

The **Problem or Nutrition Diagnosis Label** describes alterations in the patient/client's nutrition status that dietetics practitioners are responsible for treating independently. Nutrition diagnosis differs from medical diagnosis in that a nutrition diagnosis changes as the patient/client response changes. The medical diagnosis does not change as long as the disease or condition exists. A nutrition diagnosis allows the dietetics practitioner to focus on problem(s) that can be resolved and identify realistic and measurable outcomes, formulate nutrition interventions, and monitor and evaluate change.

The **Definition** of Nutrition Diagnosis Label briefly describes the Nutrition Diagnosis Label to differentiate a discrete problem area.

The **Etiology** (Cause/Contributing Risk Factors) are those factors contributing to the existence or maintenance of pathophysiological, psychosocial, situational, developmental, cultural, and/or environmental problems. It is linked to the Nutrition Diagnosis Label by the words *related to*.

The **Signs/Symptoms** (Defining Characteristics) consist of subjective and/or objective data used to determine whether the patient/client has the nutrition diagnosis specified. It is linked to the etiology by the words *as evidenced by*.

The signs and symptoms are gathered in Step 1 of the nutrition care process: nutrition assessment. There are five categories of nutrition assessment data used to cluster the information on the nutrition diagnosis reference sheet—food/nutrition history; biochemical data, medical tests, and procedures; anthropometric measurements; physical exam findings; and client history. Within each nutrition assessment category, potential indicators associated with the specific nutrition diagnosis are listed on the reference sheet.

Edition: 2008

Diagnosis

Example
Swallowing Difficulty NC-1.1

Nutrition Assessment Category	Potential Indicator of this Nutrition Diagnosis
Physical Exam Finding	• Evidence of dehydration, e.g., dry mucous membranes, poor skin turgor

These reference sheets, beginning on page 49, will assist practitioners with identifying, consistently and correctly, the nutrition diagnoses.

> **Special Note.** Laboratory parameters within the nutrition diagnosis reference sheets are provided only for guidance.
>
> Practitioners:
>
> - Should be aware that laboratory values may be different depending on the laboratory performing the test.
> - Must recognize that there may not be scientific consensus on the best measure to use for testing and evaluating a particular lab or reference standard parameter.
> - Need to evaluate laboratory findings for their significance or lack of significance depending on the patient/client population, disease severity, and/or treatment goals.
> - Are responsible for keeping abreast of national, institutional, and regulatory guidelines that impact practice and applying them as appropriate to individual patient/clients.

SUMMARY

Nutrition diagnosis is the critical link in the nutrition care process between nutrition assessment and nutrition intervention. Nutrition interventions can then be clearly targeted to address either the etiology (E) or signs and symptoms (S) of the specific nutrition diagnosis/problem identified. Using a standardized terminology for identifying the nutrition diagnosis/problem will make one aspect of the critical thinking of dietetics practitioners visible to other professionals as well as provide a clear method of communicating among dietetics practitioners. Implementation of a standard language throughout the profession, with tools to assist practitioners, is making this language a success. Ongoing study and evaluation is critical as the standardized language is utilized by the profession.

REFERENCES

1. Charney PJ.(2006). *Reliability of nutrition diagnostic codes and their defining characteristics.* (Doctoral dissertation, University of Medicine and Dentistry of New Jersey, 2006.).
2. American Dietetic Association. *Nutrition Diagnosis and Intervention: Standardized Language for the Nutrition Care Process.* Chicago, IL: American Dietetic Association; 2007.

Nutrition Diagnostic Terminology

INTAKE   NI
Defined as "actual problems related to intake of energy, nutrients, fluids, bioactive substances through oral diet or nutrition support"

Energy Balance (1)
Defined as "actual or estimated changes in energy (kcal) balance"

- ☐ *Unused*   NI-1.1
- ☐ Increased energy expenditure   NI-1.2
- ☐ *Unused*   NI-1.3
- ☐ Inadequate energy intake   NI-1.4
- ☐ Excessive energy intake   NI-1.5

Oral or Nutrition Support Intake (2)
Defined as "actual or estimated food and beverage intake from oral diet or nutrition support compared with patient goal"

- ☐ Inadequate oral food/ beverage intake   NI-2.1
- ☐ Excessive oral food/ beverage intake   NI-2.2
- ☐ Inadequate intake from enteral/parenteral nutrition   NI-2.3
- ☐ Excessive intake from enteral/parenteral nutrition   NI-2.4
- ☐ Inappropriate infusion of enteral/parenteral nutrition (use with caution)   NI-2.5

Fluid Intake (3)
Defined as "actual or estimated fluid intake compared with patient goal"

- ☐ Inadequate fluid intake   NI-3.1
- ☐ Excessive fluid intake   NI-3.2

Bioactive Substances (4)
Defined as "actual or observed intake of bioactive substances, including single or multiple functional food components, ingredients, dietary supplements, alcohol"

- ☐ Inadequate bioactive substance intake   NI-4.1
- ☐ Excessive bioactive substance intake   NI-4.2
- ☐ Excessive alcohol intake   NI-4.3

Nutrient (5)
Defined as "actual or estimated intake of specific nutrient groups or single nutrients as compared with desired levels"

- ☐ Increased nutrient needs (specify) _____   NI-5.1
- ☐ Evident protein-energy malnutrition   NI-5.2
- ☐ Inadequate protein-energy intake   NI-5.3
- ☐ Decreased nutrient needs (specify) _____   NI-5.4
- ☐ Imbalance of nutrients   NI-5.5

Fat and Cholesterol (5.6)
- ☐ Inadequate fat intake   NI-5.6.1
- ☐ Excessive fat intake   NI-5.6.2
- ☐ Inappropriate intake of food fats (specify) _____   NI-5.6.3

Protein (5.7)
- ☐ Inadequate protein intake   NI-5.7.1
- ☐ Excessive protein intake   NI-5.7.2
- ☐ Inappropriate intake of amino acids (specify) _____   NI-5.7.3

Carbohydrate and Fiber (5.8)
- ☐ Inadequate carbohydrate intake   NI-5.8.1
- ☐ Excessive carbohydrate intake   NI-5.8.2
- ☐ Inappropriate intake of types of carbohydrate (specify) _____   NI-5.8.3
- ☐ Inconsistent carbohydrate intake   NI-5.8.4
- ☐ Inadequate fiber intake   NI-5.8.5
- ☐ Excessive fiber intake   NI-5.8.6

Vitamin (5.9)
- ☐ Inadequate vitamin intake (specify) _____   NI-5.9.1
- ☐ Excessive vitamin intake (specify) _____   NI-5.9.2
  - ☐ A   ☐ Riboflavin
  - ☐ C   ☐ Niacin
  - ☐ D   ☐ Folate
  - ☐ E   ☐ B6
  - ☐ K   ☐ B12
  - ☐ Thiamin
  - ☐ Other (specify) _____

Mineral (5.10)
- ☐ Inadequate mineral intake (specify) _____   NI-5.10.1
- ☐ Excessive mineral intake (specify) _____   NI-5.10.2
  - ☐ Calcium   ☐ Phosphorus
  - ☐ Iron   ☐ Potassium
  - ☐ Magnesium   ☐ Zinc
  - ☐ Other (specify) _____

CLINICAL   NC
Defined as "nutritional findings/problems identified that relate to medical or physical conditions"

Functional (1)
Defined as "change in physical or mechanical functioning that interferes with or prevents desired nutritional consequences"

- ☐ Swallowing difficulty   NC-1.1
- ☐ Biting/Chewing (masticatory) difficulty   NC-1.2
- ☐ Breastfeeding difficulty   NC-1.3
- ☐ Altered GI function   NC-1.4

Biochemical (2)
Defined as "change in capacity to metabolize nutrients as a result of medications, surgery, or as indicated by altered lab values"

- ☐ Impaired nutrient utilization   NC-2.1
- ☐ Altered nutrition-related laboratory values (specify) _____   NC-2.2
- ☐ Food-medication interaction   NC-2.3

Weight (3)
Defined as "chronic weight or changed weight status when compared with usual or desired body weight"

- ☐ Underweight   NC-3.1
- ☐ Involuntary weight loss   NC-3.2
- ☐ Overweight/obesity   NC-3.3
- ☐ Involuntary weight gain   NC-3.4

BEHAVIORAL- ENVIRONMENTAL   NB
Defined as "nutritional findings/problems identified that relate to knowledge, attitudes/beliefs, physical environment, access to food, or food safety"

Knowledge and Beliefs (1)
Defined as "actual knowledge and beliefs as related, observed or documented"

- ☐ Food- and nutrition-related knowledge deficit   NB-1.1
- ☐ Harmful beliefs/attitudes about food- or nutrition-related topics (*use with caution*)   NB-1.2
- ☐ Not ready for diet/ lifestyle change   NB-1.3
- ☐ Self-monitoring deficit   NB-1.4
- ☐ Disordered eating pattern   NB-1.5
- ☐ Limited adherence to nutrition-related recommendations   NB-1.6
- ☐ Undesirable food choices   NB-1.7

Physical Activity and Function (2)
Defined as "actual physical activity, self-care, and quality-of-life problems as reported, observed, or documented"

- ☐ Physical inactivity   NB-2.1
- ☐ Excessive exercise   NB-2.2
- ☐ Inability or lack of desire to manage self-care   NB-2.3
- ☐ Impaired ability to prepare foods/meals   NB-2.4
- ☐ Poor nutrition quality of life   NB-2.5
- ☐ Self-feeding difficulty   NB-2.6

Food Safety and Access (3)
Defined as "actual problems with food access or food safety"

- ☐ Intake of unsafe food   NB-3.1
- ☐ Limited access to food   NB-3.2

Date Identified	Date Resolved

#1 **Problem** _____

    Etiology _____

    Signs/Symptoms _____

#2 **Problem** _____

    Etiology _____

    Signs/Symptoms _____

#3 **Problem** _____

    Etiology _____

    Signs/Symptoms _____

Edition: 2008

NUTRITION DIAGNOSIS TERMS AND DEFINITIONS

Nutrition Diagnostic Term	Term Number	Definition	Reference Sheet Page Numbers
DOMAIN: INTAKE	NI	**Actual problems related to intake of energy, nutrients, fluids, bioactive substances through oral diet or nutrition support (enteral or parenteral nutrition).**	
Class: Energy Balance (1)			
Unused	NI-1.1	Actual or estimated changes in energy (kcal) balance.	
Increased energy expenditure	NI-1.2	Resting metabolic rate (RMR) more than predicted requirements due to body composition, medications, endocrine, neurologic, or genetic changes. Note: RMR is the sum of metabolic processes of active cell mass related to the maintenance of normal body functions and regulatory balance during rest.	49
Unused	NI-1.3		
Inadequate energy intake	NI-1.4	Energy intake that is less than energy expenditure, established reference standards, or recommendations based on physiological needs. Exception: when the goal is weight loss or during end of life care.	50-51
Excessive energy intake	NI-1.5	Energy intake(e.g., oral, EN/PN, IV, medications) that exceeds energy expenditure, established reference standards, or recommendations based on physiological needs. Exception: when weight gain is desired.	52-53

NUTRITION DIAGNOSIS TERMS AND DEFINITIONS

Nutrition Diagnostic Term	Term Number	Definition	Reference Sheet Page Numbers
Class: Oral or Nutrition Support Intake (2)		Actual or estimated food and beverage intake from oral diet or nutrition support compared with patient goal.	
Inadequate oral food/beverage intake	NI-2.1	Oral food/beverage intake that is less than established reference standards or recommendations based on physiological needs. Exception: when recommendation is weight loss or during end-of-life care.	54-55
Excessive oral food/beverage intake	NI-2.2	Oral food/beverage intake that exceeds estimated energy needs, established reference standards, or recommendations based on physiological needs. Exception: when weight gain is desired.	56-57
Inadequate intake from enteral/parenteral nutrition	NI-2.3	Enteral or parenteral infusion that provides fewer calories or nutrients compared to establish reference standards or recommendations based on physiological needs. Exception: when recommendation is for weight loss or during end-of-life care.	58-59
Excessive intake from enteral/parenteral nutrition	NI-2.4	Enteral or parenteral infusion that provides more calories or nutrients compared to established reference standards or recommendations based on physiological needs	60-61
Inappropriate infusion of enteral/parenteral nutrition USE WITH CAUTION ONLY AFTER DISCUSSION WITH OTHER MEMBERS IF THE HEALTH CARE TEAM	NI-2.5	Enteral or parenteral infusion that provides either fewer or more calories and/or nutrients or is of the wrong composition or type, parental nutrition that is not warranted because the patient is able to tolerate an enteral intake, or is unsafe because of the potential for sepsis or other complications	62-63

41

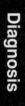

NUTRITION DIAGNOSIS TERMS AND DEFINITIONS

Nutrition Diagnostic Term	Term Number	Definition	Reference Sheet Page Numbers
Class: Fluid Intake (3)		Actual or estimated fluid intake compared with patient goal.	
Inadequate fluid intake	NI-3.1	Lower intake of fluid-containing foods or substances compared to established reference standards or recommendations based on physiological needs	64-65
Excessive fluid intake	NI-3.2	Higher intake of fluid compared to established reference standards or recommendations based on physiological needs	66-67
Class: Bioactive Substances (4)		Actual or observed intake of bioactive substances, including single or multiple functional food components, ingredients, dietary supplements, alcohol.	
Inadequate bioactive substance intake	NI-4.1	Lower intake of bioactive substances or foods containing bioactive substances compared to established reference standards or recommendations based on physiological needs	68-69
Excessive bioactive substance intake	NI-4.2	Higher intake of bioactive substances other than traditional nutrients, such as functional foods, bioactive food components, dietary supplements, or food concentrates compared to established reference standards or recommendations based on physiological needs	70-71
Excessive alcohol intake	NI-4.3	Intake more than the suggested limits for alcohol	72-73
Class: Nutrient (5)		Actual or estimated intake of specific nutrient groups or single nutrients as compared with desired levels.	
Increased nutrient needs (specify)	NI-5.1	Increased need for a specific nutrient compared to established reference standards or recommendations based on physiological needs	74-75

NUTRITION DIAGNOSIS TERMS AND DEFINITIONS

Nutrition Diagnostic Term	Term Number	Definition	Reference Sheet Page Numbers
Evident protein-energy malnutrition	NI-5.2	Inadequate intake of protein and/or energy over prolonged periods of time resulting in loss of fat stores and/or muscle wasting	76-77
Inadequate protein-energy intake	NI-5.3	Inadequate intake of protein and/or energy compared to established reference standards or recommendations based on physiological needs of short or recent duration	78-79
Decreased nutrient needs (specify)	NI-5.4	Decreased need for a specific nutrient compared to established reference standards or recommendations based on physiological needs	80-81
Imbalance of nutrients	NI-5.5	An undesirable combination of ingested nutrients, such that the amount of one nutrient ingested interferes with or alters absorption and/or utilization of another nutrient	82-83
Subclass: Fat and Cholesterol (5.6)			
Inadequate fat intake	NI-5.6.1	Lower fat intake compared to established reference standards or recommendations based on physiological needs. Exception: when recommendation is for weight loss or during end-of-life care.	84-85
Excessive fat intake	NI-5.6.2	Higher fat intake compared to established reference standards or recommendations based on physiological needs	86-87
Inappropriate intake of food fats (specify)	NI-5.6.3	Intake of wrong type or quality of food fats compared to established reference standards or recommendations based on physiological needs	88-89
Subclass: Protein (5.7)			
Inadequate protein intake	NI-5.7.1	Lower intake of protein-containing foods or substances compared to established reference standards or recommendations based on physiological needs	90-91

43

NUTRITION DIAGNOSIS TERMS AND DEFINITIONS

Nutrition Diagnostic Term	Term Number	Definition	Reference Sheet Page Numbers
Excessive protein intake	NI-5.7.2	Intake more than the recommended level of protein compared to established reference standards or recommendations based on physiological needs	92-93
Inappropriate intake of amino acids (specify)	NI-5.7.3	Intake that is more or less than recommended level and/or type of amino acids compared to established reference standards or recommendations based on physiological needs	94-95
Subclass: Carbohydrate and Fiber (5.8)			
Inadequate carbohydrate intake	NI-5.8.1	Lower intake of carbohydrate-containing foods or substances compared to established reference standards or recommendations based on physiological needs	96
Excessive carbohydrate intake	NI-5.8.2	Intake more than the recommended level and type of carbohydrate compared to established reference standards or recommendations based on physiological needs	97-98
Inappropriate intake of types of carbohydrate (specify)	NI-5.8.3	Intake or the type or amount of carbohydrate that is more or less than the established reference standards or recommendations based on physiological needs	99-100
Inconsistent carbohydrate intake	NI-5.8.4	Inconsistent timing of carbohydrate intake throughout the day, day to day, or a pattern of carbohydrate intake that is not consistent with recommended pattern based on physiological needs	101-102
Inadequate fiber intake	NI-5.8.5	Lower intake of fiber-containing foods or substances compared to established reference standards or recommendations based on physiological needs	103-104
Excessive fiber intake	NI-5.8.6	Higher intake of fiber-containing foods or substances compared to recommendations based on patient/client condition	105-106

Edition: 2008

NUTRITION DIAGNOSIS TERMS AND DEFINITIONS

Nutrition Diagnostic Term	Term Number	Definition	Reference Sheet Page Numbers
Subclass: Vitamin (5.9)			
Inadequate vitamin intake (specify)	NI-5.9.1	Lower intake of vitamin-containing foods or substances compared to established reference standards or recommendations based on physiological needs	107-109
Excessive vitamin intake (specify)	NI-5.9.2	Higher intake of vitamin-containing foods or substances compared to established reference standards or recommendations based on physiological needs	110-111
Subclass: Mineral (5.10)			
Inadequate mineral intake (specify)	NI-5.10.1	Lower intake of mineral-containing foods or substances compared to established reference standards or recommendations based on physiological needs	112-113
Excessive mineral intake (specify)	NI-5.10.2	Higher intake of mineral from foods, supplements, medications, or water, compared to established reference standards or recommendations based on physiological needs	114-115
DOMAIN: CLINICAL	NC	**Nutritional findings/problems identified that relate to medical or physical conditions.**	
Class: Functional (1)		Change in physical or mechanical functioning that interferes with or prevents desired nutritional consequences.	
Swallowing difficulty	NC-1.1	Impaired or difficult movement of food and liquid within the oral cavity to the stomach	116-117
Biting/Chewing (masticatory) difficulty	NC-1.2	Impaired ability to manipulate or masticate food for swallowing	118-120
Breastfeeding difficulty	NC-1.3	Inability to sustain nutrition through breastfeeding	121-122
Altered GI function	NC-1.4	Changes in ability to digest or absorb nutrients	123-124

Edition: 2008

NUTRITION DIAGNOSIS TERMS AND DEFINITIONS

Nutrition Diagnostic Term	Term Number	Definition	Reference Sheet Page Numbers
Class: Biochemical (2)			
Impaired nutrient utilization	NC-2.1	Change in capacity to metabolize nutrients as a result of medications, surgery, or as indicated by altered lab values.	125-126
Altered nutrition-related laboratory values (specify)	NC-2.2	Changes in ability to absorb or metabolize nutrients and bioactive substances	127-128
Food-medication interaction	NC-2.3	Undesirable/harmful interaction(s) between food and over-the-counter (OTC) medications, prescribed medications, herbals, botanicals, and/or dietary supplements that diminishes, enhances, or alters effect of nutrients and/or medications	129-130
Class: Weight (3)			
Underweight	NC-3.1	Chronic weight or changed weight status when compared with usual or desired body weight.	131-132
Involuntary weight loss	NC-3.2	Low body weight compared to established reference standards or recommendations	133-134
Overweight/obesity	NC-3.3	Decrease in body weight that is not planned or desired	135-137
Involuntary weight gain	NC-3.4	Increased adiposity compared to established reference standards or recommendations, ranging from overweight to morbid obesity.	138-139
		Weight gain more than that which is desired or expected	

Edition: 2008

NUTRITION DIAGNOSIS TERMS AND DEFINITIONS

Nutrition Diagnostic Term	Term Number	Definition	Reference Sheet Page Numbers
DOMAIN: BEHAVIORAL-ENVIRONMENTAL	NB	**Nutritional findings/problems identified that relate to knowledge, attitudes/beliefs, physical environment, access to food, or food safety.**	
Class: Knowledge and Beliefs (1)		Actual knowledge and beliefs as reported, observed, ordocumented	
Food- and nutrition-related knowledge deficit	NB-1.1	Incomplete or inaccurate knowledge about food, nutrition, or nutrition-related information and guidelines, e.g., nutrient requirements, consequences of food behaviors, life stage requirements, nutrition recommendations, diseases and conditions, physiological function, or products	140-141
Harmful beliefs/attitudes about food or nutrition-related topics USE WITH CAUTION TO BE SENSITIVE TO PATIENT CONCERNS	NB-1.2	Beliefs/attitudes and practices about food, nutrition, and nutrition-related topics that are incompatible with sound nutrition principles, nutrition care, or disease/condition	142-143
Not ready for diet/lifestyle change	NB-1.3	Lack of perceived value of nutrition-related behavior change compared to costs (consequences or effort required to make changes); conflict with personal value system; antecedent to behavior change	144-145
Self-monitoring deficit	NB-1.4	Lack of data recording to track personal progress	146-147
Disordered eating pattern	NB-1.5	Beliefs, attitudes, thoughts, and behaviors related to food, eating, and weight management, including classic eating disorders as well as less severe, similar conditions that negatively impact health	148-150
Limited adherence to nutrition-related recommendations	NB-1.6	Lack of nutrition-related changes as per intervention agreed upon by client or population	151-152
Undesirable food choices	NB-1.7	Food and/or beverage choices that are inconsistent with DRIs, US Dietary Guidelines, or MyPyramid, or with targets defined in the nutrition prescription or nutrition care process.	153-154

47

NUTRITION DIAGNOSIS TERMS AND DEFINITIONS

Nutrition Diagnostic Term	Term Number	Definition	Reference Sheet Page Numbers
Class: Physical Activity and Function (2)			
Physical inactivity	NB-2.1	Actual physical activity, self-care, and quality-of-life problems as reported, observed, or documented	155-156
Excessive exercise	NB-2.2	Low level of activity or sedentary behavior to the extent that it reduces energy expenditure and impacts health	157-158
Inability or lack of desire to manage self-care	NB-2.3	An amount of exercise that exceeds that which is necessary to improve health and/or athletic performance	159-160
Impaired ability to prepare foods/meals	NB-2.4	Lack of capacity or unwillingness to implement methods to support healthful food- and nutrition-related behavior	161-162
Poor nutrition quality of life	NB-2.5	Cognitive or physical impairment that prevents preparation of foods/meals	163-164
Self-feeding difficulty	NB-2.6	Diminished patient/client perception of quality of life in response to nutrition problems and recommendations.	165-166
Class: Food Safety and Access (3)		Impaired ability to place food in mouth	
		Actual problems with food access or food safety.	
Intake of unsafe food	NB-3.1	Intake of food and/or fluids intentionally or unintentionally contaminated with toxins, poisonous products, infectious agents, microbial agents, additives, allergens, and/or agents of bioterrorism	167-168
Limited access to food	NB-3.2	Diminished ability to acquire a sufficient quantity and variety of healthful food based upon the U.S. Dietary Guidelines or MyPyramid. Limitation to food because of concerns about weight or aging.	169-170

48

Edition: 2008

INCREASED ENERGY EXPENDITURE (NI-1.2)

Definition

Resting metabolic rate (RMR) more than predicted requirements due to body composition, medications, endocrine, neurologic, or genetic changes. Note: RMR is the sum of metabolic processes of active cell mass related to the maintenance of normal body functions and regulatory balance during rest.

Etiology (Cause/Contributing Risk Factors)

Factors gathered during the nutrition assessment process that contribute to the existence or the maintenance of pathophysiological, psychosocial, situational, developmental, cultural, and/or environmental problems:

- Anabolism or growth
- Voluntary or involuntary physical activity/movement

Signs/Symptoms (Defining Characteristics)

A typical cluster of subjective and objective signs and symptoms gathered during the nutrition assessment process that provide evidence that a problem exists; quantify the problem and describe its severity.

Nutrition Assessment Category	Potential Indicators of this Nutrition Diagnosis (one or more must be present)
Biochemical Data, Medical Tests and Procedures	
Anthropometric Measurements	▪ Unintentional weight loss of ≥ 10% in 6 months, ≥ 5% in 1 month (adults and pediatrics) and > 2% in 1 week (pediatrics) ▪ Evidence of need for accelerated or catch-up growth or weight gain in children; absence of normal growth ▪ Increased proportional lean body mass
Physical Examination Findings	▪ Fever ▪ Measured RMR > estimated or expected RMR ▪ Increased physical activity, e.g., endurance athlete
Food/Nutrition History	
Client History	▪ Conditions associated with a diagnosis or treatment, e.g., Parkinson's disease, cerebral palsy, Alzheimer's disease, cystic fibrosis, chronic obstructive pulmonary disease (COPD) ▪ Medications that increase energy expenditure

References

1. Frankenfield D, Roth-Yousey L, Compher C. Comparison of predictive equations to measured resting metabolic rate in healthy nonobese and obese individuals, a systematic review. *J Am Diet Assoc.* 2005;105:775-789.

Updated: 2008 Edition

Edition: 2008

Intake

INTAKE DOMAIN • Energy Balance

INADEQUATE ENERGY INTAKE (NI-1.4)

Definition

Energy intake that is less than energy expenditure, established reference standards, or recommendations based on physiological needs. Exception: when the goal is weight loss or during end-of-life care.

Etiology (Cause/Contributing Risk Factors)

Factors gathered during the nutrition assessment process that contribute to the existence or the maintenance of pathophysiological, psychosocial, situational, developmental, cultural, and/or environmental problems:

- Pathologic or physiological causes that result in increased energy requirements or decreased ability to consume sufficient energy, e.g., increased nutrient needs due to prolonged catabolic illness
- Lack of access to food or artificial nutrition, e.g., economic constraints, cultural, or religious practices restricting food given to elderly and/or children
- Food- and nutrition-related knowledge deficit
- Psychological causes, e.g., depression or disordered eating

Signs/Symptoms (Defining Characteristics)

A typical cluster of subjective and objective signs and symptoms gathered during the nutrition assessment process that provide evidence that a problem exists; quantify the problem and describe its severity.

Nutrition Assessment Category	Potential Indicators of this Nutrition Diagnosis (one or more must be present)
Biochemical Data, Medical Tests and Procedures	
Anthropometric Measurements	
Physical Examination Findings	▪ Failure to gain or maintain appropriate weight ▪ Poor dentition

Edition: 2008

INADEQUATE ENERGY INTAKE (NI-1.4)

Food/Nutrition History	Reports or observations of: ▪ Insufficient energy intake from diet compared to needs based on estimated or measured resting metabolic rate ▪ Restriction or omission of energy-dense foods from diet ▪ Food avoidance and/or lack of interest in food ▪ Inability to independently consume foods/fluids (diminished joint mobility of wrist, hand, or digits) ▪ Parenteral or enteral nutrition insufficient to meet needs based on estimated or measured resting metabolic rate
Client History	▪ Excessive consumption of alcohol or other drugs that reduce hunger ▪ Conditions associated with diagnosis or treatment, e.g., mental illness, eating disorders, dementia, alcoholism, substance abuse, and acute or chronic pain management ▪ Medications that affect appetite

References

1 National Academy of Sciences, Institute of Medicine. *Dietary Reference Intakes for Energy, Carbohydrate, Fiber, Fat, Fatty Acids, Cholesterol, Protein, and Amino Acids.* Washington, DC: National Academy Press; 2002.

Updated: 2008 Edition

51

INTAKE DOMAIN • Energy Balance

EXCESSIVE ENERGY INTAKE (NI-1.5)

Definition

Energy intake (e.g., oral, EN/PN, IV, medications) that exceeds energy expenditure, established reference standards, or recommendations based on physiological needs. Exception: when weight gain is desired.

Etiology (Cause/Contributing Risk Factors)

Factors gathered during the nutrition assessment process that contribute to the existence or the maintenance of pathophysiological, psychosocial, situational, developmental, cultural, and/or environmental problems:

- Harmful beliefs/attitudes about food, nutrition, and nutrition-related topics
- Food- and nutrition-related knowledge deficit
- Lack of access to healthful food choices, e.g., healthful food choices not provided as an option by caregiver or parent, homeless
- Lack of value for behavior change, competing values
- Medications that increase appetite, e.g., steroids, antidepressants
- Overfeeding of parenteral/enteral nutrition (PN/EN)
- Calories unaccounted for from IV infusion and/or medications
- Unwilling or uninterested in reducing energy intake
- Failure to adjust for lifestyle changes and decreased metabolism (e.g., aging)
- Resolution of prior hypermetabolism without reduction in intake

Signs/Symptoms (Defining Characteristics)

A typical cluster of subjective and objective signs and symptoms gathered during the nutrition assessment process that provide evidence that a problem exists; quantify the problem and describe its severity.

Nutrition Assessment Category	Potential Indicators of this Nutrition Diagnosis (one or more must be present)
Biochemical Data, Medical Tests and Procedures	• Abnormal liver function tests after prolonged exposure (3-6 weeks) • Respiratory quotient >1.0

52

INTAKE DOMAIN• Energy Balance

EXCESSIVE ENERGY INTAKE (NI-1.5)

Anthropometric Measurements	▪ Body fat percentage > 25% for men and > 32% for women
	▪ BMI > 25 (adults), BMI > 95th percentile (pediatrics)
	▪ Weight gain
Physical Exam Findings	▪ Increased body adiposity
	▪ Increased respiratory rate
Food/Nutrition History	Reports or observations of:
	▪ Intake of high caloric density or large portions of foods/beverages
	▪ EN/PN more than estimated or measured (e.g., indirect calorimetry) energy expenditure
Client History	

References

1. McClave SA, Lowen CC, Kleber MJ, McConnell JW, Jung LY, Goldsmith LJ. Clinical use of the respiratory quotient obtained from indirect calorimetry. *JPEN J Parenter Enteral Nutr.* 2003;27:21-26.

2. McClave SA, Lowen CC, Kleber MJ, Nicholson JF, Jimmerson SC, McConnell JW, Jung LY. Are patients fed appropriately according to their caloric requirements? *JPEN J Parenter Enteral Nutr.* 1998;22:375-381.

3. Overweight and Obesity: Health Consequences. www.surgeongeneral.gov/topics/obesity/calltoaction/fact_consequences.htm. Accessed August 28, 2004.

Updated: 2008 Edition

Edition: 2008

INTAKE DOMAIN • Oral or Nutrition Support Intake

INADEQUATE ORAL FOOD/BEVERAGE INTAKE (NI-2.1)

Definition

Oral food/beverage intake that is less than established reference standards or recommendations based on physiological needs. Exception: when the goal is weight loss or during end-of-life care.

Etiology (Cause/Contributing Risk Factors)

Factors gathered during the nutrition assessment process that contribute to the existence or the maintenance of pathophysiological, psychosocial, situational, developmental, cultural, and/or environmental problems:

- Physiological causes, e.g., increased nutrient needs due to prolonged catabolic illness
- Lack of access to food, e.g., economic constraints, cultural or religious practices, restricting food given to elderly and/or children
- Food- and nutrition-related knowledge deficit concerning sufficient oral food/beverage intake
- Psychological causes, e.g., depression or disordered eating

Signs/Symptoms (Defining Characteristics)

A typical cluster of subjective and objective signs and symptoms gathered during the nutrition assessment process that provide evidence that a problem exists; quantify the problem and describe its severity.

Nutrition Assessment Category	Potential Indicators of this Nutrition Diagnosis (one or more must be present)
Biochemical Data, Medical Tests and Procedures	
Anthropometric Measurements	▪ Weight loss, insufficient growth velocity
Physical Examination Findings	▪ Dry skin, mucous membranes, poor skin turgor
Food/Nutrition History	Reports or observations of: ▪ Insufficient intake of energy or high-quality protein from diet when compared to requirements ▪ Economic constraints that limit food availability ▪ Anorexia, nausea, or vomiting ▪ Change in appetite or taste

54

INADEQUATE ORAL FOOD/BEVERAGE INTAKE (NI-2.1)

Client History
▪ Conditions associated with a diagnosis or treatment of catabolic illness such as AIDS, tuberculosis, anorexia nervosa, sepsis or infection from recent surgery, depression, acute or chronic pain
▪ Protein and/or nutrient malabsorption
▪ Excessive consumption of alcohol or other drugs that reduce hunger
▪ Medications that cause anorexia

References

1. National Academy of Sciences, Institute of Medicine. *Dietary Reference Intakes for Energy, Carbohydrate, Fiber, Fat, Fatty Acids, Cholesterol, Protein, and Amino Acids.* Washington, DC: National Academy Press; 2002.
2. National Academy of Sciences, Institute of Medicine. *Dietary Reference Intakes for Water, Potassium, Sodium, Chloride, and Sulfate.* Washington, DC: National Academy Press; 2002.

Intake

Edition: 2008

INTAKE DOMAIN • Oral or Nutrition Support Intake

EXCESSIVE ORAL FOOD/BEVERAGE INTAKE (NI-2.2)

Definition

Oral food/beverage intake that exceeds estimated energy needs, established reference standards, or recommendations based on physiological needs. Exception: when weight gain is desired.

Etiology (Cause/Contributing Risk Factors)

Factors gathered during the nutrition assessment process that contribute to the existence or the maintenance of pathophysiological, psychosocial, situational, developmental, cultural, and/or environmental problems:

- Harmful beliefs/attitudes about food, nutrition, and nutrition-related topics
- Food- and nutrition-related knowledge deficit
- Lack of access to healthful food choices, e.g., healthful food choices not provided as an option by caregiver or parent, homeless
- Lack of value for behavior change, competing values
- Inability to limit or refuse offered foods
- Lack of food planning, purchasing, and preparation skills
- Loss of appetite awareness
- Medications that increase appetite, e.g., steroids, antidepressants
- Mental illness, depression
- Unwilling or uninterested in reducing intake

Signs/Symptoms (Defining Characteristics)

A typical cluster of subjective and objective signs and symptoms gathered during the nutrition assessment process that provide evidence that a problem exists; quantify the problem and describe its severity.

Nutrition Assessment Category	Potential Indicators of this Nutrition Diagnosis (one or more must be present)
Biochemical Data, Medical Tests and Procedures	
Anthropometric Measurements	▪ Weight gain not attributed to fluid retention or normal growth
Physical Exam Findings	

Edition: 2008

56

EXCESSIVE ORAL FOOD/BEVERAGE INTAKE (NI-2.2)

Food/Nutrition History	Reports or observations of: ■ Intake of high caloric-density foods/beverages (juice, soda, or alcohol) at meals and/or snacks ■ Intake of large portions of foods/beverages, food groups, or specific food items ■ Intake that exceeds estimated or measured energy needs ■ Highly variable daily energy intake ■ Binge eating patterns ■ Frequent, excessive fast food or restaurant intake
Client History	■ Conditions associated with a diagnosis or treatment, e.g., obesity, overweight, or metabolic syndrome, depression, anxiety disorder

References

1. Overweight and Obesity: Health Consequences. www.surgeongeneral.gov/topics/obesity/calltoaction/fact_consequences.htm. Accessed August 28, 2004.
2. Position of the American Dietetic Association: Weight management. *J Am Diet Assoc.* 2002;102:1145-1155.
3. Position of the American Dietetic Association: Total diet approach to communicating food and nutrition information. *J Am Diet Assoc.* 2007;107(in press)..
4. Position of the American Dietetic Association: The role of dietetics professionals in health promotion and disease prevention. *J Am Diet Assoc.* 2006;106:1875-1884.

Updated: 2008 Edition

Intake

57

Edition: 2008

INTAKE DOMAIN • Oral or Nutrition Support Intake

INADEQUATE INTAKE FROM ENTERAL/PARENTERAL (EN/PN) NUTRITION (NI-2.3)

Definition

Enteral or parenteral infusion that provides fewer calories or nutrients compared to established reference standards or recommendations based on physiological needs. Exception: when recommendation is for weight loss or during end-of-life care.

Etiology (Cause/Contributing Risk Factors)

Factors gathered during the nutrition assessment process that contribute to the existence or the maintenance of pathophysiological, psychosocial, situational, developmental, cultural, and/or environmental problems:

- Altered absorption or metabolism of nutrients, e.g., medications
- Food- and nutrition-related knowledge deficit (patient/client, caregiver, supplier)-- incorrect formula/formulation given, e.g., wrong enteral feeding, missing component of PN
- Lack of, compromised, or incorrect access for delivering EN/PN
- Increased biological demand of nutrients, e.g., accelerated growth, wound healing, chronic infection, multiple fractures
- Intolerance of EN/PN
- Infusion volume not reached or schedule for infusion interrupted

Signs/Symptoms (Defining Characteristics)

A typical cluster of subjective and objective signs and symptoms gathered during the nutrition assessment process that provide evidence that a problem exists; quantify the problem and describe its severity.

Nutrition Assessment Category	Potential Indicators of this Nutrition Diagnosis (one or more must be present)

Biochemical Data, Medical Tests and Procedures	▪ Metabolic cart/indirect calorimetry measurement, e.g., respiratory quotient < 0.7
	 ▪ Vitamin/mineral abnormalities:
	   • Calcium < 9.2 mg/dL (2.3 mmol/L)
	   • Vitamin K—abnormal international normalized ratio (INR)
	   • Copper < 70 µg/dL (11 µmol/L)
	   • Zinc < 78 µg/dL (12 µmol/L)
	   • Iron < 50 µg/dL (nmol/L); iron-binding capacity < 250 µg/dL (44.8 µmol/L)

Edition: 2008

INADEQUATE INTAKE FROM ENTERAL/PARENTERAL (EN/PN) NUTRITION (NI-2.3)

Anthropometric Measurements	▪ Growth failure, based on National Center for Health Statistics (NCHS) growth standards and fetal growth failure ▪ Insufficient maternal weight gain ▪ Lack of planned weight gain ▪ Unintentional weight loss of ≥ 5% in 1 month or ≥ 10% in 6 months (not attributed to fluid) in adults ▪ Any weight loss in infants or children ▪ Underweight (BMI < 18.5)
Physical Exam Findings	▪ Clinical evidence of vitamin/mineral deficiency (e.g., hair loss, bleeding gums, pale nail beds, neurologic changes) ▪ Evidence of dehydration, e.g., dry mucous membranes, poor skin turgor ▪ Loss of skin integrity, delayed wound healing, or pressure ulcers ▪ Loss of muscle mass and/or subcutaneous fat ▪ Nausea, vomiting, diarrhea
Food/Nutrition History	Reports or observations of: ▪ Inadequate EN/PN volume compared to estimated or measured (indirect calorimetry) requirements
Client History	▪ Conditions associated with a diagnosis or treatment, e.g., intestinal resection, Crohn's disease, HIV/AIDS, burns, pre-term birth, malnutrition ▪ Feeding tube or venous access in wrong position or removed ▪ Altered capacity for desired levels of physical activity or exercise, easy fatigue with increased activity

References

1. McClave SA, Spain DA, Skolnick JL, Lowen CC, Kieber MJ, Wickerham PS, Vogt JR, Looney SW. Achievement of steady state optimizes results when performing indirect calorimetry. *JPEN J Parenter Enteral Nutr.* 2003;27:16-20.
2. McClave SA, Lowen CC, Kieber MJ, McConnell JW, Jung LY, Goldsmith LJ. Clinical use of the respiratory quotient obtained from indirect calorimetry. *JPEN J Parenter Enteral Nutr.* 2003;27:21-26.
3. McClave SA, Snider HL. Clinical use of gastric residual volumes as a monitor for patients on enteral tube feeding. *JPEN J Parenter Enteral Nutr.* 2002;26(Suppl):S43-S48; discussion S49-S50.
4. McClave SA, DeMeo MT, DeLegge MH, DiSario JA, Heyland DK, Maloney JP, Metheny NA, Moore FA, Scolapio JS, Spain DA, Zaloga GP. North American Summit on Aspiration in the Critically Ill Patient: consensus statement. *JPEN J Parenter Enteral Nutr.* 2002;26(Suppl):S80-S85.
5. McClave SA, McClain CJ, Snider HL. Should indirect calorimetry be used as part of nutritional assessment? *J Clin Gastroenterol.* 2001;33:14-19.
6. McClave SA, Sexton LK, Spain DA, Adams JL, Owens NA, Sullins MB, Blandford BS, Snider HL. Enteral tube feeding in the intensive care unit: factors impeding adequate delivery. *Crit Care Med.* 1999;27:1252-1256.
7. McClave SA, Lowen CC, Kieber MJ, Nicholson JF, Jimmerson SC, McConnell JW, Jung LY. Are patients fed appropriately according to their caloric requirements? *JPEN J Parenter Enteral Nutr.* 1998;22:375-381.
8. Spain DA, McClave SA, Sexton LK, Adams JL, Blanford BS, Sullins ME, Owens NA, Snider HL. Infusion protocol improves delivery of enteral tube feeding in the critical care unit. *JPEN J Parenter Enteral Nutr.* 1999;23:288-292.

Updated: 2008 Edition

Edition: 2008

Intake

INTAKE DOMAIN • Oral or Nutrition Support Intake

EXCESSIVE INTAKE FROM ENTERAL OR PARENTERAL NUTRITION (NI-2.4)

Definition

Enteral or parenteral infusion that provides more calories or nutrients compared to established reference standards or recommendations based on physiological needs.

Etiology *(Cause/Contributing Risk Factors)*

Factors gathered during the nutrition assessment process that contribute to the existence or the maintenance of pathophysiological, psychosocial, situational, developmental, cultural, and/or environmental problems:

- Physiological causes, e.g., decreased needs related to low activity levels with critical illness or organ failure
- Food- and nutrition-related knowledge deficit on the part of the caregiver, patient/client, or clinician

Signs/Symptoms *(Defining Characteristics)*

A typical cluster of subjective and objective signs and symptoms gathered during the nutrition assessment process that provide evidence that a problem exists; quantify the problem and describe its severity.

Nutrition Assessment Category	Potential Indicators of this Nutrition Diagnosis (one or more must be present)
Biochemical Data, Medical Tests and Procedures	▪ Elevated BUN:creatinine ratio (protein) ▪ Hyperglycemia (carbohydrate) ▪ Hypercapnia ▪ Elevated liver enzymes
Anthropometric Measurements	▪ Weight gain in excess of lean tissue accretion
Physical Examination Findings	▪ Edema with excess fluid administration
Food/Nutrition History	Reports or observations of: ▪ Documented intake from enteral or parenteral nutrients that is consistently more than recommended intake for carbohydrate, protein, and fat (e.g., 36 kcal/kg for well, active adults, 25 kcal/kg or as measured by indirect calorimetry for critically ill adults, 0.8 g/kg protein for well adults, 1.5 g/kg protein for critically ill adults, 1.2 g/kg lipid for adults, or 3 g/kg for children)*

* When entering weight (i.e., gram) information into the medical record, use institution or Joint Commission approved abbreviation list.

Edition: 2008

EXCESSIVE INTAKE FROM ENTERAL OR PARENTERAL NUTRITION (NI-2.4)

Client History	• Use of drugs that reduce requirements or impair metabolism of energy, protein, fat, or fluid.
	• Unrealistic expectations of weight gain or ideal weight

References

1. National Academy of Sciences, Institute of Medicine. *Dietary Reference Intakes for Energy, Carbohydrate, Fiber, Fat, Fatty Acids, Cholesterol, Protein, and Amino Acids*. Washington, DC: National Academy Press, 2002.
2. National Academy of Sciences, Institute of Medicine. *Dietary Reference Intakes for Water, Potassium, Sodium, Chloride, and Sulfate*. Washington, DC: National Academy Press, 2004.
3. Aarsland A, Chinkes D, Wolfe RR. Hepatic and whole-body fat synthesis in humans during carbohydrate overfeeding. *Am J Clin Nutr*. 1997;65:1774-1782.
4. McClave SA, Lowen CC, Kleber MJ, Nicholson JF, Jimmerson SC, McConnell JW, Jung LY. Are patients fed appropriately according to their caloric requirements? *JPEN J Parenter Enteral Nutr*. 1998;22:375-381.
5. McClave SA, Lowen CC, Kleber MJ, McConnell JW, Jung LY, Goldsmith LJ. Clinical use of the respiratory quotient obtained from indirect calorimetry. *JPEN J Parenter Enteral Nutr*. 2003;27:21-26.
6. Wolfe RR, O'Donnell TF Jr, Stone MD, Richmand DA, Burke JF. Investigation of factors determining the optimal glucose infusion rate in total parenteral nutrition. *Metabolism*. 1980;29:892-900.
7. Jensen GL, Mascioli EA, Seidner DL, Istfan NW, Domnitch AM, Selleck K, Babayan VK, Blackburn GL, Bistrian BR. Parenteral infusion of long- and medium-chain triglycerides and reticulothelial system function in man. *JPEN J Parenter Enteral Nutr*. 1990;14:467-471.
8. Joint Commission Official "Do not use" list of abbreviations. Available: http://www.jointcommission.org/PatientSafety/DoNotUseList. Accessed May 2007.

Intake

Edition: 2008

INTAKE DOMAIN • Oral or Nutrition Support Intake

INAPPROPRIATE INFUSION OF ENTERAL OR PARENTERAL NUTRITION (NI-2.5)

Use with caution–only after discussion with other health team members

Definition

Enteral or parenteral infusion that provides either fewer or more calories and/or nutrients or is of the wrong composition or type, parenteral or enteral nutrition that is not warranted because the patient/client is able to tolerate an enteral intake, or is unsafe because of the potential for sepsis or other complications.

Etiology (*Cause/Contributing Risk Factors*)

Factors gathered during the nutrition assessment process that contribute to the existence or the maintenance of pathophysiological, psychosocial, situational, developmental, cultural, and/or environmental problems:

- Physiological causes, e.g., improvement in patient/client status, allowing return to total or partial oral diet; changes in the course of disease resulting in changes in nutrient requirements
- Product or knowledge deficit on the part of the caregiver or clinician
- End-of-life care if patient/client or family do not desire nutrition support

Signs/Symptoms (*Defining Characteristics*)

A typical cluster of subjective and objective signs and symptoms gathered during the nutrition assessment process that provide evidence that a problem exists; quantify the problem and describe its severity.

Nutrition Assessment Category	Potential Indicators of this Nutrition Diagnosis (one or more must be present)
Biochemical Data, Medical Tests and Procedures	▪ Abnormal liver function tests in patient/client on long-term (more than 3-6 weeks) feeding ▪ Abnormal levels of markers specific for various nutrients, e.g., hyperphosphatemia in patient/client receiving feedings with a high phosphorus content, hypokalemia in patient/client receiving feedings with low potassium content
Anthropometric Measurements	▪ Weight gain in excess of lean tissue accretion ▪ Weight loss
Physical Examination Findings	▪ Edema with excess fluid administration ▪ Loss of subcutaneous fat and muscle stores

Edition: 2008

INAPPROPRIATE INFUSION OF ENTERAL OR PARENTERAL NUTRITION (NI-2.5)

Food/Nutrition History	Reports or observations of:
	▪ Documented intake from enteral or parenteral nutrients that is consistently more or less than recommended intake for carbohydrate, protein, and/or fat– especially related to patient/client's ability to consume an oral diet that meets needs at this point in time
	▪ Documented intake of other nutrients that is consistently more or less than recommended
	▪ Nausea, vomiting, diarrhea, high gastric residual volume
Client History	▪ History of enteral or parenteral nutrition intolerance
	▪ Complications such as fatty liver in the absence of other causes

References

1. Aarsland A, Chinkes D, Wolfe RR. Hepatic and whole-body fat synthesis in humans during carbohydrate overfeeding. *Am J Clin Nutr.* 1997;65:1774-1782.
2. McClave SA, Lowen CC, Kleber MJ, Nicholson JF, Jimmerson SC, McConnell JW, Jung LY. Are patients fed appropriately according to their caloric requirements? *JPEN J Parenter Enteral Nutr.* 1998;22:375-381.
3. McClave SA, Lowen CC, Kleber MJ, McConnell JW, Jung LY, Goldsmith LJ. Clinical use of the respiratory quotient obtained from indirect calorimetry. *JPEN J Parenter Enteral Nutr.* 2003;27:21-26.
4. National Academy of Sciences, Institute of Medicine. *Dietary Reference Intakes for Energy, Carbohydrate, Fiber, Fat, Fatty Acids, Cholesterol, Protein, and Amino Acids.* Washington, DC: National Academy Press; 2002.
5. National Academy of Sciences, Institute of Medicine. *Dietary Reference Intakes for Water, Potassium, Sodium, Chloride, and Sulfate.* Washington DC: National Academy Press; 2004.
6. National Academy of Sciences, Institute of Medicine. *Dietary Reference Intakes for Calcium, Phosphorus, Magnesium, Vitamin D, and Fluoride.* Washington, DC: National Academy Press; 1997.
7. National Academy of Sciences, Institute of Medicine. *Dietary Reference Intakes for Vitamin C, Vitamin E, Selenium, and Carotenoids.* Washington, DC: National Academy Press; 2000.
8. Wolfe RR, O'Donnell TF, Jr., Stone MD, Richmand DA, Burke JF. Investigation of factors determining the optimal glucose infusion rate in total parenteral nutrition. *Metabolism.* 1980;29:892-900.

Edition: 2008

INTAKE DOMAIN • Fluid Intake

INADEQUATE FLUID INTAKE (NI-3.1)

Definition

Lower intake of fluid-containing foods or substances compared to established reference standards or recommendations based on physiological needs.

Etiology (Cause/Contributing Risk Factors)

Factors gathered during the nutrition assessment process that contribute to the existence or the maintenance of pathophysiological, psychosocial, situational, developmental, cultural, and/or environmental problems:

- Physiological causes, e.g., increased fluid needs due to climate/temperature change; increased exercise or conditions leading to increased fluid losses; fever causing increased insensible losses, decreased thirst sensation, use of drugs that reduce thirst
- Lack of access to fluid, e.g., economic constraints, cultural or religious practices, unable to access fluid independently such as elderly or children
- Food- and nutrition-related knowledge deficit
- Psychological causes, e.g., depression or disordered eating; dementia resulting in decreased recognition of thirst

Signs/Symptoms (Defining Characteristics)

A typical cluster of subjective and objective signs and symptoms gathered during the nutrition assessment process that provide evidence that a problem exists; quantify the problem and describe its severity.

Nutrition Assessment Category	Potential Indicators of this Nutrition Diagnosis (one or more must be present)
Biochemical Data, Medical Tests and Procedures	• Plasma or serum osmolality greater than 290 mOsm/kg • ↑ BUN, ↑ Na
Anthropometric Measurements	• Acute weight loss
Physical Examination Findings	• Dry skin and mucous membranes, poor skin turgor • Urine output <30 mL/hr
Food/Nutrition History	Reports or observations of: • Insufficient intake of fluid compared to requirements (e.g., per body surface area for pediatrics) • Thirst • Difficulty swallowing

Edition: 2008

INADEQUATE FLUID INTAKE (NI-3.1)

Client History	• Conditions associated with a diagnosis or treatment, e.g., Alzheimer's disease or other dementia resulting in decreased recognition of thirst, diarrhea
	• Use of drugs that reduce thirst

References

1. National Academy of Sciences, Institute of Medicine. *Dietary Reference Intakes for Water; Potassium, Sodium, Chloride, and Sulfate*, Washington, DC: National Academy Press; 2004.
2. Grandjean AC, Campbell, SM. *Hydration: Fluids for Life*. Monograph Series. Washington DC: International Life Sciences Institute North America; 2004.
3. Grandjean AC, Reimers KJ, Buyckx ME: Hydration: Issues for the 21st Century. *Nutr Rev.* 2003;61:261-271.

Updated: 2008 Edition

Intake

65

INTAKE DOMAIN • Fluid Intake

EXCESSIVE FLUID INTAKE (NI-3.2)

Definition

Higher intake of fluid compared to established reference standards or recommendations based on physiological needs.

Etiology (Cause/Contributing Risk Factors)

Factors gathered during the nutrition assessment process that contribute to the existence or the maintenance of pathophysiological, psychosocial, situational, developmental, cultural, and/or environmental problems:

- Physiological causes, e.g., decreased fluid losses due to kidney, liver or cardiac failure; diminished water and sodium losses due to changes in exercise or climate, syndrome of inappropriate antidiuretic hormone (SIADH)

- Food- and nutrition-related knowledge deficit

- Psychological causes, e.g., depression or disordered eating

Signs/Symptoms (Defining Characteristics)

A typical cluster of subjective and objective signs and symptoms gathered during the nutrition assessment process that provide evidence that a problem exists; quantify the problem and describe its severity.

Nutrition Assessment Category	Potential Indicators of this Nutrition Diagnosis (one or more must be present)
Biochemical Data, Medical Tests and Procedures	▪ Lowered plasma osmolarity (270-280 mOsm/kg), only if positive fluid balance is in excess of positive sodium balance
	▪ Decreased serum sodium in SIADH
Anthropometric Measurements	▪ Weight gain
Physical Examination Findings	▪ Edema in the skin of the legs, sacral area, or diffusely; weeping of fluids from lower legs
	▪ Ascites
	▪ Pulmonary edema as evidenced by shortness of breath; orthopnea; crackles or rales
Food/Nutrition History	Reports or observations of:
	▪ Excessive intake of fluid compared to requirements (e.g., per body surface area for pediatrics)
	▪ Excessive salt intake

Edition: 2008

EXCESSIVE FLUID INTAKE (NI-3.2)

Client History	
	▪ Conditions associated with a diagnosis or treatment, e.g., end-stage renal disease, nephrotic syndrome, heart failure, or liver disease
	▪ Nausea, vomiting, anorexia, headache, muscle spasms, convulsions, coma (SIADH)
	▪ Shortness of breath or dyspnea with exertion or at rest
	▪ Providing medications in large amounts of fluid
	▪ Use of drugs that impair fluid excretion

References

1. National Academy of Sciences, Institute of Medicine. *Dietary Reference Intakes for Water, Potassium, Sodium, Chloride, and Sulfate.* Washington DC. National Academy Press; 2004.
2. Schirer, R.W. ed. *Renal and Electrolyte Disorders.* Philadelphia, PA: Lipincott Williams and Willkins; 2003.
3. SIADH: http://www.nlmnih.gov/medlineplus/ency/article/000394.htm. Accessed May 30, 2006.

Updated: 2008 Edition

Intake

67

Edition: 2008

INTAKE DOMAIN • Bioactive Substances

INADEQUATE BIOACTIVE SUBSTANCE INTAKE (NI-4.1)

Definition

Lower intake of bioactive substances or foods containing bioactive substances compared to established reference standards or recommendations based on physiological needs.

*Bioactive substances are the physiologically active components of foods

Etiology (Cause/Contributing Risk Factors)

Factors gathered during the nutrition assessment process that contribute to the existence or the maintenance of pathophysiological, psychosocial, situational, developmental, cultural, and/or environmental problems:

- Food- and nutrition-related knowledge deficit
- Limited access to a food that contains the substance
- Altered GI function, e.g., pain or discomfort

Signs/Symptoms (Defining Characteristics)

A typical cluster of subjective and objective signs and symptoms gathered during the nutrition assessment process that provide evidence that a problem exists; quantify the problem and describe its severity.

Nutrition Assessment Category	Potential Indicators of this Nutrition Diagnosis (one or more must be present)
Biochemical Data, Medical Tests and Procedures	
Anthropometric Measurements	
Physical Exam Findings	
Food/Nutrition History	Reports or observations of: ▪ Low intake of plant foods containing: ▪ Soluble fiber, e.g., psyllium (↓ total and LDL cholesterol) ▪ Soy protein (↓ total and LDL cholesterol) ▪ β-glucan, e.g., whole oat products (↓ total and LDL cholesterol) ▪ Plant sterol and stanol esters, e.g., fortified margarines (↓ total and LDL cholesterol)

Edition: 2008

INADEQUATE BIOACTIVE SUBSTANCE INTAKE (NI-4.1)

Client History
▪ Conditions associated with a diagnosis or treatment, e.g., cardiovascular disease, elevated cholesterol

References

1. Position of the American Dietetic Association: Functional foods. *J Am Diet Assoc.* 2004;104:814-826.

Updated: 2008 Edition

INTAKE DOMAIN • Bioactive Substances

EXCESSIVE BIOACTIVE SUBSTANCE INTAKE (NI-4.2)

Definition

Higher intake of bioactive substances other than traditional nutrients, such as functional foods, bioactive food components, dietary supplements, food concentrates compared to established reference standards or recommendations based on physiological needs.

*Bioactive substances are the physiologically active components of foods

Etiology (Cause/Contributing Risk Factors)

Factors gathered during the nutrition assessment process that contribute to the existence or the maintenance of pathophysiological, psychosocial, situational, developmental, cultural, and/or environmental problems:

- Food- and nutrition-related knowledge deficit
- Contamination, misname, mislabel, misuse, recent brand change, recent dose increase, recent formulation change of substance consumed
- Frequent intake of foods containing bioactive substances
- Altered GI function, e.g., pain or discomfort

Signs/Symptoms (Defining Characteristics)

A typical cluster of subjective and objective signs and symptoms gathered during the nutrition assessment process that provide evidence that a problem exists; quantify the problem and describe its severity.

Nutrition Assessment Category	Potential Indicators of this Nutrition Diagnosis (one or more must be present)
Biochemical Data, Medical Tests and Procedures	▪ Lab values indicating excessive intake of the specific substance, such as rapid decrease in cholesterol from intake of stanol or sterol esters and a statin drug and related dietary changes or medications ▪ Increased hepatic enzyme reflecting hepatocellular damage
Anthropometric Measurements	▪ Weight loss as a result of malabsorption or maldigestion
Physical Exam Findings	▪ Constipation or diarrhea related to excessive intake ▪ Neurologic changes, e.g., anxiety, mental status changes ▪ Cardiovascular changes, e.g., heart rate, EKG changes, blood pressure

EXCESSIVE BIOACTIVE SUBSTANCE INTAKE (NI-4.2)

Food/Nutrition History	Reports or observations of:
	▪ High intake of plant foods containing:
	▪ Soy protein ($\downarrow$ total and LDL cholesterol)
	▪ β-glucan, e.g., whole oat products ($\downarrow$ total and LDL cholesterol)
	▪ Plant sterol and stanol esters, e.g., fortified margarines ($\downarrow$ total and LDL cholesterol) or other foods based on dietary substance, concentrate, metabolite, constituent, extract, or combination
	▪ Substances that interfere with digestion or absorption of foodstuffs
	▪ Ready access to available foods/products with bioactive substance, e.g., as from dietary supplement vendors
	▪ Attempts to use supplements or bioactive substances for weight loss, to treat constipation, or to prevent or cure chronic or acute disease
Client History	▪ Conditions associated with a diagnosis or treatment, e.g., cardiovascular disease, elevated cholesterol, hypertension
	▪ Discomfort or pain associated with intake of foods rich in bioactive substances, e.g., soluble fiber, β-glucan, soy protein

References

1. National Academy of Sciences, Institute of Medicine. *Dietary Supplements: A framework for evaluating safety.* Washington, DC: National Academy Press; 2004.
2. Position of the American Dietetic Association: Functional foods. *J Am Diet Assoc.* 2004;104:814-826.

Updated: 2008 Edition

Intake

71

INTAKE DOMAIN • Bioactive Substances

EXCESSIVE ALCOHOL INTAKE (NI-4.3)

Definition

Intake more than the suggested limits for alcohol.

Etiology (Cause/Contributing Risk Factors)

Factors gathered during the nutrition assessment process that contribute to the existence or the maintenance of pathophysiological, psychosocial, situational, developmental, cultural, and/or environmental problems:

- Harmful beliefs/attitudes about food, nutrition, and nutrition-related topics
- Food- and nutrition-related knowledge deficit
- Lack of value for behavior change, competing values
- Alcohol addiction

Signs/Symptoms (Defining Characteristics)

A typical cluster of subjective and objective signs and symptoms gathered during the nutrition assessment process that provide evidence that a problem exists; quantify the problem and describe its severity.

Nutrition Assessment Category	Potential Indicators of this Nutrition Diagnosis (one or more must be present)
Biochemical Data, Medical Tests and Procedures	▪ Elevated aspartate aminotransferase (AST), gamma-glutamyl transferase (GGT), carbohydrate-deficient transferrin, mean corpuscular volume, blood alcohol levels
Anthropometric Measurements	
Physical Exam Findings	
Food/Nutrition History	Reports or observations of: ▪ Intake of > 2 drinks*/day (men) ▪ Intake of > 1 drink*/day (women) ▪ Binge drinking ▪ Consumption of any alcohol when contraindicated *1 drink = 5 oz wine, 12 oz beer, 1 oz distilled alcohol

Edition: 2008

EXCESSIVE ALCOHOL INTAKE (NI-4.3)

Client History	▪ Conditions associated with a diagnosis or treatment, e.g., severe hypertriglyceridemia, elevated blood pressure, depression, liver disease, pancreatitis ▪ New medical diagnosis or change in existing diagnosis or condition ▪ History of excessive alcohol intake ▪ Giving birth to an infant with fetal alcohol syndrome ▪ Drinking during pregnancy despite knowledge of risk

References

1. Position of the American Dietetic Association: The role of dietetics professionals in health promotion and disease prevention. *J Am Diet Assoc.* 2006;106:1875-1884.

Updated: 2008 Edition

73

INTAKE DOMAIN • Nutrient

INCREASED NUTRIENT NEEDS (SPECIFY) (NI-5.1)

Definition

Increased need for a specific nutrient compared to established reference standards or recommendations based on physiological needs.

Etiology (Cause/Contributing Risk Factors)

Factors gathered during the nutrition assessment process that contribute to the existence or the maintenance of pathophysiological, psychosocial, situational, developmental, cultural, and/or environmental problems:

- Altered absorption or metabolism of nutrient, e.g., from medications
- Compromise of organs related to GI function, e.g., pancreas, liver
- Decreased functional length of intestine, e.g., short-bowel syndrome
- Decreased or compromised function of intestine, e.g., celiac disease, Crohn's disease
- Food- and nutrition-related knowledge deficit
- Increased demand for nutrient, e.g., accelerated growth, wound healing, chronic infection

Signs/Symptoms (Defining Characteristics)

A typical cluster of subjective and objective signs and symptoms gathered during the nutrition assessment process that provide evidence that a problem exists; quantify the problem and describe its severity.

Nutrition Assessment Category	Potential Indicators of this Nutrition Diagnosis (one or more must be present)
Biochemical Data, Medical Tests and Procedures	▪ Decreased total cholesterol < 160 mg/dL, albumin, prealbumin, C-reactive protein, indicating increased stress and increased metabolic needs
	▪ Electrolyte/mineral (e.g., potassium, magnesium, phosphorus) abnormalities
	▪ Urinary or fecal losses of specific or related nutrient (e.g., fecal fat, d-xylose test)
	▪ Vitamin and/or mineral deficiency
Anthropometric Measurements	▪ Growth failure, based on National Center for Health Statistics (NCHS) growth standards and fetal growth failure
	▪ Unintentional weight loss of ≥5% in 1 month or ≥10% in 6 months
	▪ Loss of muscle mass, subcutaneous fat
	▪ Underweight (BMI < 18.5)

74

INCREASED NUTRIENT NEEDS (SPECIFY) (NI-5.1)

Physical Examination Findings	▪ Clinical evidence of vitamin/mineral deficiency (e.g., hair loss, bleeding gums, pale nail beds) ▪ Loss of skin integrity, delayed wound healing, or pressure ulcers
Food/Nutrition History	Reports or observations of: ▪ Inadequate intake of foods/supplement containing needed nutrient as compared to estimated requirements ▪ Intake of foods that do not contain sufficient quantities of available nutrient (e.g., overprocessed, overcooked, or stored improperly) ▪ Food- and nutrition-related knowledge deficit (e.g., lack of information, incorrect information or noncompliance with intake of needed nutrient)
Client History	▪ Conditions associated with a diagnosis or treatment, e.g., intestinal resection, Crohn's disease, HIV/AIDS, burns, pre-term birth, malnutrition ▪ Medications affecting absorption or metabolism of needed nutrient

References

1. Beyer P. Gastrointestinal disorders: Roles of nutrition and the dietetics practitioner. *J Am Diet Assoc.* 1998;98:272-277.
2. Position of the American Dietetic Association and Dietitians of Canada: Nutrition intervention in the care of persons with human immunodeficiency virus infection. *J Am Diet Assoc.* 2004;104:1425-1441.

Updated: 2008 Edition

Intake

INTAKE DOMAIN • Nutrient

EVIDENT PROTEIN–ENERGY MALNUTRITION (NI-5.2)

Definition

Inadequate intake of protein and/or energy over prolonged periods of time resulting in loss of fat stores and/or muscle wasting.

Etiology (Cause/Contributing Risk Factors)

Factors gathered during the nutrition assessment process that contribute to the existence or the maintenance of pathophysiological, psychosocial, situational, developmental, cultural, and/or environmental problems:

- Physiological causes, e.g., altered nutrient needs due to prolonged catabolic illness, malabsorption
- Lack of access to food, e.g., economic constraints, cultural or religious practices, restricting food given to elderly and/or children
- Food- and nutrition-related knowledge deficit, e.g., avoidance of high-quality protein foods
- Psychological causes, e.g., depression or eating disorders

Signs/Symptoms (Defining Characteristics)

A typical cluster of subjective and objective signs and symptoms gathered during the nutrition assessment process that provide evidence that a problem exists; quantify the problem and describe its severity.

Nutrition Assessment Category	Potential Indicators of this Nutrition Diagnosis (one or more must be present)
Biochemical Data, Medical Tests and Procedures	▪ Normal serum albumin level (uncomplicated malnutrition)
	▪ Albumin < 3.4 mg/dL (disease/trauma related malnutrition)
Anthropometric Measurements	▪ BMI < 18.5 indicates underweight
	▪ Failure to thrive, e.g., failure to attain desirable growth rates
	▪ Inadequate maternal weight gain
	▪ Weight loss of > 10% in 6 months
	▪ Underweight with muscle wasting
	▪ Normal or slightly underweight, stunted growth in children

Edition: 2008

EVIDENT PROTEIN–ENERGY MALNUTRITION (NI-5.2)

Physical Exam Findings	▪ Uncomplicated malnutrition: Thin, wasted appearance; severe muscle wasting; minimal body fat; sparse, thin, dry, easily pluckable hair; dry, thin skin; obvious bony prominences, occipital wasting; lowered body temperature, blood pressure, heart rate; changes in hair or nails consistent with insufficient protein intake
	▪ Disease/trauma related malnutrition: Thin to normal appearance, with peripheral edema, ascites, or anasarca; edema of the lower extremities; some muscle wasting with retention of some body fat; dyspigmentation of hair (flag sign) and skin
	▪ Delayed wound healing
Food/Nutrition History	Reports or observations of:
	▪ Insufficient energy intake from diet compared to estimated or measured RMR
	▪ Insufficient intake of high-quality protein when compared to requirements
	▪ Food avoidance and/or lack of interest in food
Client History	▪ Chronic or acute disease or trauma, geographic location and socioeconomic status associated with altered nutrient intake of indigenous phenomenon
	▪ Severe protein and/or nutrient malabsorption (e.g., extensive bowel resection)
	▪ Excessive consumption of alcohol or other drugs that reduce hunger
	▪ Enlarged fatty liver

References

1. Wellcome Trust Working Party. Classification of infantile malnutrition. *Lancet.* 1970;2:302-303.
2. Seres DS. Resurrection, LB. Kwashiorkor: Dysmetabolism versus malnutrition. *Nutr Clin Pract.* 2003;18:297-301.
3. Jelliffe DB, Jelliffe EF. Causation of kwashiorkor: Toward a multifactoral consensus. *Pediatrics.* 1992;90:110-113.
4. Centers for Disease Control and Prevention web site: http://www.cdc.gov/nccdphp/dnpa/bmi/bmi-adult.htm. Accessed October 5, 2004.
5. Fuhrman MP, Charney P, Mueller CM. Hepatic proteins and nutrition assessment. *J Am Diet Assoc.* 2004;104:1258-1264.
6. American Medical Association. *AMA ICD-9-CM 2007: Physician, International Classification of Diseases:Clinical Modification, 9th Revised Ed.* Chicago, IL: American Medical Association Press; 2006.

77

INTAKE DOMAIN • Nutrient

INADEQUATE PROTEIN–ENERGY INTAKE (NI-5.3)

Definition

Inadequate intake of protein and/or energy compared to established reference standards or recommendations based on physiological needs of short or recent duration.

Etiology (*Cause/Contributing Risk Factors*)

Factors gathered during the nutrition assessment process that contribute to the existence or the maintenance of pathophysiological, psychosocial, situational, developmental, cultural, and/or environmental problems:

- Short-term physiological causes, e.g., increased nutrient needs due to catabolic illness, malabsorption
- Recent lack of access to food, e.g., economic constraints, cultural or religious practices, restricting food given or food selected
- Food- and nutrition-related knowledge deficit, e.g., avoidance of all fats for new dieting pattern
- Recent onset of psychological causes, e.g., depression or eating disorders

Signs/Symptoms (*Defining Characteristics*)

A typical cluster of subjective and objective signs and symptoms gathered during the nutrition assessment process that provide evidence that a problem exists; quantify the problem and describe its severity.

Nutrition Assessment Category	Potential Indicators of this Nutrition Diagnosis (one or more must be present)
Biochemical Data, Medical Tests and Procedures	• Normal albumin (in the setting of normal liver function despite decrease protein-energy intake)
Anthropometric Measurements	• Inadequate maternal weight gain (mild but not severe) • Weight loss of 5%-7% during past 3 months in adults, any weight loss in children • Normal or slightly underweight • Growth failure in children
Physical Exam Findings	• Slow wound healing in pressure ulcer or surgical patient/client

Edition: 2008

INADEQUATE PROTEIN–ENERGY INTAKE (NI-5.3)

Food/Nutrition History	Reports or observations of:
	▪ Insufficient energy intake from diet compared to estimated or measured RMR or recommended levels
	▪ Restriction or omission of food groups such as dairy or meat group foods (protein); bread or milk group foods (energy)
	▪ Recent food avoidance and/or lack of interest in food
	▪ Lack of ability to prepare meals
Client History	▪ Conditions associated with a diagnosis or treatment of mild protein-energy malnutrition, recent illness, e.g., pulmonary or cardiac failure, flu, infection, surgery
	▪ Nutrient malabsorption (e.g., bariatric surgery, diarrhea, steatorrhea)
	▪ Excessive consumption of alcohol or other drugs that reduce hunger
	▪ Patient/client reports of hunger in the face of inadequate access to food supply
	▪ Patient/client reports lack of ability to prepare meals
	▪ Patient/client reports lack of funds for purchase of appropriate foods

References

1. Centers for Disease Control and Prevention web site: http://www.cdc.gov/nccdphp/dnpa/bmi/bmi-adult.htm. Accessed October 5, 2004.
2. Fuhrman MP, Charney P, Mueller CM. Hepatic proteins and nutrition assessment. *J Am Diet Assoc.* 2004;104:1258-1264.
3. American Medical Association. *AMA ICD-9-CM 2007: Physician, International Classification of Diseases:Clinical Modification, 9th Revised Ed.* Chicago, IL: American Medical Association Press; 2006.

Intake

INTAKE DOMAIN • Nutrient

DECREASED NUTRIENT NEEDS (SPECIFY) (NI-5.4)

Definition

Decreased need for a specific nutrient compared to established reference standards or recommendations based on physiological needs.

Etiology (Cause/Contributing Risk Factors)

Factors gathered during the nutrition assessment process that contribute to the existence or the maintenance of pathophysiological, psychosocial, situational, developmental, cultural, and/or environmental problems:

- Renal dysfunction
- Liver dysfunction
- Altered cholesterol metabolism/regulation
- Heart failure
- Food intolerances, e.g., irritable bowel syndrome

Signs/Symptoms (Defining Characteristics)

A typical cluster of subjective and objective signs and symptoms gathered during the nutrition assessment process that provide evidence that a problem exists; quantify the problem and describe its severity.

Nutrition Assessment Category	Potential Indicators of this Nutrition Diagnosis (one or more must be present)
Biochemical Data, Medical Tests and Procedures	▪ Total cholesterol > 200 mg/dL (5.2 mmol/L), LDL cholesterol > 100 mg/dL (2.59 mmol/L), HDL cholesterol < 40 mg/dL (1.036 mmol/L), triglycerides > 150 mg/dL (1.695 mmol/L)
	▪ Phosphorus > 5.5 mg/dL (1.78 mmol/L)
	▪ Glomerular filtration rate (GFR) < 90 mL/min/1.73 m2
	▪ Elevated BUN, creatinine, potassium
	▪ Liver function tests indicating severe liver disease
Anthropometric Measurements	▪ Interdialytic weight gain greater than expected
Physical Exam Findings	▪ Edema/fluid retention
Food/Nutrition History	Reports or observations of:
	▪ Intake higher than recommended for fat, phosphorus, sodium, protein, fiber

Edition: 2008

DECREASED NUTRIENT NEEDS (SPECIFY) (NI-5.4)

Client History	• Conditions associated with a diagnosis or treatment that require a specific type and/or amount of nutrient, e.g., cardiovascular disease (fat), early renal disease (protein, phos), ESRD (phos, sodium, potassium, fluid), advanced liver disease (protein), heart failure (sodium, fluid), irritable bowel disease/Crohn's flare up (fiber) • Diagnosis of hypertension, confusion related to liver disease

References

1. Aparicio M, Chauveau P, Combe C. Low protein diets and outcomes of renal patients. *J Nephrol.* 2001;14:433-439.
2. Beto JA, Bansal VK. Medical nutrition therapy in chronic kidney failure: Integrating clinical practice guidelines. *J Am Diet Assoc.* 2004;104:404-409.
3. Cupisti A, Morelli E, D'Alessandro C, Lupetti S, Barsotti G. Phosphate control in chronic uremia: don't forget diet. *J Nephrol.* 2003;16:29-33.
4. Durose CL, Holdsworth M, Watson V, Przygrodzka F. Knowledge of dietary restrictions and the medical consequences of noncompliance by patients on hemodialysis are not predictive of dietary compliance. *J Am Diet Assoc.* 2004;104:35-41.
5. Floch MH, Narayan R. Diet in the irritable bowel syndrome. *Clin Gastroenterol.* 2002;35:S45-S52.
6. Kato J, Kobune M, Nakamura T, Kurojwa G, Takada K, Takimoto R, Sato Y, Fujikawa K, Takahashi M, Takayama T, Ikeda T, Niitsu Y. Normalization of elevated hepatic 8-hydroxy-2'-deoxyguanosine levels in chronic hepatitis C patients by phlebotomy and low iron diet. *Cancer Res.* 2001;61:8697-8702.
7. Lee SH, Molassiotis A. Dietary and fluid compliance in Chinese hemodialysis patients. *Int J Nurs Stud.* 2002;39:695-704.
8. Poduval RD, Wolgemuth C, Ferrell J, Hammes MS. Hyperphosphatemia in dialysis patients: is there a role for focused counseling? *J Ren Nutr.* 2003;13:219-223.
9. Tandon N, Thakur V, Guptan RK, Sarin SK. Beneficial influence of an indigenous low-iron diet on serum indicators of iron status in patients with chronic liver disease. *Br J Nutr.* 2000;83:235-239.
10. Zrinyi M, Juhasz M, Balla J, Katona E, Ben T, Kakuk G, Pall D. Dietary self-efficacy: determinant of compliance behaviours and biochemical outcomes in haemodialysis patients. *Nephrol Dial Transplant.* 2003;19:1869-1873.

INTAKE DOMAIN • Nutrient

IMBALANCE OF NUTRIENTS (NI-5.5)

Definition

An undesirable combination of ingested nutrients, such that the amount of one nutrient ingested interferes with or alters absorption and/or utilization of another nutrient.

Etiology (Cause/Contributing Risk Factors)

Factors gathered during the nutrition assessment process that contribute to the existence or the maintenance of pathophysiological, psychosocial, situational, developmental, cultural, and/or environmental problems:

- Consumption of high-dose nutrient supplements
- Food- and nutrition-related knowledge deficit
- Harmful beliefs/attitudes about food, nutrition, and nutrition-related information
- Food faddism
- Insufficient electrolyte replacement when initiating feeding (PN/EN, including oral)

Signs/Symptoms (Defining Characteristics)

A typical cluster of subjective and objective signs and symptoms gathered during the nutrition assessment process that provide evidence that a problem exists; quantify the problem and describe its severity.

Nutrition Assessment Category	Potential Indicators of this Nutrition Diagnosis (one or more must be present)
Biochemical Data, Medical Tests and Procedures	▪ Severe hypophosphatemia (↑ carbohydrate) ▪ Severe hypokalemia (↑ protein) ▪ Severe hypomagnesemia (↑carbohydrate) ▪ Refeeding syndrome
Anthropometric Data	
Physical Exam Findings	

INTAKE DOMAIN • Nutrient

INTAKE DOMAIN • Nutrient

IMBALANCE OF NUTRIENTS (NI-5.5)

Food/Nutrition History	Reports or observations of:
	▪ High intake of iron supplements (↓ zinc absorption)
	▪ High intake of zinc supplements (↓ copper status)
	▪ High intake of manganese (↓ iron status)
Client History	▪ Diarrhea or constipation (iron supplements)
	▪ Epigastric pain, nausea, vomiting, diarrhea (zinc supplements)
	▪ Contributes to the development of anemia (manganese supplements)

References

1. National Academy of Sciences, Institute of Medicine. *Dietary Reference Intakes for Vitamin A, Vitamin K, Arsenic, Boron, Chromium, Copper, Iodine, Iron, Manganese, Molybdenum, Nickel, Silicon, Vanadium, Zinc.* Washington, DC: National Academy Press; 2001.
2. National Academy of Sciences, Institute of Medicine. *Dietary Reference Intakes for Calcium, Phosphorus, Magnesium, Vitamin D, and Fluoride.* Washington, DC: National Academy Press; 1997.

Updated: 2008 Edition

Intake

83

INTAKE DOMAIN • Fat and Cholesterol

INADEQUATE FAT INTAKE (NI-5.6.1)

Definition

Lower fat intake compared to established reference standards or recommendations based on physiological needs. Exception: when the goal is weight loss or during end-of-life care.

Etiology (Cause/Contributing Risk Factors)

Factors gathered during the nutrition assessment process that contribute to the existence or the maintenance of pathophysiological, psychosocial, situational, developmental, cultural, and/or environmental problems:

- Inappropriate food choices, e.g., economic constraints, cultural or religious practices, restricting food given to elderly and/or children, specific food choices
- Food- and nutrition-related knowledge deficit, e.g., prolonged adherence to a very-low-fat diet
- Psychological causes, e.g., depression or disordered eating

Signs/Symptoms (Defining Characteristics)

A typical cluster of subjective and objective signs and symptoms gathered during the nutrition assessment process that provide evidence that a problem exists; quantify the problem and describe its severity.

Nutrition Assessment Category	Potential Indicators of this Nutrition Diagnosis (one or more must be present)
Biochemical Data, Medical Tests and Procedures	▪ Triene: tetraene ratio > 0.2
Anthropometric Measurements	▪ Impaired growth ▪ Weight loss if insufficient calories consumed
Physical Examination Findings	▪ Scaly skin and dermatitis consistent with essential fatty acid deficiency
Food/Nutrition History	Reports or observations of: ▪ Intake of essential fatty acids less than 10% of energy (primarily associated with PN)
Client History	▪ Conditions associated with a diagnosis or treatment, e.g., prolonged catabolic illness (e.g., AIDS, tuberculosis, anorexia nervosa, sepsis or severe infection from recent surgery) ▪ Severe fat malabsorption with bowel resection, pancreatic insufficiency, or hepatic disease accompanied by steatorrhea

Edition: 2008

INADEQUATE FAT INTAKE (NI-5.6.1)

References

1. National Academy of Science, Institute of Medicine. *Dietary Reference Intakes for Energy, Carbohydrate, Fiber, Fat, Fatty Acids, Cholesterol, Protein, and Amino Acids.* Washington, DC: National Academy Press; 2002.

Updated: 2008 Edition

INTAKE DOMAIN • Fat and Cholesterol

EXCESSIVE FAT INTAKE (NI-5.6.2)

Definition

Higher fat intake compared to established reference standards or recommendations based on physiological needs.

Etiology (Cause/Contributing Risk Factors)

Factors gathered during the nutrition assessment process that contribute to the existence or the maintenance of pathophysiological, psychosocial, situational, developmental, cultural, and/or environmental problems:

- Food- and nutrition-related knowledge deficit
- Harmful beliefs/attitudes about food, nutrition, and nutrition-related topics
- Lack of access to healthful food choices, e.g., healthful food choices not provided as an option by caregiver or parent, homeless
- Changes in taste and appetite or preference
- Lack of value for behavior change, competing values

Signs/Symptoms (Defining Characteristics)

A typical cluster of subjective and objective signs and symptoms gathered during the nutrition assessment process that provide evidence that a problem exists; quantify the problem and describe its severity.

Nutrition Assessment Category	Potential Indicators of this Nutrition Diagnosis (one or more must be present)
Biochemical Data, Medical Tests and Procedures	• Cholesterol > 200 mg/dL (5.2 mmol/L), LDL cholesterol > 100 mg/dL (2.59 mmol/L), HDL cholesterol < 40 mg/dL (1.036 mmol/L), triglycerides > 150 mg/dL (1.695 mmol/L)
	• Elevated serum amylase and/or lipase
	• Elevated LFTs, T. Bili
	• Fecal fat > 7g/24 hours
Anthropometric Measurements	
Physical Exam Findings	• Evidence of xanthomas

Edition: 2008

EXCESSIVE FAT INTAKE (NI-5.6.2)

Food/Nutrition History	Reports or observations of: ▪ Frequent or large portions of high-fat foods ▪ Frequent food preparation with added fat ▪ Frequent consumption of high risk lipids (i.e., saturated fat, trans fat, cholesterol) ▪ Report of foods containing fat more than diet prescription
Client History	▪ Conditions associated with a diagnosis or treatment, e.g., hyperlipidemia, cystic fibrosis, angina, artherosclerosis, pancreatic, liver, and biliary diseases, post-transplantation ▪ Medication, e.g., pancreatic enzymes, cholesterol- or other lipid-lowering medications ▪ Diarrhea, cramping, steatorrhea, epigastric pain ▪ Family history of hyperlipidemia, atherosclerosis, or pancreatitis

References

1. National Academy of Sciences, Institute of Medicine. *Dietary Reference Intakes for Energy, Carbohydrate, Fiber, Fat, Fatty Acids, Cholesterol, Protein, and Amino Acids*. Washington, DC: National Academy Press; 2002.

2. Position of the American Dietetic Association. Weight management. *J Am Diet Assoc*. 2002;102:1145-1155.

3. Position of the American Dietetic Association. Total diet approach to communicating food and nutrition information. *J Am Diet Assoc*. 2007;107:(in press).

4. Position of the American Dietetic Association. The role of dietetics professionals in health promotion and disease prevention. *J Am Diet Assoc*. 2006;106:1875-1884.

Updated: 2008 Edition

Edition: 2008

INTAKE DOMAIN • Fat and Cholesterol

INAPPROPRIATE INTAKE OF FOOD FATS (SPECIFY) (NI-5.6.3)

Definition

Intake of wrong type or quality of food fats compared to established reference standards or recommendations based on physiological needs.

Etiology (Cause/Contributing Risk Factors)

Factors gathered during the nutrition assessment process that contribute to the existence or the maintenance of pathophysiological, psychosocial, situational, developmental, cultural, and/or environmental problems:

- Food- and nutrition-related knowledge deficit
- Harmful beliefs/attitudes about food, nutrition, and nutrition-related topics
- Lack of access to healthful food choices, e.g., healthful food choices not provided as an option by caregiver or parent, homeless
- Changes in taste and appetite or preference
- Lack of value for behavior change, competing values

Signs/Symptoms (Defining Characteristics)

A typical cluster of subjective and objective signs and symptoms gathered during the nutrition assessment process that provide evidence that a problem exists; quantify the problem and describe its severity.

Nutrition Assessment Category	Potential Indicators of this Nutrition Diagnosis (one or more must be present)
Biochemical Data, Medical Tests and Procedures	• Cholesterol > 200 mg/dL (5.2 mmol/L), LDL cholesterol > 100 mg/dL (2.59 mmol/L), HDL cholesterol < 40 mg/dL (1.036 mmol/L), triglycerides > 150 mg/dL (1.695 mmol/L)
	• Elevated serum amylase and/or lipase
	• Elevated LFTs, T. Bili, C-reactive protein
Anthropometric Measurements	
Physical Exam Findings	• Evidence of dermatitis
Food/Nutrition History	Reports or observations of:
	• Frequent food preparation with added fat that is not of desired type for condition
	• Frequent consumption of fats that are undesirable for condition (i.e., saturated fat, trans fat, cholesterol, Ω-6 fatty acids)
	• Inadequate intake of monounsaturated, polyunsaturated, or Ω-3 fatty acids

Edition: 2008

INAPPROPRIATE INTAKE OF FOOD FATS (SPECIFY) (NI-5.6.3)

Client History	• Conditions associated with a diagnosis or treatment of diabetes, cardiac diseases, obesity, liver or biliary disorders
	• Diarrhea, cramping, steatorrhea, epigastric pain
	• Family history of diabetes-related heart disease, hyperlipidemia, atherosclerosis, or pancreatitis

References

1. de Lorgeril M, Salen P, Martin J-L, Monjaud I, Delaye J, Mamelle N. Mediterranean diet, traditional risk factors, and the rate of cardiovascular complications after myocardial infarction. Final report of the Lyon Diet Heart Study. *Circulation.* 1999; 99:779-785.

2. Franz MJ, Bantle JP, Beebe CA, Brunzell JD, Chiasson J-L, Garg A, Holzmeister LA, Hoogwerf B, Mayer-Davis E, Mooradian AD, Purnell JQ, Wheeler M. Technical review. Evidence-based nutrition principles and recommendations for the treatment and prevention of diabetes and related complications. *Diabetes Care.* 2002;202:148-198.

3. Knoops KTB, de Grott LCPGM, Kromhout D, Perrin A-E, Varela M-V, Menotti A, van Staveren WA. Mediterranean diet, lifestyle factors, and 10-year mortality in elderly European men and women. *JAMA.* 2004;292:1433-1439.

4. Kris-Etherton PM, Harris WS, Appel LJ, for the Nutrition Committee. AHA scientific statement. Fish consumption, fish oil, omega-3 fatty acids, and cardiovascular disease. *Circulation.* 2002;106:2747-2757.

5. Panagiotakos DB, Pitsavos C, Polychronopoulos E, Chrysohoou C, Zampelas A, Trichopoulou A. Can a Mediterranean diet moderate the development and clinical progression of coronary heart disease? A systematic review. *Med Sci Monit.* 2004;10:RA193-RA198.

6. Position of the American Dietetic Association. Weight management. *J Am Diet Assoc.* 2002;102:1145-1155.

7. Position of the American Dietetic Association. Total diet approach to communicating food and nutrition information. *J Am Diet Assoc.* 2007;107(in press).

8. Position of the American Dietetic Association. The role of dietetics professionals in health promotion and disease prevention. *J Am Diet Assoc.* 2006;106:1875-1884.

9. Zhao G, Etherton TD, Martin KR, West SG, Gilles PJ, Kris-Etherton PM. Dietary alpha-linolenic acid reduces inflammatory and lipid cardiovascular risk factors in hypercholesterolemic men and women. *J Nutr.* 2004;134:2991-2997.

Updated: 2008 Edition

INTAKE DOMAIN • Protein

INADEQUATE PROTEIN INTAKE (NI-5.7.1)

Definition

Lower intake of protein-containing foods or substances compared to established reference standards or recommendations based on physiological needs.

Etiology (Cause/Contributing Risk Factors)

Factors gathered during the nutrition assessment process that contribute to the existence or the maintenance of pathophysiological, psychosocial, situational, developmental, cultural, and/or environmental problems:

- Physiological causes, e.g., increased nutrient needs due to prolonged catabolic illness, malabsorption, age, or condition
- Lack of access to food, e.g., economic constraints, cultural or religious practices, restricting food given to elderly and/or children
- Food- and nutrition-related knowledge deficit
- Psychological causes, e.g., depression or disordered eating

Signs/Symptoms (Defining Characteristics)

A typical cluster of subjective and objective signs and symptoms gathered during the nutrition assessment process that provide evidence that a problem exists; quantify the problem and describe its severity.

Nutrition Assessment Category	Potential Indicators of this Nutrition Diagnosis (one or more must be present)
Biochemical Data, Medical Tests and Procedures	
Anthropometric Measurements	
Physical Examination Findings	
Food/Nutrition History	Reports or observation of: ■ Insufficient intake of protein to meet requirements ■ Cultural or religious practices that limit protein intake ■ Economic constraints that limit food availability ■ Prolonged adherence to a very–low-protein weight-loss diet
Client History	■ Conditions associated with a diagnosis or treatment, e.g., severe protein malabsorption such as bowel resection

90

Edition: 2008

INTAKE DOMAIN • Protein

INADEQUATE PROTEIN INTAKE (NI-5.7.1)

References

1. National Academy of Sciences, Institute of Medicine. *Dietary Reference Intakes for Energy, Carbohydrate, Fiber, Fat, Fatty Acids, Cholesterol, Protein, and Amino Acids.* Washington DC: National Academy Press; 2002.

INTAKE DOMAIN • Protein

EXCESSIVE PROTEIN INTAKE (NI-5.7.2)

Definition

Intake more than the recommended level of protein compared to established reference standards or recommendations based on physiological needs.

Etiology (Cause/Contributing Risk Factors)

Factors gathered during the nutrition assessment process that contribute to the existence or the maintenance of pathophysiological, psychosocial, situational, developmental, cultural, and/or environmental problems:

- Liver dysfunction
- Renal dysfunction
- Harmful beliefs/attitudes about food, nutrition, and nutrition-related topics
- Lack of access to specialized protein products
- Metabolic abnormality
- Food faddism

Signs/Symptoms (Defining Characteristics)

A typical cluster of subjective and objective signs and symptoms gathered during the nutrition assessment process that provide evidence that a problem exists; quantify the problem and describe its severity.

Nutrition Assessment Category	Potential Indicators of this Nutrition Diagnosis (one or more must be present)
Biochemical Data, Medical Tests and Procedures	▪ Altered laboratory values, e.g., ↑ BUN, ↓ glomerular filtration rate (altered renal status)
Anthropometric Measurements	▪ Growth stunting or failure based on National Center for Health Statistics growth charts (metabolic disorders)
Physical Exam Findings	
Food/Nutrition History	Reports or observations of: ▪ Higher than recommended total protein intake, e.g., early renal disease, advanced liver disease with confusion ▪ Inappropriate supplementation
Client History	▪ Conditions associated with a diagnosis or treatment, e.g., early renal disease or advanced liver disease with confusion

Edition: 2008

EXCESSIVE PROTEIN INTAKE (NI-5.7.2)

References

1. Position of the American Dietetic Association. Food and nutrition misinformation. *J Am Diet Assoc.* 2006;106:601-607.
2. Beto JA, Bansal VK. Medical nutrition therapy in chronic kidney failure: Integrating clinical practice guidelines. *J Am Diet Assoc.* 2004;104:404-409.
3. Brandle E, Sieberth HG, Hautmann RE. Effect of chronic dietary protein intake on the renal function in healthy subjects. *Eur J Clin Nutr.* 1996;50:734-740.
4. Frassetto LA, Todd KM, Morris RC Jr, Sebastian A. Estimation of net endogenous noncarbonic acid production in humans from diet, potassium and protein contents. *Am J Clin Nutr.* 1998;68:576-583.
5. Friedman N, ed. *Absorption and Utilization of Amino Acids, Vol. I.* Boca Raton, FL: CRC Press; 1989: 229-242.
6. Hoogeveen EK, Kostense PJ, Jager A, Heine RJ, Jakobs C, Bouter LM, Donker AJ, Stehower CD. Serum homocysteine level and protein intake are related to risk of microalbuminuria: the Hoorn study. *Kidney Int.* 1998;54:203-209.
7. Rudman D, DiFulco TJ, Galambos JT, Smith RB 3rd, Salam AA, Warren WD. Maximum rate of excretion and synthesis of urea in normal and cirrhotic subjects. *J Clin Invest.* 1973;52:2241-2249.

93

INTAKE DOMAIN • Protein

INAPPROPRIATE INTAKE OF AMINO ACIDS (SPECIFY) (NI-5.7.3)

Definition

Intake that is more or less than recommended level and/or type of amino acids compared to established reference standards or recommendations based on physiological needs.

Etiology (Cause/Contributing Risk Factors)

Factors gathered during the nutrition assessment process that contribute to the existence or the maintenance of pathophysiological, psychosocial, situational, developmental, cultural, and/or environmental problems:

- Liver dysfunction
- Renal dysfunction
- Harmful beliefs/attitudes about food, nutrition, and nutrition-related topics
- Misused specialized protein products
- Metabolic abnormality
- Food faddism
- Inborn errors of metabolism

Signs/Symptoms (Defining Characteristics)

A typical cluster of subjective and objective signs and symptoms gathered during the nutrition assessment process that provide evidence that a problem exists; quantify the problem and describe its severity.

Nutrition Assessment Category	Potential Indicators of this Nutrition Diagnosis (one or more must be present)
Biochemical Data, Medical Tests and Procedures	▪ Altered laboratory values, e.g., ↑ BUN, ↓ glomerular filtration rate (altered renal status); increased urinary 3-methyl-histidine
	▪ Elevated specific amino acids (inborn errors of metabolism)
	▪ Elevated homocysteine or ammonia
Anthropometric Measurements	
Physical Exam Findings	▪ Physical or neurological changes (inborn errors of metabolism)

INAPPROPRIATE INTAKE OF AMINO ACIDS (SPECIFY) (NI-5.7.3)

Food/Nutrition History	Reports or observation of:
	▪ Higher than recommended amino acid intake, e.g., early renal disease, advanced liver disease, inborn error of metabolism
	▪ Higher than recommended type of amino acids for prescribed parenteral and enteral nutrition therapy
	▪ Inappropriate amino acid or protein supplementation, as for athletes
	▪ Higher than recommended amino acid intake, e.g., excess phenylalanine intake
Client History	▪ Conditions associated with a diagnosis or treatment of illness that requires PEN therapy
	▪ History of inborn error of metabolism
	▪ Uremia, azotemia (renal patients)

References

1. Beto JA, Bansal VK. Medical nutrition therapy in chronic kidney failure: Integrating clinical practice guidelines. *J Am Diet Assoc.* 2004;104:404-409.
2. Brandle E, Sieberth HG, Hautmann RE. Effect of chronic dietary protein intake on the renal function in healthy subjects. *Eur J Clin Nutr.* 1996;50 :734-740.
3. Cohn RM, Roth KS. Hyperammonia, bane of the brain. *Clin Pediatr.* 2004;43:683.
4. Frassetto LA, Todd KM, Morris RC Jr, Sebastian A. Estimation of net endogenous noncarbonic acid production in humans from diet, potassium and protein contents. *Am J Clin Nutr.* 1998;68:576-583.
5. Friedman N, ed. *Absorption and Utilization of Amino Acids, Vol. I.* Boca Raton, FL: CRC Press; 1989:229-242.
6. Hoogeveen EK, Kostense PJ, Jager A, Heine RJ, Jakobs C, Bouter LM, Donker AJ, Stehower CD. Serum homocysteine level and protein intake are related to risk of microalbuminuria: the Hoorn study. *Kidney Int.* 1998;54:203-209.
7. Position of the American Dietetic Association: Food and nutrition misinformation. *J Am Diet Assoc.* 2006;106:601-607.
8. Rudman D, DiFulco TJ, Galambos JT, Smith RB 3rd, Salam AA, Warren WD. Maximal rate of excretion and synthesis of urea in normal and cirrhotic subjects. *J Clin Invest.* 1973;52:2241-2249.

Edition: 2008

INTAKE DOMAIN • Carbohydrate and Fiber

INADEQUATE CARBOHYDRATE INTAKE (NI-5.8.1)

Definition

Lower intake of carbohydrate-containing foods or substances compared to established reference standards or recommendations based on physiological needs.

Etiology (Cause/Contributing Risk Factors)

Factors gathered during the nutrition assessment process that contribute to the existence or the maintenance of pathophysiological, psychosocial, situational, developmental, cultural, and/or environmental problems:

- Physiological causes, e.g., increased energy needs due to increased activity level or metabolic change, malabsorption
- Lack of access to food, e.g., economic constraints, cultural or religious practices, restricting food given to elderly and/or children
- Food- and nutrition-related knowledge deficit
- Psychological causes, e.g., depression or disordered eating

Signs/Symptoms (Defining Characteristics)

A typical cluster of subjective and objective signs and symptoms gathered during the nutrition assessment process that provide evidence that a problem exists; quantify the problem and describe its severity.

Nutrition Assessment Category	Potential Indicators of this Nutrition Diagnosis (one or more must be present)
Biochemical Data, Medical Tests and Procedures	
Anthropometric Measurements	
Physical Examination Findings	• Ketone smell on breath
Food/Nutrition History	Reports or observation of: • Carbohydrate intake less than recommended amounts • Inability to independently consume foods/fluids, e.g., diminished mobility in hand, wrist, or digits
Client History	• Conditions associated with a diagnosis or treatment, e.g., pancreatic insufficiency, hepatic disease, celiac disease, seizure disorder, or carbohydrate malabsorption

References

1. National Academy of Sciences, Institute of Medicine. *Dietary Reference Intakes for Energy, Carbohydrate, Fiber, Fat, Fatty Acids, Cholesterol, Protein, and Amino Acids.* Washington, DC: National Academy Press; 2002.

EXCESSIVE CARBOHYDRATE INTAKE (NI-5.8.2)

Definition

Intake more than the recommended level and type of carbohydrate compared to established reference standards or recommendations based on physiological needs.

Etiology (Cause/Contributing Risk Factors)

Factors gathered during the nutrition assessment process that contribute to the existence or the maintenance of pathophysiological, psychosocial, situational, developmental, cultural, and/or environmental problems:

- Physiological causes requiring modified carbohydrate intake, e.g., diabetes mellitus, lactase deficiency, sucrase-isomaltase deficiency, aldolase-B deficiency

- Cultural or religious practices that interfere with the ability to reduce carbohydrate intake

- Food- and nutrition-related knowledge deficit, e.g., inability to access sufficient information concerning appropriate carbohydrate intake

- Food and nutrition compliance limitations, e.g., lack of willingness or failure to modify carbohydrate intake in response to recommendations from a dietitian or physician

- Psychological causes, e.g., depression or disordered eating

Signs/Symptoms (Defining Characteristics)

A typical cluster of subjective and objective signs and symptoms gathered during the nutrition assessment process that provide evidence that a problem exists; quantify the problem and describe its severity.

Nutrition Assessment Category	Potential Indicators of this Nutrition Diagnosis (one or more must be present)
Biochemical Data, Medical Tests and Procedures	▪ Hyperglycemia (fasting blood sugar > 126 mg/dL) ▪ Hemoglobin A1C > 6% ▪ Abnormal oral glucose tolerance test (2-hour post load glucose > 200 mg/dL)
Anthropometric Measurements	
Physical Examination Findings	▪ Dental caries ▪ Diarrhea in response to carbohydrate feeding

97

INTAKE DOMAIN • Carbohydrate and Fiber

EXCESSIVE CARBOHYDRATE INTAKE (NI-5.8.2)

Food/Nutrition History	Reports or observation of:
	▪ Cultural or religious practices that do not support modification of dietary carbohydrate intake
	▪ Economic constraints that limit availability of appropriate foods
	▪ Carbohydrate intake that is consistently more than recommended amounts
Client History	▪ Conditions associated with a diagnosis or treatment of, e.g., diabetes mellitus, inborn errors of carbohydrate metabolism, lactase deficiency, severe infection, sepsis, or obesity
	▪ Chronic use of medications that cause hyperglycemia, e.g., steroids
	▪ Pancreatic insufficiency resulting in reduced insulin production

References

1. Bowman BA, Russell RM. *Present Knowledge in Nutrition. 8th Ed.* Washington, DC: ILSI Press; 2001.
2. Clement S, Braithwaite SS, Magee MF, Ahmann A, Smith EP, Schafer RG, Hirsch IB, American Diabetes Association Diabetes in Hospitals Writing Committee. Management of diabetes in hospitals. *Diabetes Care.* 2004;27:553-592.
3. National Academy of Sciences, Institute of Medicine. *Dietary Reference Intakes for Energy, Carbohydrate, Fiber, Fat, Fatty Acids, Cholesterol, Protein, and Amino Acids.* Washington, DC: National Academy Press; 2002.
4. The Expert Committee on the Diagnosis and Classification of Diabetes Mellitus. Diagnosis and classification of diabetes mellitus. *Diabetes Care.* 2004;27:S5-S10.

INAPPROPRIATE INTAKE OF TYPES OF CARBOHYDRATES (SPECIFY) (NI-5.8.3)

Definition

Intake of the type or amount of carbohydrate that is more or less than the established reference standards or recommendations based on physiological needs.

Etiology (Cause/Contributing Risk Factors)

Factors gathered during the nutrition assessment process that contribute to the existence or the maintenance of pathophysiological, psychosocial, situational, developmental, cultural, and/or environmental problems:

- Physiological causes requiring careful use of modified carbohydrate, e.g., diabetes mellitus, metabolic syndrome, hypoglycemia, celiac disease, allergies, obesity
- Cultural or religious practices that interfere with the ability to regulate types of carbohydrate consumed
- Food- and nutrition-related knowledge deficit, e.g., inability to access sufficient information concerning more appropriate carbohydrate types and/or amounts
- Food and nutrition compliance limitations, e.g., lack of willingness or failure to modify carbohydrate intake in response to recommendations from a dietitian, physician, or caregiver
- Psychological causes, e.g., depression or disordered eating

Signs/Symptoms (Defining Characteristics)

A typical cluster of subjective and objective signs and symptoms gathered during the nutrition assessment process that provide evidence that a problem exists; quantify the problem and describe its severity.

Nutrition Assessment Category	Potential Indicators of this Nutrition Diagnosis (one or more must be present)
Biochemical Data, Medical Tests and Procedures	▪ Hypoglycemia or hyperglycemia documented on regular basis when compared with goal of maintaining glucose levels at or less than 140 mg/dL throughout the day
Anthropometric Measurements	
Physical Examination Findings	

INTAKE DOMAIN • Carbohydrate and Fiber

INAPPROPRIATE INTAKE OF TYPES OF CARBOHYDRATES (SPECIFY) (NI-5.8.3)

Food/Nutrition History	Reports or observations of:
	▪ Diarrhea in response to high intake of refined carbohydrates
	▪ Economic constraints that limit availability of appropriate foods
	▪ Carbohydrate intake that is different from recommended types
	▪ Allergic reactions to certain carbohydrate foods or food groups
	▪ Limited knowledge of carbohydrate composition of foods or of carbohydrate metabolism
Client History	▪ Conditions associated with a diagnosis or treatment, e.g., diabetes mellitus, obesity, metabolic syndrome, hypoglycemia
	▪ Chronic use of medications that cause altered glucose levels, e.g., steroids, antidepressants, antipsychotics

References

1. Bowman BA, Russell RM. *Present Knowledge in Nutrition. 8th Ed.* Washington, DC: ILSI Press, 2001.
2. Clement S, Braithwaite SS, Magee MF, Ahmann A, Smith EP, Schafer RG, Hirsch IB, American Diabetes Association Diabetes in Hospitals Writing Committee. Management of diabetes in hospitals. *Diabetes Care.* 2004;27:553-592.
3. Franz MJ, Bantle JP, Beebe CA, Brunzell JD, Chiasson J-L, Garg A, Holzmeister LA, Hoogwerf B, Mayer-Davis E, Mooradian AD, Purnell JQ, Wheeler M. Technical review. Evidence-based nutrition principles and recommendations for the treatment and prevention of diabetes and related complications. *Diabetes Care.* 2002:202:148-198.
4. Sheard NF, Clark NG, Brand-Miller JC, Franz MJ, PJ-Sunyer FX, Mayer-Davis E, Kulkarni K, Geil P. A statement by the American Diabetes Association. Dietary carbohydrate (amount and type) in the prevention and management of diabetes. *Diabetes Care* 2004:27:2266-2271.
5. Gross LS, Li L, Ford ES, Liu S. Increased consumption of refined carbohydrates and epidemic or type 2 diabetes in the United States: an ecologic assessment. *Am J Clin Nutr.* 2004;79:774-779.
6. French S, Lin B-H, Gutherie JF. National trends in soft drink consumption among children and adolescents age 6 to17 years: prevalence, amounts, and sources, 1977/1978 to 1994/1998. *J Am Diet Assoc.* 2003;103L1326-1331,
7. National Academy of Sciences, Institute of Medicine. *Dietary Reference Intakes for Energy, Carbohydrate, Fiber, Fat, Fatty Acids, Cholesterol, Protein, and Amino Acids.* Washington, DC: National Academy Press; 2002.
8. Teff KL, Elliott SS, Tschöp M, Kieffer TJ, Rader D, Heiman M, Townsend RR, Keim NL, D'Alessio D, Havel PJ. Dietary fructose reduces circulating insulin and leptin, attenuates postprandial suppression of ghrelin, and increases triglycerides in women. *J Clin Endocrinol Metab.* 2004;89:2963-2972.
9. The Expert Committee on the Diagnosis and Classification of Diabetes Mellitus. Diagnosis and classification of diabetes mellitus. *Diabetes Care.* 2004:27:S5-S10.

INCONSISTENT CARBOHYDRATE INTAKE (NI-5.8.4)

Definition

Inconsistent timing of carbohydrate intake throughout the day, day to day, or a pattern of carbohydrate intake that is not consistent with recommended pattern based on physiological or medication needs.

Etiology (Cause/Contributing Risk Factors)

Factors gathered during the nutrition assessment process that contribute to the existence or the maintenance of pathophysiological, psychosocial, situational, developmental, cultural, and/or environmental problems:

- Physiological causes requiring careful timing and consistency in the amount of carbohydrate, e.g., diabetes mellitus, hypoglycemia
- Cultural or religious practices or lifestyle factors that interfere with the ability to regulate timing of carbohydrate consumption
- Food- and nutrition-related knowledge deficit, e.g., inability to access sufficient information concerning more appropriate timing of carbohydrate intake
- Food and nutrition compliance limitations, e.g., lack of willingness or failure to modify carbohydrate timing in response to recommendations from a dietitian, physician, or caregiver
- Psychological causes, e.g., depression or disordered eating

Signs/Symptoms (Defining Characteristics)

A typical cluster of subjective and objective signs and symptoms gathered during the nutrition assessment process that provide evidence that a problem exists; quantify the problem and describe its severity.

Nutrition Assessment Category	Potential Indicators of this Nutrition Diagnosis (one or more must be present)
Biochemical Data, Medical Tests and Procedures	▪ Hypoglycemia or hyperglycemia documented on regular basis associated with inconsistent carbohydrate intake ▪ Wide variations in blood glucose levels
Anthropometric Measurements	
Physical Examination Findings	
Food/Nutrition History	Reports or observations of: ▪ Economic constraints that limit availability of appropriate foods ▪ Carbohydrate intake that is different from recommended types or ingested on an irregular basis

101

INTAKE DOMAIN • Carbohydrate and Fiber

INCONSISTENT CARBOHYDRATE INTAKE (NI-5.8.4)

Client History	▪ Conditions associated with a diagnosis or treatment, e.g., diabetes mellitus, obesity, metabolic syndrome, hypoglycemia ▪ Use of insulin or insulin secretagogues ▪ Chronic use of medications that cause altered glucose levels, e.g., steroids, antidepressants, antipsychotics

References

1. Bowman BA, Russell RM. *Present Knowledge in Nutrition. 8th Ed.* Washington, DC: ILSI Press; 2001.

2. Clement S, Braithwaite SS, Magee MF, Ahmann A, Smith EP, Schafer RG, Hirsch IB, American Diabetes Association Diabetes in Hospitals Writing Committee. Management of diabetes in hospitals. *Diabetes Care.* 2004;27:553-592.

3. Cryer PE, Davis SN, Shamoon H. Technical review. Hypoglycemia in diabetes. *Diabetes Care.* 2003;26L1902-1912.

4. Franz MJ, Bantle JP, Beebe CA, Brunzell JD, Chiasson J-L, Garg A, Holzmeister LA, Hoogwerf B, Mayer-Davis E, Mooradian AD, Purnell JQ, Wheeler M. Technical review. Evidence-based nutrition principles and recommendations for the treatment and prevention of diabetes and related complications. *Diabetes Care.* 2002:202:148-198.

5. National Academy of Sciences, Institute of Medicine. *Dietary Reference Intakes for Energy, Carbohydrate, Fiber, Fat, Fatty Acids, Cholesterol, Protein, and Amino Acids.* Washington, DC: National Academy Press; 2002.

6. Rabasa-Lhoret R, Garon J, Langelier H, Poisson D, Chiasson J-L. The effects of meal carbohydrate content on insulin requirements in type 1 patients with diabetes treated intensively with the basal bolus (ultralente-regular) insulin regimen. *Diabetes Care.* 1999;22:667-673.

7. Savoca MR, Miller CK, Ludwig DA. Food habits are related to glycemic control among people with type 2 diabetes mellitus. *J Am Diet Assoc.* 2004;104:560-566.

8. The Expert Committee on the Diagnosis and Classification of Diabetes Mellitus. Diagnosis and classification of diabetes mellitus. *Diabetes Care.* 2004:27:S5-S10.

9. Wolever TMS, Hamad S, Chiasson J-L, Josse RG, Leiter LA, Rodger NW, Ross SA, Ryan EA. Day-to-day consistency in amount and source of carbohydrate intake associated with improved glucose control in type 1 diabetes. *J Am Coll Nutr.* 1999; 18:242-247.

Edition: 2008

INTAKE DOMAIN • Carbohydrate and Fiber

INADEQUATE FIBER INTAKE (NI-5.8.5)

Definition
Lower intake of fiber-containing foods or substances compared to established reference standards or recommendations based on physiological needs.

Etiology (Cause/Contributing Risk Factors)
Factors gathered during the nutrition assessment process that contribute to the existence or the maintenance of pathophysiological, psychosocial, situational, developmental, cultural, and/or environmental problems:

- Lack of access to fiber-containing foods
- Food- and nutrition-related knowledge deficit
- Psychological causes, e.g., depression or disordered eating
- Prolonged adherence to a low-fiber or low-residue diet
- Difficulty chewing or swallowing high-fiber foods
- Economic constraints that limit availability of appropriate foods
- Inability or unwillingness to purchase or consume fiber-containing foods
- Inappropriate food preparation practices, e.g., reliance on overprocessed, overcooked foods

Signs/Symptoms (Defining Characteristics)
A typical cluster of subjective and objective signs and symptoms gathered during the nutrition assessment process that provide evidence that a problem exists; quantify the problem and describe its severity.

Nutrition Assessment Category	Potential Indicators of this Nutrition Diagnosis (one or more must be present)
Biochemical Data, Medical Tests and Procedures	
Anthropometric Measurements	
Physical Examination Findings	
Food/Nutrition History	Reports or observations of: • Insufficient intake of fiber when compared to recommended amounts (38 g/day for men and 25 g/day for women)

Edition: 2008

INTAKE DOMAIN • Carbohydrate and Fiber

INADEQUATE FIBER INTAKE (NI-5.8.5)

Client History	• Conditions associated with a diagnosis or treatment, e.g., ulcer disease, inflammatory bowel disease, or short-bowel syndrome treated with a low-fiber diet • Low stool volume, constipation

References

1. DiPalma JA. Current treatment options for chronic constipation. *Rev Gastroenterol Disord.* 2004;2:S34-S42.
2. Higgins PD, Johanson JF. Epidemiology of constipation in North America: a systematic review. *Am J Gastroenterol.* 2004;99:750-759.
3. Lembo A, Camilieri M. Chronic constipation. *New Engl J Med.* 2003;349:360-368.
4. National Academy of Sciences, Institute of Medicine. *Dietary Reference Intakes for Energy, Carbohydrate, Fiber, Fat, Fatty Acids, Cholesterol, Protein, and Amino Acids.* Washington, DC: National Academy Press; 2002.
5. Talley NJ. Definition, epidemiology, and impact of chronic constipation. *Rev Gastroenterol Disord.* 2004;2:S3-S10.

Updated: 2008 Edition

EXCESSIVE FIBER INTAKE (NI-5.8.6)

Definition

Higher intake of fiber-containing foods or substances compared to recommendations based on patient/client condition.

Etiology (Cause/Contributing Risk Factors)

Factors gathered during the nutrition assessment process that contribute to the existence or the maintenance of pathophysiological, psychosocial, situational, developmental, cultural, and/or environmental problems:

- Food- and nutrition-related knowledge deficit about desirable quantities of fiber for individual condition
- Harmful beliefs or attitudes about food- or nutrition-related topics, e.g., obsession with bowel frequency and habits
- Lack of knowledge about appropriate fiber intake for condition
- Food preparation or eating patterns that involve only high-fiber foods to the exclusion of other nutrient-dense foods

Signs/Symptoms (Defining Characteristics)

A typical cluster of subjective and objective signs and symptoms gathered during the nutrition assessment process that provide evidence that a problem exists; quantify the problem and describe its severity.

Nutrition Assessment Category	Potential Indicators of this Nutrition Diagnosis (one or more must be present)
Biochemical Data, Medical Tests and Procedures	
Anthropometric Measurements	
Physical Examination Findings	
Food/Nutrition History	Reports or observations of: • Fiber intake higher than tolerated or generally recommended for current medical condition
Client History	• Conditions associated with a diagnosis or treatment, e.g., ulcer disease, irritable bowel syndrome, inflammatory bowel disease, short-bowel syndrome, diverticulitis, obstructive constipation, prolapsing hemorrhoids, gastrointestinal stricture, eating disorders, or mental illness with obsessive-compulsive tendencies • Nausea, vomiting, excessive flatulence, diarrhea, abdominal cramping, high stool volume or frequency that causes discomfort to the individual; obstruction; phytobezoar

105

Intake

INTAKE DOMAIN • Carbohydrate and Fiber

EXCESSIVE FIBER INTAKE (NI-5.8.6)

References

1. DiPalma JA. Current treatment options for chronic constipation. *Rev Gastroenterol Disord.* 2004;2:S34-S42.

2. Higgins PD, Johanson JF. Epidemiology of constipation in North America: a systematic review. *Am J Gastroenterol.* 2004;99:750-759.

3. Lembo A, Camilieri M. Chronic constipation. *New Engl J Med.* 2003;349:360-368.

4. National Academy of Sciences, Institute of Medicine. *Dietary Reference Intakes for Energy, Carbohydrate, Fiber, Fat, Fatty Acids, Cholesterol, Protein, and Amino Acids.* Washington, DC: National Academy Press; 2002.

5. Position of the American Dietetic Association: Health implications of dietary fiber. *J Am Diet Assoc.* 2002;102:993-1000.

6. Talley NJ. Definition, epidemiology, and impact of chronic constipation. *Rev Gastroenterol Disord.* 2004;2:S3-S10.

7. van den Berg H, van der Gaag M, Hendriks H. Influence of lifestyle on vitamin bioavailability. *Int J Vitam Nutr Res.* 2002;72:53-55.

8. Wald A. Irritable bowel syndrome. *Curr Treat Options Gastroenterol.* 1999;2:13-19.

Updated: 2008 Edition

INADEQUATE VITAMIN INTAKE (SPECIFY) (NI-5.9.1)

Definition

Lower intake of vitamin-containing foods or substances compared to established reference standards or recommendations based on physiological needs.

Etiology (Cause/Contributing Risk Factors)

Factors gathered during the nutrition assessment process that contribute to the existence or the maintenance of pathophysiological, psychosocial, situational, developmental, cultural, and/or environmental problems:

- Physiological causes, e.g., increased nutrient needs due to prolonged catabolic illness, disease state, malabsorption, or medications
- Lack of access to food, e.g., economic constraints, cultural or religious practices, restricting food given to elderly and/or children
- Food- and nutrition-related knowledge deficit concerning food sources of vitamins
- Psychological causes, e.g., depression or eating disorders

Signs/Symptoms (Defining Characteristics)

A typical cluster of subjective and objective signs and symptoms gathered during the nutrition assessment process that provide evidence that a problem exists; quantify the problem and describe its severity.

107

INTAKE DOMAIN • Vitamin

INADEQUATE VITAMIN INTAKE (SPECIFY) (NI-5.9.1)

Nutrition Assessment Category	Potential Indicators of this Nutrition Diagnosis (one or more must be present)
Biochemical Data, Medical Tests and Procedures	▪ Vitamin A: serum retinol < 10 µg/dL (0.35 µmol/L)
	▪ Vitamin C: plasma concentrations < 0.2 mg/dL (11.4 µmol/L)
	▪ Vitamin D: ionized calcium < 3.9 mg/dL (0.98 mmol/L) with elevated parathyroid hormone, normal serum calcium, and serum phosphorus < 2.6 mg/dL (0.84 mmol/L)
	▪ Vitamin E: plasma alpha-tocopherol < 18 µmol/g (41.8 µmol/L)
	▪ Vitamin K: elevated prothrombin time; altered INR (without anticoagulation therapy)
	▪ Thiamin: erythrocyte transketolase activity > 1.20 µg/mL/h
	▪ Riboflavin: erythrocyte glutathione reductase > 1.2 IU/g hemoglobin
	▪ Niacin: N¹methyl-nicotinamide excretion < 5.8 µmol/day
	▪ Vitamin B-6: plasma pryrdoxal 5' phosphate <5 ng/mL (20 nmol/L)
	▪ Vitamin B-12: serum concentration < 24.4 ng/dL (180 pmol/L); elevated homocysteine
	▪ Folic acid—serum concentration < 0.3 µg/dL (7 nmol/L); red cell folate < 315 nmol/L
Anthropometric Measurements	
Physical Exam Findings	▪ Vitamin A: night blindness, Bitot's spots, xerophthalmia, follicular hyperkeratosis
	▪ Vitamin C: follicular hyperkeratosis, petichiae, ecchymosis, coiled hairs, inflamed and bleeding gums, perifolicular hemorrhages, joint effusions, arthralgia, and impaired wound healing
	▪ Vitamin D: widening at ends of long bones
	▪ Riboflavin: sore throat, hyperemia, edema of pharyngeal and oral mucous membranes, cheilosis, angular stomatitis, glossitis, magenta tongue, seborrheic dermatitis, and normochromic, normocytic anemia with pure erythrocyte cytoplasia of the bone marrow
	▪ Niacin: symmetrical, pigmented rash on areas exposed to sunlight; bright red tongue
	▪ Vitamin B-6: seborrheic dermatitis, stomatitis, cheilosis, glossitis, confusion, depression
	▪ Vitamin B-12: tingling and numbness in extremities, diminished vibratory and position sense, motor disturbances including gait disturbances

Edition: 2008

INADEQUATE VITAMIN INTAKE (SPECIFY) (NI-5.9.1)

Food/Nutrition History	Reports or observations of:
	▪ Dietary history reflects inadequate intake of foods containing specific vitamins as compared to requirements or recommended level
	▪ Dietary history reflects excessive consumption of foods that do not contain available vitamins, e.g., over processed, overcooked, or improperly stored foods
	▪ Prolonged use of substances known to increase vitamin requirements or reduce vitamin absorption
	▪ Lack of interest in foods
	▪ Vitamin/mineral deficiency
Client History	▪ Conditions associated with a diagnosis or treatment, e.g., malabsorption as a result of celiac disease, short-bowel syndrome, or inflammatory bowel
	▪ Certain environmental conditions, e.g., infants exclusively fed breast milk with limited exposure to sunlight (Vitamin D)
	▪ Rachitic rosary in children, rickets, osteomalacia
	▪ Pellegra

References

1. National Academy of Sciences, Institute of Medicine. *Dietary Reference Intakes for Vitamin A, Vitamin K, Arsenic, Boron, Chromium, Copper, Iodine, Iron, Manganese, Molybdenum, Nickel, Silicon, Vanadium, and Zinc.* Washington, DC: National Academy Press; 2000.
2. National Academy of Sciences, Institute of Medicine. *Dietary Reference Intakes for Thiamine, Riboflavin, Niacin, Vitamin B6, Folate, Vitamin B12, Pantothenic Acid, Biotin, and Choline.* Washington, DC: National Academy Press; 2000.
3. National Academy of Sciences, Institute of Medicine. *Dietary Reference Intakes for Vitamin C, Vitamin E, Selenium, and Carotenoids.* Washington, DC: National Academy Press; 2000.
4. National Academy of Sciences, Institute of Medicine. *Dietary Reference Intakes for Calcium, Phosphorus, Magnesium, Vitamin D, and Fluoride.* Washington, DC: National Academy Press; 1997.

Edition: 2008

INTAKE DOMAIN • Vitamin

EXCESSIVE VITAMIN INTAKE (SPECIFY) (NI-5.9.2)

Definition

Higher intake of vitamin-containing foods or substances compared to established reference standards or recommendations based on physiological needs.

Etiology (Cause/Contributing Risk Factors)

Factors gathered during the nutrition assessment process that contribute to the existence or the maintenance of pathophysiological, psychosocial, situational, developmental, cultural, and/or environmental problems:

- Physiological causes, e.g., decreased nutrient needs due to prolonged immobility or chronic renal disease
- Access to foods and supplements in excess of needs, e.g., cultural or religious practices, inappropriate food and supplements given to pregnant women, elderly, or children
- Food- and nutrition-related knowledge deficit concerning food and supplemental sources of vitamins
- Psychological causes, e.g., depression or eating disorders
- Accidental overdose from oral and supplemental forms, enteral or parenteral sources

Signs/Symptoms (Defining Characteristics)

A typical cluster of subjective and objective signs and symptoms gathered during the nutrition assessment process that provide evidence that a problem exists; quantify the problem and describe its severity.

Nutrition Assessment Category	Potential Indicators of this Nutrition Diagnosis (one or more must be present)
Biochemical Data, Medical Tests and Procedures	• Vitamin D: ionized calcium > 5.4 mg/dL (1.35 mmol/L) with elevated parathyroid hormone, normal serum calcium, and serum phosphorus > 2.6 mg/dL (0.84 mmol/L)
	• Vitamin K: slowed prothrombin time or altered INR
	• Niacin: N' methyl-nicotinamide excretion > 7.3 μmol/day
	• Vitamin B-6: plasma prydoxal 5' phosphate > 15.7 ng/mL (94 noml/L)
	• Vitamin A: serum retinol concentration > 60 μg/dL (2.09 μmol/L)
Anthropometric Measurements	• Vitamin D: growth retardation

110

EXCESSIVE VITAMIN INTAKE (SPECIFY) (NI-5.9.2)

Physical Exam Findings	• Vitamin A: changes in the skin and mucous membranes; dry lips (cheilitis); early—dryness of the nasal mucosa and eyes; later—dryness, erythema, scaling and peeling of the skin, hair loss, and nail fragility. Headache, nausea, and vomiting. Infants may have bulging fontanelle; children may develop bone alterations.
	• Vitamin D: elevated serum calcium (hypercalcemia) and phosphorus (hyperphosphatemia) levels; calcification of soft tissues (calcinosis), including the kidney, lungs, heart, and even the tympanic membrane of the ear, which can result in deafness. Headache and nausea. Infants given excessive amounts of vitamin D may have gastrointestinal upset, bone fragility.
	• Vitamin K: hemolytic anemia in adults or severe jaundice in infants have been noted on rare occasions
	• Niacin: histamine release, which causes flushing, aggravation of asthma, or liver disease
Food/Nutrition History	Reports or observations of:
	• History or measured intake reflects excessive intake of foods and supplements containing vitamins as compared to estimated requirements, including fortified cereals, meal replacements, vitamin-mineral supplements, other dietary supplements (e.g., fish liver oils or capsules), tube feeding, and/or parenteral solutions
	• Intake > Tolerable Upper Limit (UL) for vitamin A (as retinol ester, not as -carotene) is 600 µg/d for infants and toddlers; 900 µg/d for children 4-8 y, 1700 µg/d for children 9-13 y, 2800 for children 14-18 y, and 3000 µg/d for adults
	• Intake more than UL for vitamin D is 25 µg/d for infants and 50 µg/d for children and adults
	• Niacin: clinical, high-dose niacinamide (NA), 1-2 g, three times per day, can have side effects
Client History	• Conditions associated with a diagnosis or treatment, e.g., chronic liver or kidney diseases, heart failure, cancer

References

1. Allen LH, Haskell M. Estimating the potential for vitamin A toxicity in women and young children. *J Nutr.* 2002;132:S2907-S2919.
2. Croquet V, Pilette C, Lespine A, Vuillemin E, Rousselet MC, Oberti F, Saint Andre JP, Periquet B, Francois S, Ifrah N, Cales P. Hepatic hyper-vitaminosis A: importance of retinyl ester level determination. *Eur J Gastroenterol Hepatol.* 2000;12:361-364.
3. Krasinski SD, Russell RM, Otradovec CL, Sadowski JA, Hartz SC, Jacob RA, McGandy RB. Relationship of vitamin A and vitamin E intake to fasting plasma retinol, retinol-binding protein, retinyl esters, carotene, alpha-tocopherol, and cholesterol among elderly people and young adults: increased plasma retinyl esters among vitamin A-supplement users. *Am J Clin Nutr.* 1989;49:112-120.
4. National Academy of Sciences, Institute of Medicine. *Dietary Reference Intakes for Vitamin A, Vitamin K, Arsenic, Boron, Chromium, Copper, Iodine, Iron, Manganese, Molybdenum, Nickel, Silicon, Vanadium, and Zinc.* Washington, DC: National Academy Press;2000.
5. National Academy of Sciences, Institute of Medicine. *Dietary Reference Intakes for Thiamine, Riboflavin, Niacin, Vitamin B6, Folate, Vitamin B12, Pantothenic Acid, Biotin, and Choline* Washington, DC: National Academy Press;2000.
6. National Academy of Sciences, Institute of Medicine. *Dietary Reference Intakes for Vitamin C, Vitamin E, Selenium, and Carotenoids.* Washington, DC: National Academy Press;2000.
7. Russell RM. New views on RDAs for older adults. *J Am Diet Assoc.* 1997;97:515-518.

Edition: 2008

INTAKE DOMAIN • Mineral

INADEQUATE MINERAL INTAKE (SPECIFY) (NI-5.10.1)

Definition

Lower intake of mineral-containing foods or substances compared to established reference standards or recommendations based on physiological needs.

Etiology (*Cause/Contributing Risk Factors*)

Factors gathered during the nutrition assessment process that contribute to the existence or the maintenance of pathophysiological, psychosocial, situational, developmental, cultural, and/or environmental problems:

- Physiological causes, e.g., increased nutrient needs due to prolonged catabolic illness, malabsorption, hyperexcretion, nutrient/drug and nutrient/nutrient interaction, growth and maturation
- Lack of access to food, e.g., economic constraints, cultural or religious practices, restricting food given to elderly and/or children
- Food- and nutrition-related knowledge deficit concerning food sources of minerals; misdiagnosis of lactose intolerance/lactase deficiency; perception of conflicting nutrition messages from health professionals; inappropriate reliance on supplements
- Psychological causes, e.g., depression or eating disorders
- Environmental causes, e.g., inadequately tested nutrient bioavailability of fortified foods, beverages, and supplements; inappropriate marketing of fortified foods/beverages/supplements as a substitute for natural food source of nutrient(s)

Signs/Symptoms (*Defining Characteristics*)

A typical cluster of subjective and objective signs and symptoms gathered during the nutrition assessment process that provide evidence that a problem exists; quantify the problem and describe its severity.

Nutrition Assessment Category	Potential Indicators of this Nutrition Diagnosis (one or more must be present)
Biochemical Data, Medical Tests and Procedures	• Calcium: bone mineral content (BMC) below the young adult mean. Hypocalciuria, serum 25(OH)D < 32 ng/mL
	• Phosphorus < 2.6 mg/dL (0.84 mmol/L)
	• Magnesium <1.8 mg/dL (0.7 mmol/L)
	• Iron: hemoglobin < 13 g/L (2 mmol/L) (males); < 12 g/L (1.86 mmol/L) (females)
	• Iodine: urinary excretion < 100 µg/L (788 nmol/L)
	• Copper, serum copper < 64 µg/dL (10 µmol/L)
Anthropometric Measurements	• Height loss
Physical Exam Findings	• Calcium: diminished bone mineral density, hypertension, obesity

INADEQUATE MINERAL INTAKE (SPECIFY) (NI-5.10.1)

Food/Nutrition History	Reports or observations of insufficient mineral intake from diet compared to recommended intake: ▪ Food avoidance and/or elimination of whole food group(s) from diet ▪ Lack of interest in food ▪ Inappropriate food choices and/or chronic dieting behavior ▪ Vitamin/mineral deficiency
Client History	▪ Conditions associated with a diagnosis or treatment, e.g., malabsorption as a result of celiac disease, short bowel syndrome, inflammatory bowel disease, or post-menopausal women without estrogen supplementation and increased calcium need ▪ Polycystic ovary syndrome, premenstrual syndrome, kidney stones, colon polyps ▪ Other significant medical diagnoses and therapies ▪ Geographic latitude and history of Ultraviolet-B exposure/use of sunscreen ▪ Change in living environment/independence

References

1. Appel LJ, Moore TJ, Obarzanek E, Vollmer WM, Svetkey LP, Sacks FM, Bray GA, Vogt TM, Cutler JA, Windhauser MM, Lin P-H, Karanja N. A clinical trial of the effects of dietary patterns on blood pressure. *N Engl J Med.* 1997;336:1117-1124.

2. Heaney RP. Role of dietary sodium in osteoporosis. *J Am Coll Nutr.* 25(3 suppl):S271-S276. 2006.

3. Heaney RP. Nutrients, interactions, and foods. The Importance of Source. In Burckhardt P, Dawson-Hughes B, Heaney RP, Eds. *Nutritional Aspects of Osteoporosis 2nd Ed.* San Diego, CA: Elsevier, 2004:61-76.

4. Heaney RP. Nutrients, interactions, and foods. Serum 25-hydroxy-vitamin D and the health of the calcium economy. In Burckhardt P, Dawson-Hughes B, Heaney RP, Eds. *Nutritional Aspects of Osteoporosis 2nd Ed.* San Diego, CA: Elsevier, 2004:227-244.

5. Heaney RP, Rafferty K, Bierman J. Not all calcium-fortified beverages are equal. *Nutr Today.* 2005;40:39-41.

6. Heaney RP, Dowell MS, Hale CA, Bendich A. Calcium absorption varies within the reference range for serum 25-hydroxyvitamin D. *J Am Coll Nutr.* 2003;22:142-146.

7. Heaney RP, Dowell MS, Rafferty K, Bierman J. Bioavailability of the calcium in fortified soy imitation milk, with some observations on method. *Am J Clin Nutr.* 2000;71:1166-1169.

8. Holick MF. Functions of vitamin D: importance for prevention of common cancers, Type I diabetes and heart Disease. *Nutritional Aspects of Osteoporosis, 2nd Edition.* Burckhardt P, Dawson-Hughes B, Heaney RP, eds. San Diego, CA: Elsevier Inc.;2004:181-201

9. Massey LK, Whiting SJ. Dietary salt, urinary calcium, and bone loss. *J Bone Miner Res.* 1996; 11:731-736.

10. Suaraz FL, Savaiano D, Arbisi P, Levitt MD. Tolerance to the daily ingestion of two cups of milk by individuals claiming lactose intolerance. *Am J Clin Nutr.* 1997;65:1502-1506.

11. Thys-Jacobs S, Donovan D, Papadopoulos A, Sarrel P. Bilezikian JP. Vitamin D and calcium dysregulation in the polycystic ovarian syndrome. *Steroids.* 1999; 64:430-435.

12. Thys-Jacobs S, Starkey P, Bernstein D, Tian J. Calcium carbonate and the premenstrual syndrome: Effects on premenstrual and menstrual symptomatology. *Am J Obstet Gynecol.* 1998;179:444-452.

13. Zemel MB, Thompson W, Milstead A, Morris K, Campbell P. Calcium and dairy acceleration of weight and fat loss during energy restriction in obese adults. *Obesity Res.* 2004;12:582-590.

Updated: 2008 Edition

Intake

Edition: 2008

INTAKE DOMAIN • Mineral

EXCESSIVE MINERAL INTAKE (SPECIFY) (NI-5.10.2)

Definition

Higher intake of mineral from foods, supplements, medications or water, compared to established reference standards or recommendations based on physiological needs.

Etiology (Cause/Contributing Risk Factors)

Factors gathered during the nutrition assessment process that contribute to the existence or the maintenance of pathophysiological, psychosocial, situational, developmental, cultural, and/or environmental problems:

- Food- and nutrition-related knowledge deficit
- Harmful beliefs/attitudes about food, nutrition, and nutrition-related topics
- Food faddism
- Accidental oversupplementation
- Overconsumption of a limited variety of foods
- Lack of knowledge about management of diagnosed genetic disorder altering mineral homeostasis [hemochromatosis (iron), Wilson's disease (copper)]
- Lack of knowledge about management of diagnosed disease state requiring mineral restriction [cholestatic liver disease (copper and manganese), renal insufficiency (phosphorus, magnesium, potassium)]

Signs/Symptoms (Defining Characteristics)

A typical cluster of subjective and objective signs and symptoms gathered during the nutrition assessment process that provide evidence that a problem exists; quantify the problem and describe its severity.

Nutrition Assessment Category	Potential Indicators of this Nutrition Diagnosis (one or more must be present)
Biochemical Data, Medical Tests and Procedures	Changes in appropriate laboratory values, such as: • ↑ TSH (iodine supplementation) • ↓ HDL (zinc supplementation) • ↑ Serum ferritin and transferrin saturation (iron overload) • Hyperphosphatemia • Hypermagnesemia

EXCESSIVE MINERAL INTAKE (SPECIFY) (NI-5.10.2)

Anthropometric Measurements	
Physical Exam Findings	▪ Hair and nail changes (selenium)
Food/Nutrition History	Reports or observations of:
	▪ High intake of foods or supplements containing mineral compared to DRIs
	▪ Anorexia (zinc supplementation)
Client History	▪ GI disturbances (iron, magnesium, copper, zinc, selenium)
	▪ Copper deficiency anemia (zinc)
	▪ Liver damage (copper, iron), enamel or skeletal fluorosis (fluoride)

References

1. Bowman BA, Russell RM, eds. *Present Knowledge in Nutrition. 8th Ed.* Washington, DC: ILSI Press; 2001.
2. National Academy of Sciences, Institute of Medicine. *Dietary Reference Intakes for Vitamin A, Vitamin K, Arsenic, Boron, Chromium, Copper, Iodine, Iron, Manganese, Molybdenum, Nickel, Silicon, Vanadium, Zinc.* Washington, DC: National Academy Press; 2001.
3. National Academy of Sciences, Institute of Medicine. *Dietary Reference Intakes for Calcium, Phosphorus, Magnesium, Vitamin D, and Fluoride.* Washington, DC: National Academy Press; 1997.
4. Position of the American Dietetic Association: Food and nutrition misinformation. *J Am Diet Assoc.* 2006;106:601-607.

115

SWALLOWING DIFFICULTY (NC-1.1)

Definition

Impaired or difficult movement of food and liquid within the oral cavity to the stomach

Etiology (Cause/Contributing Risk Factors)

Factors gathered during the nutrition assessment process that contribute to the existence or the maintenance of pathophysiological, psychosocial, situational, developmental, cultural, and/or environmental problems:

- Mechanical causes, e.g., inflammation, surgery, stricture, or oral, pharyngeal and esophageal tumors, mechanical ventilation
- Motor causes, e.g., neurological or muscular disorders, such as, cerebral palsy, stroke, multiple sclerosis, scleroderma, prematurity

Signs/Symptoms (Defining Characteristics)

A typical cluster of subjective and objective signs and symptoms gathered during the nutrition assessment process that provide evidence that a problem exists; quantify the problem and describe its severity.

Nutrition Assessment Category	Potential Indicators of this Nutrition Diagnosis (one or more must be present)
Biochemical Data, Medical Tests and Procedures	• Radiological findings, e.g., abnormal swallowing studies
Anthropometric Measurements	
Physical Exam Findings	• Evidence of dehydration, e.g., dry mucous membranes, poor skin turgor • Non-normal findings in cranial nerves and (CN VII) muscles of facial expression, (Nerve IX) gag reflex, swallow (Nerve X) and tongue range of motions (Nerve XII), cough reflex, drooling, facial weakness and ability to perform and wet and dry swallow
Food/Nutrition History	Reports or observations of: • Coughing, choking, prolonged chewing, pouching of food, regurgitation, facial expression changes during eating, prolonged feeding time, drooling, noisy wet upper airway sounds, feeling of "food getting stuck," pain while swallowing • Decreased food intake • Avoidance of foods • Mealtime resistance

Edition: 2008

SWALLOWING DIFFICULTY (NC-1.1)

| *Client History* | ▪ Conditions associated with a diagnosis or treatment, e.g., dysphagia, achalasia |
| | ▪ Repeated upper respiratory infections and or pneumonia |

References

1. Braunwald E, Fauci AS, Kasper DL, Hauser SL, Longo DL, Jameson JL, ed. *Harrison's Principles of Internal Medicine, 15th Edition.* New York, NY: McGraw-Hill; 2001.
2. Brody R, Touger-Decker R, O'Sullivan-Maillet J. The effectiveness of dysphagia screening by an RD on the determination of dysphagia risk. *J Am Diet Assoc.* 2000;100:1029-1037.
3. Huhmann M, Touger-Decker R, Byham-Gray L, O'Sullivan-Maillet J, Von Hagen S. Comparison of dysphagia screening by a registered dietitian in acute stroke patients to speech language pathologist's evaluation. Topics in Clinical Nutrition. 2004;19:239-249.
4. Groher ME. *Dysphagia Diagnosis and Management,* 3rd ed. Boston: Butterworth-Heinemann 1997.

Updated: 2008 Edition

Clinical

117

CLINCAL DOMAIN • Functional

BITING/CHEWING (MASTICATORY) DIFFICULTY (NC-1.2)

Definition

Impaired ability to bite or chew food in preparation for swallowing.

Etiology (Cause/Contributing Risk Factors)

Factors gathered during the nutrition assessment process that contribute to the existence or the maintenance of pathophysiological, psychosocial, situational, developmental, cultural, and/or environmental problems:

- Craniofacial malformations
- Oral surgery
- Neuromuscular dysfunction
- Partial or complete edentulism
- Soft tissue disease (primary or oral manifestations of a systemic disease)
- Xerostomia

Signs/Symptoms (Defining Characteristics)

A typical cluster of subjective and objective signs and symptoms gathered during the nutrition assessment process that provide evidence that a problem exists; quantify the problem and describe its severity.

Nutrition Assessment Category	Potential Indicators of this Nutrition Diagnosis (one or more must be present)
Biochemical Data, Medical Tests and Procedures	
Anthropometric Measurements	
Physical Exam Findings	▪ Partial or complete edentulism
	▪ Alterations in cranial nerve function (V, VII, IX, X, XII)
	▪ Dry mouth
	▪ Oral lesions interfering with eating ability
	▪ Impaired tongue movement
	▪ Ill-fitting dentures or broken dentures

BITING/CHEWING (MASTICATORY) DIFFICULTY (NC-1.2)

Food/Nutrition History	Reports or observations of:
	▪ Decreased intake of food
	▪ Alterations in food intake from usual
	▪ Decreased intake or avoidance of food difficult to form into a bolus, e.g., nuts, whole pieces of meat, poultry, fish, fruits, vegetables
	▪ Avoidance of foods of age-appropriate texture
	▪ Spitting food out or prolonged feeding time
Client History	▪ Conditions associated with a diagnosis or treatment, e.g., alcoholism; Alzheimer's; head, neck or pharyngeal cancer; cerebral palsy; cleft lip/palate; oral soft tissue infections (e.g., candidiasis, leukoplakia); lack of developmental readiness; oral manifestations of systemic disease (e.g., rheumatoid arthritis, lupus, Crohn's disease, penphigus vulgaris, HIV, diabetes)
	▪ Recent major oral surgery
	▪ Wired jaw
	▪ Chemotherapy with oral side effects
	▪ Radiation therapy to oral cavity

References

1. Bailey R, Ledikwe JH, Smiciklas-Wright H, Mitchell DC, Jensen GL. Persistent oral health problems associated with comorbidity and impaired diet quality in older adults. *J Am Diet Assoc.* 2004;104:1273-1276.
2. Chernoff R, ed. Oral health in the elderly. *Geriatric Nutrition.* Gaithersburg, MD: Aspen Publishers; 1999.
3. Dormenval V, Mojon P, Budtz-Jorgensen E. Association between self-assessed masticatory ability, nutritional status and salivary flow rate in hospitalized elderly. *Oral Diseases.* 1999;5:32-38.
4. Hildebrand GH, Dominguez BL, Schork MA, Loesche WJ. Functional units, chewing, swallowing and food avoidance among the elderly. *J Prosthet Dent.* 1997;77:585-595.
5. Hirano H, Ishiyama N, Watanabe I, Nasu I. Masticatory ability in relation to oral status and general health in aging. *J Nutr Health Aging.* 1999;3:48-52.
6. Huhmann M, Touger-Decker R, Byham-Gray L, O'Sullivan-Maillet J, Von Hagen S. Comparison of dysphagia screening by a registered dietitian in acute stroke patients to speech language pathologist's evaluation. *Top Clin Nutr.* 2004;19:239-249.
7. Kademani D, Glick M. Oral ulcerations in individuals infected with human immunodeficiency virus: clinical presentations, diagnosis, management and relevance to disease progression. *Quintessence International.* 1998;29:1103-1108.
8. Keller HH, Ostbye T, Bright-See E. Predictors of dietary intake in Ontario seniors. *Can J Public Health.* 1997;88:303-309.
9. Krall E, Hayes C, Garcia R. How dentition status and masticatory function affect nutrient intake. *J Am Dent Assoc.* 1998;129:1261-1269.
10. Joshipura K, Willett WC, Douglass CW. The impact of edentulousness on food and nutrient intake. *J Am Dent Assoc.* 1996;127:459-467.
11. Mackle T, Touger-Decker R, O'Sullivan Maillet J, Holland, B. Registered Dietitians' use of physical assessment parameters in practice. *J Am Diet Assoc.* 2004;103:1632-1638.
12. Mobley C, Saunders M. Oral health screening guidelines for nondental healthcare providers. *J Am Diet Assoc.* 1997;97:S123-S126.
13. Morse D. Oral and pharyngeal cancer. In: R Touger-Decker et al eds. *Nutrition and Oral Medicine.* Totowa NJ: Humana Press, Inc; 2005, 205-222.
14. Moynihan P, Butler T, Thomason J, Jepson N. Nutrient intake in partially dentate patients: the effect of prosthetic rehabilitation. *J Dent.* 2000;28:557-563.
15. Position of the American Dietetic Association: Oral health and nutrition. *J Am Diet Assoc.* 2007;107(in press).

CLINCAL DOMAIN • Functional

BITING/CHEWING (MASTICATORY) DIFFICULTY (NC-1.2)

16. Sayhoun NR Lin CL, Krall E. Nutritional status of the older adult is associated with dentition status. *J Am Diet Assoc.* 2003;103:61-66.
17. Sheiham A, Steele JG. The impact of oral health on stated ability to eat certain foods; finding from the national diet and nutrition survey of older people in Great Britain. *Gerodontology.* 1999;16:11-20.
18. Ship J, Duffy V, Jones J, Langmore S. Geriatric oral health and its impact on eating. *J Am Geriatr Soc.* 1996;44:456-464.
19. Touger-Decker R. Clinical and laboratory assessment of nutrition status. *Dent Clin North Am.* 2003;47:259-278.
20. Touger-Decker R, Sirois D, Mobley C (eds). *Nutrition and Oral Medicine.* Totowan, NJ: Humana Press; 2004.
21. Walls AW, Steele JG, Sheiham A, Marcenes W, Moynihan PJ. Oral health and nutrition in older people. *J Public Health Dent.* 2000;60:304-307.

Updated: 2008 Edition

BREASTFEEDING DIFFICULTY (NC-1.3)

Definition

Inability to sustain infant nutrition through breastfeeding.

Etiology (Cause/Contributing Risk Factors)

Factors gathered during the nutrition assessment process that contribute to the existence or the maintenance of pathophysiological, psychosocial, situational, developmental, cultural, and/or environmental problems:

Infant:

- Difficulty latching on, e.g., tight frenulum
- Poor sucking ability
- Oral pain
- Malnutrition/malabsorption
- Lethargy, sleepiness
- Irritability
- Swallowing difficulty

Mother:

- Painful breasts, nipples
- Breast or nipple abnormality
- Mastitis
- Perception of inadequate milk supply
- Lack of social, cultural, or environmental support

Signs/Symptoms (Defining Characteristics)

A typical cluster of subjective and objective signs and symptoms gathered during the nutrition assessment process that provide evidence that a problem exists; quantify the problem and describe its severity.

Nutrition Assessment Category	Potential Indicators of this Nutrition Diagnosis (one or more must be present)
Biochemical Data, Medical Tests and Procedures	▪ Laboratory evidence of dehydration (infant)
Anthropometric Measurements	▪ Any weight loss or poor weight gain (infant)
Physical Exam Findings	▪ Frenulum abnormality (infant)
	▪ Vomiting or diarrhea (infant)

121

CLINCAL DOMAIN • Functional

BREASTFEEDING DIFFICULTY (NC-1.3)

Food/Nutrition History	Reports or observations of (infant):
	▪ Coughing
	▪ Crying, latching on and off, pounding on breasts
	▪ Decreased feeding frequency/duration, early cessation of feeding, and/or feeding resistance
	▪ Lethargy
	▪ Hunger, lack of satiety after feeding
	▪ Fewer than six wet diapers in 24 hours
	Reports or observations of (mother):
	▪ Small amount of milk when pumping
	▪ Lack of confidence in ability to breastfeed
	▪ Doesn't hear infant swallowing
	▪ Concerns regarding mother's choice to breastfeed/lack of support
	▪ Insufficient knowledge of breastfeeding or infant hunger/satiety signals
	▪ Lack of facilities or accommodations at place of employment or in community for breastfeeding
Client History	▪ Conditions associated with a diagnosis or treatment of (infant), e.g., cleft lip/palate, thrush, premature birth, malabsorption, infection
	▪ Conditions associated with a diagnosis or treatment of (mother), e.g., mastitis, candidiasis, engorgement, history of breast surgery

References

1. Barron SP, Lane HW, Hannan TE, Struempler B, Williams JC. Factors influencing duration of breast feeding among low-income women. *J Am Diet Assoc.* 1988;88:1557-1561.
2. Bryant C, Coreil J, D'Angelo SL, Bailey DFC, Lazarov MA. A strategy for promoting breastfeeding among economically disadvantaged women and adolescents. *NAACOGs Clin Issu Perinat Womens Health Nurs.* 1992;3:723-730.
3. Bentley ME, Caulfield LE, Gross SM, Bronner Y, Jensen J, Kessler LA, Paige DM. Sources of influence on intention to breastfeed among African-American women at entry to WIC. *J Hum Lact.* 1999;15:27-34.
4. Moreland JC, Lloyd L, Braun SB, Heins JN. A new teaching model to prolong breastfeeding among Latinos. *J Hum Lact.* 2000;16:337-341.
5. Position of the American Dietetic Association: Promoting and supporting breastfeeding. *J Am Diet Assoc.* 2005;105:810-818.
6. Wooldrige MS, Fischer C. Colic, "overfeeding" and symptoms of lactose malabsorption in the breast-fed baby. *Lancet.* 1988;2:382-384.

122

ALTERED GASTROINTESTINAL (GI) FUNCTION (NC-1.4)

Definition
Changes in ability to digest or absorb nutrients.

Etiology (Cause/Contributing Risk Factors)
Factors gathered during the nutrition assessment process that contribute to the existence or the maintenance of pathophysiological, psychosocial, situational, developmental, cultural, and/or environmental problems:

- Alterations in GI anatomical structure, e.g., gastric bypass, Roux En Y
- Changes in the GI tract motility, e.g., gastroparesis
- Compromised GI tract function, e.g., celiac disease, Crohn's disease, infection, radiation therapy
- Compromised function of related GI organs, e.g., pancreas, liver
- Decreased functional length of the GI tract, e.g., short-bowel syndrome

Signs/Symptoms (Defining Characteristics)
A typical cluster of subjective and objective signs and symptoms gathered during the nutrition assessment process that provide evidence that a problem exists; quantify the problem and describe its severity.

Nutrition Assessment Category	Potential Indicators of this Nutrition Diagnosis (one or more must be present)
Biochemical Data, Medical Tests and Procedures	• Abnormal digestive enzyme and fecal fat studies
	• Abnormal hydrogen breath test, d-xylose test, stool culture, and gastric emptying and/or small bowel transit time
	• Endoscopic or colonoscopic examination results, biopsy results
Anthropometric Measurements	• Wasting due to malnutrition in severe cases
Physical Exam Findings	• Abdominal distension
	• Increased (or sometimes decreased) bowel sounds
Food/Nutrition History	Reports or observations of:
	• Avoidance or limitation of total intake or intake of specific foods/food groups due to GI symptoms, e.g., bloating, cramping, pain, diarrhea, steatorrhea (greasy, floating, foul-smelling stools) especially following ingestion of food

Clinical

CLINCAL DOMAIN • Functional

ALTERED GASTROINTESTINAL (GI) FUNCTION (NC-1.4)

Client History	▪ Anorexia, nausea, vomiting, diarrhea, steatorrhea, constipation, abdominal pain
	▪ Conditions associated with a diagnosis or treatment, e.g., malabsorption, maldigestion, steatorrhea, constipation, diverticulitis, Crohn's disease, inflammatory bowel disease, cystic fibrosis, celiac disease, irritable bowel syndrome, infection
	▪ Surgical procedures, e.g., esophagectomy, dilatation, gastrectomy, vagotomy, gastric bypass, bowel resections

References

1. Braunwald E, Fauci AS, Kasper DL, Hauser SL, Longo DL, Jameson JL, ed. *Harrison's Principles of Internal Medicine. 15th Edition.* New York, NY: McGraw-Hill; 2001.

Updated: 2008 Edition

IMPAIRED NUTRIENT UTILIZATION (NC-2.1)

Definition

Changes in ability to absorb or metabolize nutrients and bioactive substances.

Etiology (Cause/Contributing Risk Factors)

Factors gathered during the nutrition assessment process that contribute to the existence or the maintenance of pathophysiological, psychosocial, situational, developmental, cultural, and/or environmental problems:

- Alterations in gastrointestinal anatomical structure
- Compromised function of the GI tract
- Compromised function of related GI organs, e.g., pancreas, liver
- Decreased functional length of the GI tract
- Metabolic disorders

Signs/Symptoms (Defining Characteristics)

A typical cluster of subjective and objective signs and symptoms gathered during the nutrition assessment process that provide evidence that a problem exists; quantify the problem and describe its severity.

Nutrition Assessment Category	Potential Indicators of this Nutrition Diagnosis (one or more must be present)
Biochemical Data, Medical Tests and Procedures	- Abnormal digestive enzyme and fecal fat studies - Abnormal hydrogen breath test, d-xylose test - Abnormal tests for inborn errors of metabolism
Anthropometric Measurements	- Weight loss of $\geq 5\%$ in one month, $\geq 10\%$ in six months - Growth stunting or failure
Physical Exam Findings	- Abdominal distension - Increased or decreased bowel sounds - Evidence of vitamin and/or mineral deficiency, e.g., glossitis, cheilosis, mouth lesions

CLINCAL DOMAIN • Biochemical

IMPAIRED NUTRIENT UTILIZATION (NC-2.1)

Food/Nutrition History	Reports or observations of:
	▪ Avoidance or limitation of total intake or intake of specific foods/food groups due to GI symptoms, e.g., bloating, cramping, pain, diarrhea, steatorrhea (greasy, floating, foul-smelling stools) especially following ingestion of food
Client History	▪ Diarrhea, steatorrhea, abdominal pain
	▪ Endoscopic or colonoscopic examination results, biopsy results
	▪ Conditions associated with a diagnosis or treatment, e.g., malabsorption, maldigestion, cystic fibrosis, celiac disease, Crohn's disease, infection, radiation therapy, inborn errors of metabolism
	▪ Surgical procedures, e.g., gastric bypass, bowel resection

References

1. Beyer P. Gastrointestinal disorders: Roles of nutrition and the dietetics practitioner. *J Am Diet Assoc.* 1998;98:272-277.
2. Position of the American Dietetic Association: Health implications of dietary fiber. *J Am Diet Assoc.* 2002;102:993-1000.

ALTERED NUTRITION-RELATED LABORATORY VALUES (SPECIFY) (NC-2.2)

Definition

Changes due to body composition, medications, body system changes or genetics, or changes in ability to eliminate byproducts of digestive and metabolic processes.

Etiology (Cause/Contributing Risk Factors)

Factors gathered during the nutrition assessment process that contribute to the existence or the maintenance of pathophysiological, psychosocial, situational, developmental, cultural, and/or environmental problems:

- Kidney, liver, cardiac, endocrine, neurologic, and/or pulmonary dysfunction
- Other organ dysfunction that leads to biochemical changes

Signs/Symptoms (Defining Characteristics)

A typical cluster of subjective and objective signs and symptoms gathered during the nutrition assessment process that provide evidence that a problem exists; quantify the problem and describe its severity.

Nutrition Assessment Category	Potential Indicators of this Nutrition Diagnosis (one or more must be present)
Biochemical Data, Medical Tests and Procedures	■ Increased AST, ALT, T. bili, serum ammonia (liver disorders)
	■ Abnormal BUN, Cr, K, phosphorus, glomerular filtration rate (GFR) (kidney disorders)
	■ Altered pO_2 and pCO_2 (pulmonary disorders)
	■ Abnormal serum lipids
	■ Abnormal plasma glucose and/or HgbA1c levels
	■ Inadequate blood glucose control
	■ Other findings of acute or chronic disorders that are abnormal and of nutritional origin or consequence
Anthropometric Measurements	■ Rapid weight changes
	■ Other anthropometric measures that are altered
Physical Exam Findings	■ Jaundice, edema, ascites, itching (liver disorders)
	■ Edema, shortness of breath (cardiac disorders)
	■ Blue nail beds, clubbing (pulmonary disorders)

Clinical

127

CLINCAL DOMAIN • Biochemical

Clinical

ALTERED NUTRITION-RELATED LABORATORY VALUES (SPECIFY) (NC-2.2)

Food/Nutrition History	Reports or observations of:
	▪ Anorexia, nausea, vomiting
	▪ Intake of foods high in or overall excess intake of protein, potassium, phosphorus, sodium, fluid
	▪ Inadequate intake of micronutrients
	▪ Food- and nutrition-related knowledge deficit, e.g., lack of information, incorrect information, or noncompliance with modified diet
Client History	▪ Conditions associated with a diagnosis or treatment, e.g., renal or liver disease, alcoholism, cardiopulmonary disorders, diabetes

References

1. Beto JA, Bansal VK. Medical nutrition therapy in chronic kidney failure: integrating clinical practice guidelines. *J Am Diet Assoc.* 2004;104:404-409.
2. Davern II TJ, Scharschmidt BF. Biochemical liver tests. In Feldman M, Scharschmidt BF, Sleisenger MH (eds): *Sleisenger and Fordtran's Gasrointestinal and Liver Disease, ed 6, vol 2*, Philadelphia, PA: WB Saunders; 1998: 1112-1122.
3. Durose CL, Holdsworth M, Watson V, Przygrodzka F. Knowledge of dietary restrictions and the medical consequences of noncompliance by patients on hemodialysis are not predictive of dietary compliance. *J Am Diet Assoc.* 2004;104:35-41.
4. Kassiske BL, Lakatua JD, Ma JZ, Louis TA. A meta-analysis of the effects of dietary protein restriction on the rate of decline in renal function. *Am J Kidney Dis.* 1998;31;954-961.
5. Knight EL, Stampfer MJ, Hankinson SE, Spiegelman D, Curhan GC. The impact of protein intake on renal function decline in women with normal renal function or mild renal insufficiency. *Ann Intern Med.* 2003;138:460-467.
6. Nakao T, Matsumoto, Okada T, Kanazawa Y, Yoshino M, Nagaoka Y, Takeguchi F. Nutritional management of dialysis patients: balancing among nutrient intake, dialysis dose, and nutritional status. *Am J Kidney Dis.* 2003;41:S133-S136.
7. National Kidney Foundation, Inc. Part 5. Evaluation of laboratory measurements for clinical assessment of kidney disease. *Am J Kidney Dis.* 2002;39:S76-S92.
8. National Kidney Foundation, Inc. Guideline 9. Association of level of GFR with nutritional status. *Am J Kidney Dis.* 2002;39:S128-S142.

Updated: 2008 Edition

FOOD–MEDICATION INTERACTION (NC-2.3)

Definition

Undesirable/harmful interaction(s) between food and over-the-counter (OTC) medications, prescribed medications, herbals, botanicals, and/or dietary supplements that diminishes, enhances, or alters effect of nutrients and/or medications.

Etiology (Cause/Contributing Risk Factors)

Factors gathered during the nutrition assessment process that contribute to the existence or the maintenance of pathophysiological, psychosocial, situational, developmental, cultural, and/or environmental problems:

- Combined ingestion or administration of medication and food that results in undesirable/harmful interaction

Signs/Symptoms (Defining Characteristics)

A typical cluster of subjective and objective signs and symptoms gathered during the nutrition assessment process that provide evidence that a problem exists; quantify the problem and describe its severity.

Nutrition Assessment Category	Potential Indicators of this Nutrition Diagnosis (one or more must be present)
Biochemical Data, Medical Tests and Procedures	▪ Alterations of biochemical tests based on medication affect and patient/client condition
Anthropometric Measurements	▪ Alterations of anthropometric measurements based on medication affect and patient/client conditions, e.g., weight gain and corticosteroids
Physical Exam Findings	

Edition: 2008

CLINCAL DOMAIN • Biochemical

FOOD–MEDICATION INTERACTION (NC-2.3)

Food/Nutrition History	Reports or observations of:
	▪ Intake that is problematic or inconsistent with OTC, prescribed drugs, herbals, botanicals, and dietary supplements, such as:
	● fish oils and prolonged bleeding
	● coumadin, vitamin K–rich foods
	● high-fat diet while on cholesterol-lowering medications
	● iron supplements, constipation and low-fiber diet
	▪ Intake that does not support replacement or mitigation of OTC, prescribed drugs, herbals, botanicals, and dietary supplements affects such as potassium-wasting diuretics
	▪ Changes in appetite or taste
Client History	▪ Multiple drugs (OTC, prescribed drugs, herbals, botanicals, and dietary supplements) that are known to have food–medication interactions
	▪ Medications that require nutrient supplementation that can not be accomplished via food intake, e.g., isoniazid and vitamin B-6

References

1. Position of the American Dietetic Association: Integration of nutrition and pharmacotherapy. *J Am Diet Assoc.* 2003;103:1363-1370.

130

UNDERWEIGHT (NC-3.1)

Definition

Low body weight compared to established reference standards or recommendations.

Etiology (*Cause/Contributing Risk Factors*)

Factors gathered during the nutrition assessment process that contribute to the existence or the maintenance of pathophysiological, psychosocial, situational, developmental, cultural, and/or environmental problems:

- Disordered eating pattern
- Excessive physical activity
- Harmful beliefs/attitudes about food, nutrition, and nutrition-related topics
- Inadequate energy intake
- Increased energy needs
- Limited access to food

Signs/Symptoms (*Defining Characteristics*)

A typical cluster of subjective and objective signs and symptoms gathered during the nutrition assessment process that provide evidence that a problem exists; quantify the problem and describe its severity.

Nutrition Assessment Category	Potential Indicators of this Nutrition Diagnosis (one or more must be present)
Biochemical Data, Medical Tests and Procedures	▪ Measured resting metabolic rate (RMR) measurement higher than expected and/or estimated RMR
Anthropometric Measurements	▪ Weight for age less than 5th percentile for infants younger than 12 months
	▪ Decreased skinfold thickness and MAMC
	▪ BMI < 18.5 (most adults)
	▪ BMI for older adults (older than 65 years) < 23
	▪ BMI < 5th percentile (children, 2-19 years)
Physical Exam Findings	▪ Decreased muscle mass, muscle wasting (gluteal and temporal)

131

CLINCAL DOMAIN • Weight

UNDERWEIGHT (NC-3.1)

Food/Nutrition History	Reports or observations of:
	▪ Inadequate intake of food compared to estimated or measured needs
	▪ Limited supply of food in home
	▪ Dieting, food faddism
	▪ Hunger
	▪ Refusal to eat
	▪ Physical activity more than recommended amount
	▪ Vitamin/mineral deficiency
Client History	▪ Malnutrition
	▪ Illness or physical disability
	▪ Mental illness, dementia, confusion
	▪ Medications that affect appetite, e.g., stimulants for ADHD
	▪ Athlete, dancer, gymnast

References

1. Assessment of nutritional status. In: Kleinman R (ed.). *Pediatric Nutrition Handbook*, 5th ed. Elk Grove Village, IL: American Academy of Pediatrics; 2004:407-423.
2. Beck AM, Ovesen LW. At which body mass index and degree of weight loss should hospitalized elderly patients be considered at nutritional risk? *Clin Nutr*. 1998;17:195-198.
3. Blaum CS, Fries BE, Fiatarone MA. Factors associated with low body mass index and weight loss in nursing home residents. *J Gerontol A Biol Sci Med Sci*. 1995;50A:M162-M168.
4. Cook Z, Kirk S, Lawrenson S, Sandford S. Use of BMI in the assessment of undernutrition in older subjects: reflecting on practice. Proceedings of the Nutrition Society. Aug 2005;64:313-317.
5. Position of the American Dietetic Association: Food insecurity and hunger in the United States. *J Am Diet Assoc*. 2006;106:446-458.
6. Position of the American Dietetic Association: Addressing world hunger, malnutrition, and food insecurity. *J Am Diet Assoc*. 2003;103:1046-1057.
7. Position of the American Dietetic Association: Nutrition intervention in the treatment of anorexia nervosa, bulimia nervosa, and eating disorder not otherwise specified (EDNOS). *J Am Diet Assoc*. 2006;106:2073-2082.
8. Ranhoff AH, Gjoen AU, Mowe M. Screening for malnutrition in elderly acute medical patients: the usefulness of MNA-SF. *J Nutr Health Aging*. Jul-Aug 2005;9:221-225.
9. Reynolds MW, Fredman L, Langenberg P, Magaziner J. Weight, weight change, and mortality in a random sample of older community-dwelling women. *J Am Geriatr Soc*. 1999;47:1409-1414.
10. Schneider SM, Al-Jaouni R, Pivot X, Braulio VB, Rampal P, Hebuerne X. Lack of adaptation to severe malnutrition in elderly patients. *Clin Nutr*. 2002;21:499-504.
11. Spear BA. Adolescent growth and development. *J Am Diet Assoc*. 2002 (suppl);102:S23- S29.
12. Sullivan DH, Walls RC. Protein-energy undernutrition and the risk of mortality within six years of hospital discharge. *J Am Coll Nutr*. 1998;17:571-578.

Updated: 2008 Edition

INVOLUNTARY WEIGHT LOSS (NC-3.2)

Definition

Decrease in body weight that is not planned or desired.

Etiology *(Cause/Contributing Risk Factors)*

Factors gathered during the nutrition assessment process that contribute to the existence or the maintenance of pathophysiological, psychosocial, situational, developmental, cultural, and/or environmental problems:

- Physiological causes, e.g., prolonged catabolic illness, trauma, malabsorption
- Lack of access to food, e.g., economic constraints, cultural or religious practices, restricting food given to elderly and/or children
- Prolonged hospitalization
- Psychological issues
- Lack of self-feeding ability

Signs/Symptoms *(Defining Characteristics)*

A typical cluster of subjective and objective signs and symptoms gathered during the nutrition assessment process that provide evidence that a problem exists; quantify the problem and describe its severity.

Nutrition Assessment Category	Potential Indicators of this Nutrition Diagnosis (one or more must be present)
Biochemical Data, Medical Tests and Procedures	
Anthropometric Measurements	▪ Weight loss of $\geq 5\%$ within 30 days, $\geq 7.5\%$ in 90 days, or $\geq 10\%$ in 180 days
Physical Examination Findings	▪ Fever
	▪ Decreased senses, i.e., smell, taste, vision
	▪ Increased heart rate
	▪ Increased respiratory rate
	▪ Loss of subcutaneous fat and muscle stores

133

CLINCAL DOMAIN • Weight

INVOLUNTARY WEIGHT LOSS (NC-3.2)

Food/Nutrition History	Reports or observations of:
	▪ Normal or usual intake in face of illness
	▪ Poor intake, change in eating habits, early satiety, skipped meals
	▪ Change in way clothes fit
Client History	▪ Conditions associated with a diagnosis or treatment, e.g., AIDS/HIV, burns, chronic obstructive pulmonary disease, dysphagia, hip/long bone fracture, infection, surgery, trauma, hyperthyroidism (pre- or untreated), some types of cancer or metastatic disease (specify), substance abuse
	▪ Changes in mental status or function (e.g., depression)
	▪ Medications associated with weight loss, such as certain antidepressants or cancer chemotherapy

References

1. Collins N. Protein-energy malnutrition and involuntary weight loss: Nutritional and pharmacologic strategies to enhance wound healing. *Expert Opin Pharmacother.* 2003;7:1121-1140.
2. Splett PL, Roth-Yousey LL, Vogelzang JL. Medical nutrition therapy for the prevention and treatment of unintentional weight loss in residential healthcare facilities. *J Am Diet Assoc.* 2003;103:352-362.
3. Wallace JL, Schwartz RS, LaCroix AZ, Uhlmann RF, Pearlman RA. Involuntary weight loss in older patients: incidence and clinical significance. *J Am Geriatr Soc.* 1995;43:329-337.

Updated: 2008 Edition

OVERWEIGHT/OBESITY (NC-3.3)

Definition

Increased adiposity compared to established reference standards or recommendations, ranging from overweight to morbid obesity.

Etiology (*Cause/Contributing Risk Factors*)

Factors gathered during the nutrition assessment process that contribute to the existence or the maintenance of pathophysiological, psychosocial, situational, developmental, cultural, and/or environmental problems:

- Decreased energy needs
- Disordered eating pattern
- Excess energy intake
- Food- and nutrition-related knowledge deficit
- Not ready for diet/lifestyle change
- Physical inactivity
- Increased psychological/life stress

Signs/Symptoms (*Defining Characteristics*)

A typical cluster of subjective and objective signs and symptoms gathered during the nutrition assessment process that provide evidence that a problem exists; quantify the problem and describe its severity.

Nutrition Assessment Category	Potential Indicators of this Nutrition Diagnosis (one or more must be present)
Biochemical Data, Medical Tests and Procedures	▪ Measured resting metabolic rate (RMR) measurement less than expected and/or estimated RMR

Anthropometric Measurements	▪ BMI more than normative standard for age and gender
	   • Overweight 25-29.9
	   • Obesity-grade I 30-34.9
	   • Obesity-grade II 35-39.9
	   • Obesity-grade III 40+

CLINCAL DOMAIN • Weight

OVERWEIGHT/OBESITY (NC-3.3)

Anthropometric Measurements cont'd	▪ Waist circumference more than normative standard for age and sex ▪ Increased skinfold thickness ▪ Weight for height more than normative standard for age and sex
Physical Exam Findings	▪ Increased body adiposity
Food/Nutrition History	Reports or observations of: ▪ Overconsumption of high-fat and/or calorie-density food or beverage ▪ Large portions of food (portion size more than twice than recommended) ▪ Excessive energy intake ▪ Infrequent, low-duration and/or low-intensity physical activity ▪ Large amounts of sedentary activities, e.g., TV watching, reading, computer use in both leisure and work/school ▪ Uncertainty regarding nutrition-related recommendations ▪ Inability to apply nutrition-related recommendations ▪ Inability to maintain weight or regain of weight ▪ Unwillingness or disinterest in applying nutrition-related recommendations
Client History	▪ Conditions associated with a diagnosis or treatment, e.g., hypothyroidism, metabolic syndrome, eating disorder not otherwise specified, depression ▪ Physical disability or limitation ▪ History of familial obesity ▪ History of childhood obesity ▪ History of physical, sexual, or emotional abuse ▪ Inability to lose a significant amount of excess weight through conventional weight loss intervention ▪ Medications that impact RMR, e.g., midazolam, propranolol, glipizide

References

1. Crawford S. Promoting dietary change. *Can J Cardiol.* 1995;11(suppl A):14A-15A.
2. Dickerson RN, Roth-Yousey L. Medication effects on metabolic rate: A systematic review. *J Am Diet Assoc.* 2005;105:835-843.
3. Kumanyika SK, Van Horn L, Bowen D, Perri MG, Rolls BJ, Czajkowski SM, Schron E. Maintenance of dietary behavior change. *Health Psychol.* 2000;19(1 suppl):S42-S56.
4. NHLBI Clinical Guidelines on the Identification, Evaluation, and Treatment of Overweight and Obesity in Adults—Executive Summary. Available at: http://www.nhlbi.nih.gov/guidelines/obesity/ob_tbl2.htm. Accessed January 29, 2007.

Edition: 2008

OVERWEIGHT/OBESITY (NC-3.3)

5. Position of the American Dietetic Association: Weight management. *J Am Diet Assoc.* 2002;102:1145-1155.

6. Position of the American Dietetic Association: Total diet approach to communicating food and nutrition information. *J Am Diet Assoc.* 2007;107(in press).

7. Position of the American Dietetic Association: The role of dietetics professionals in health promotion and disease prevention. *J Am Diet Assoc.* 2006;106:1875-1884.

8. Position of the American Dietetic Association: Nutrition intervention in the treatment of anorexia nervosa, bulimia nervosa, and eating disorder not otherwise specified (EDNOS). *J Am Diet Assoc.* 2006;106:2073-2082.

9. Shepherd R. Resistance to changes in diet. *Proc Nutr Soc.* 2002;61:267-272.

10. U.S. Preventive Services Task Force. Behavioral counseling in primary care to promote a healthy diet. *Am J Prev Med.* 2003;24:93-100.

Updated: 2008 Edition

Clinical

CLINCAL DOMAIN • Weight

INVOLUNTARY WEIGHT GAIN (NC-3.4)

Definition

Weight gain more than that which is desired or planned.

Etiology (Cause/Contributing Risk Factors)

Factors gathered during the nutrition assessment process that contribute to the existence or the maintenance of pathophysiological, psychosocial, situational, developmental, cultural, and/or environmental problems:

- Illness causing unexpected weight gain because of head trauma, immobility, paralysis or related condition
- Chronic use of medications known to cause weight gain, such as use of certain antidepressants, antipsychotics, corticosteroids, certain HIV medications
- Condition leading to excessive fluid weight gains

Signs/Symptoms (Defining Characteristics)

A typical cluster of subjective and objective signs and symptoms gathered during the nutrition assessment process that provide evidence that a problem exists; quantify the problem and describe its severity.

Nutrition Assessment Category	Potential Indicators of this Nutrition Diagnosis (one or more must be present)
Biochemical Data, Medical Tests and Procedures	▪ Decrease in serum albumin, hyponatremia, elevated fasting serum lipid levels, elevated fasting glucose levels, fluctuating hormone levels
Anthropometric Measurements	▪ Increased weight, any increase in weight more than planned or desired, such as 10% in 6 months ▪ Noticeable change in body fat distribution
Physical Examination Findings	▪ Fat accumulation, excessive subcutaneous fat stores ▪ Lipodystrophy associated with HIV diagnosis: increase in dorsocervial fat, breast enlargement, increased abdominal girth ▪ Edema ▪ Shortness of breath

138

Edition: 2008

INVOLUNTARY WEIGHT GAIN (NC-3.4)

Food/Nutrition History	Reports or observations of: ▪ Intake consistent with estimated or measured energy needs ▪ Changes in recent food intake level ▪ Fluid administration more than requirements ▪ Use of alcohol, narcotics ▪ Extreme hunger with or without palpitations, tremor, and sweating ▪ Physical inactivity or change in physical activity level
Client History	▪ Conditions associated with a diagnosis or treatment of asthma, psychiatric illnesses, rheumatic conditions, HIV/AIDS, Cushing's syndrome, obesity, Prader-Willi syndrome, hypothyroidism ▪ Muscle weakness ▪ Fatigue ▪ Medications associated with increased appetite

References

1. Lichtenstein K, Delaney K, Ward D, Palella F. Clinical factors associated with incidence and prevalence of fat atrophy and accumulation (abstract P64). *Antivir Ther*. 2000;5:61-62
2. Heath KV, Hogg RS, Chan KJ, Harris M, Montessori V, O'Shaughnessy MV, Montaner JS. Lipodystrophy-associated morphological, cholesterol and triglyceride abnormalities in a population-based HIV/AIDS treatment database. *AIDS*. 2001;15:231-239.
3. Safri S, Grunfeld C. Fat distribution and metabolic changes in patients with HIV infection. *AIDS*. 1999;13:2493-2505.
4. Sattler F. Body habitus changes related to lipodystrophy. *Clin Infect Dis*. 2003;36:S84-S90.

Updated: 2008 Edition

BEHAVIORAL-ENVIRONMENTAL DOMAIN • Knowledge and Beliefs

FOOD- AND NUTRITION-RELATED KNOWLEDGE DEFICIT (NB-1.1)

Definition

Incomplete or inaccurate knowledge about food, nutrition, or nutrition-related information and guidelines, e.g., nutrient requirements, consequences of food behaviors, life stage requirements, nutrition recommendations, diseases and conditions, physiological function, or products.

Etiology (*Cause/Contributing Risk Factors*)

Factors gathered during the nutrition assessment process that contribute to the existence or the maintenance of pathophysiological, psychosocial, situational, developmental, cultural, and/or environmental problems:

- Harmful beliefs/attitudes about food, nutrition, and nutrition-related topics
- Lack of prior exposure to information
- Language or cultural barrier impacting ability to learn information
- Learning disability, neurological or sensory impairment
- Prior exposure to incompatible information
- Prior exposure to incorrect information
- Unwilling or uninterested in learning information

Signs/Symptoms (*Defining Characteristics*)

A typical cluster of subjective and objective signs and symptoms gathered during the nutrition assessment process that provide evidence that a problem exists; quantify the problem and describe its severity.

Nutrition Assessment Category	Potential Indicators of this Nutrition Diagnosis (one or more must be present)
Biochemical Data, Medical Tests and Procedures	
Anthropometric Measurements	
Physical Exam Findings	

Edition: 2008

FOOD- AND NUTRITION-RELATED KNOWLEDGE DEFICIT (NB-1.1)

Food/Nutrition History	Reports or observations of:
	▪ Verbalizes inaccurate or incomplete information
	▪ Provides inaccurate or incomplete written response to questionnaire/written tool or is unable to read written tool
	▪ No prior knowledge of need for food- and nutrition-related recommendations
	▪ Demonstrates inability to apply food- and nutrition-related information, e.g., select food based on nutrition therapy or prepare infant feeding as instructed
	▪ Relates concerns about previous attempts to learn information
	▪ Verbalizes unwillingness or disinterest in learning information
Client History	▪ Conditions associated with a diagnosis or treatment, e.g., mental illness
	▪ New medical diagnosis or change in existing diagnosis or condition

References

1. Crawford S. Promoting dietary change. *Can J Cardiol.* 1995;11(suppl A):14A-15A.
2. Kumanyika SK, Van Horn L, Bowen D, Perri MG, Rolls BJ, Czajkowski SM, Schron E. Maintenance of dietary behavior change. *Health Psychol.* 2000;19(1 suppl):S42-S56.
3. Position of the American Dietetic Association: Weight management. *J Am Diet Assoc.* 2002;102:1145-1155.
4. Position of the American Dietetic Association: Total diet approach to communicating food and nutrition information. *J Am Diet Assoc* 2007;107(in press).
5. Position of the American Dietetic Association: The role of dietetics professionals in health promotion and disease prevention. *J Am Diet Assoc.* 2006;106:1875-1884.
6. Shepherd R. Resistance to changes in diet. *Proc Nutr Soc.* 2002;61:267-272.
7. U.S. Preventive Services Task Force. Behavioral counseling in primary care to promote a healthy diet. *Am J Prev Med.* 2003;24:93-100.

Behavioral

141

Edition: 2008

BEHAVIORAL-ENVIRONMENTAL DOMAIN • Knowledge and Beliefs

HARMFUL BELIEFS/ATTITUDES ABOUT FOOD OR NUTRITION-RELATED TOPICS (NB-1.2)

Use with caution: Be sensitive to patient concerns.

Definition

Beliefs/attitudes or practices about food, nutrition, and nutrition-related topics that are incompatible with sound nutrition principles, nutrition care, or disease/condition (excluding disordered eating patterns and eating disorders).

Etiology *(Cause/Contributing Risk Factors)*

Factors gathered during the nutrition assessment process that contribute to the existence or the maintenance of pathophysiological, psychosocial, situational, developmental, cultural, and/or environmental problems:

- Disbelief in science-based food and nutrition information
- Exposure to incorrect food and nutrition information
- Eating behavior serves a purpose other than nourishment (e.g., pica)
- Desire for a cure for a chronic disease through the use of alternative therapy

Signs/Symptoms *(Defining Characteristics)*

A typical cluster of subjective and objective signs and symptoms gathered during the nutrition assessment process that provide evidence that a problem exists; quantify the problem and describe its severity.

Nutrition Assessment Category	Potential Indicators of this Nutrition Diagnosis (one or more must be present)
Biochemical Data, Medical Tests and Procedures	
Anthropometric Measurements	
Physical Exam Findings	

HARMFUL BELIEFS/ATTITUDES ABOUT FOOD OR NUTRITION-RELATED TOPICS (NB-1.2)

Food/Nutrition History	Reports or observations of:
	▪ Food fetish, pica
	▪ Food faddism
	▪ Intake that reflects an imbalance of nutrients/food groups
	▪ Avoidance of foods/food groups (e.g., sugar, wheat, cooked foods)
Client History	▪ Conditions associated with a diagnosis or treatment, e.g., obesity, diabetes, cancer, cardiovascular disease, mental illness

References

1. Chapman GE, Beagan B. Women's perspectives on nutrition, health, and breast cancer. *J Nutr Educ Behav.* 2003;35:135-141.
2. Gonzalez VM, Vitousek KM. Feared food in dieting and non-dieting young women: a preliminary validation of the Food Phobia Survey. *Appetite.* 2004;43:155-173.
3. Jowett SL, Seal CJ, Phillips E, Gregory W, Barton JR, Welfare MR. Dietary beliefs of people with ulcerative colitis and their effect on relapse and nutrient intake. *Clin Nutr.* 2004;23:161-170.
4. Madden H, Chamberlain K. Nutritional health messages in women's magazines: a conflicted space for women readers. *J Health Psychol.* 2004;9:583-597.
5. Peters CL, Shelton J, Sharma P. An investigation of factors that influence the consumption of dietary supplements. *Health Mark Q.* 2003;21:113-135.
6. Position of the American Dietetic Association: Food and nutrition misinformation. *J Am Diet Assoc.* 2006;106:601-607.
7. Povey R, Wellens B, Conner M. Attitudes towards following meat, vegetarian and vegan diets: an examination of the role of ambivalence. *Appetite.* 2001;37:15-26.
8. Putterman E, Linden W. Appearance versus health: does the reason for dieting affect dieting behavior? *J Behav Med.* 2004;27:185-204.
9. Salminen E, Heikkila S, Poussa T, Lagstrom H, Saario R, Salminen S. Female patients tend to alter their diet following the diagnosis of rheumatoid arthritis and breast cancer. *Prev Med.* 2002;34:529-535.

Behavioral

Edition: 2008

BEHAVIORAL-ENVIRONMENTAL DOMAIN • Knowledge and Beliefs

NOT READY FOR DIET/LIFESTYLE CHANGE (NB-1.3)

Definition

Lack of perceived value of nutrition-related behavior change compared to costs (consequences or effort required to make changes); conflict with personal value system; antecedent to behavior change.

Etiology (Cause/Contributing Risk Factors)

Factors gathered during the nutrition assessment process that contribute to the existence or the maintenance of pathophysiological, psychosocial, situational, developmental, cultural, and/or environmental problems:

- Harmful beliefs/attitudes about food, nutrition, and nutrition-related topics
- Cognitive deficits or inability to focus on dietary changes
- Lack of social support for implementing changes
- Denial of need to change
- Perception that time, interpersonal, or financial constraints prevent changes
- Unwilling or uninterested in learning information
- Lack of self-efficacy for making change or demoralization from previous failures at change

Signs/Symptoms (Defining Characteristics)

A typical cluster of subjective and objective signs and symptoms gathered during the nutrition assessment process that provide evidence that a problem exists; quantify the problem and describe its severity.

Nutrition Assessment Category	Potential Indicators of this Nutrition Diagnosis (one or more must be present)
Biochemical Data, Medical Tests and Procedures	
Anthropometric Measurements	
Physical Exam Findings	• Negative body language, e.g., frowning, lack of eye contact, defensive posture, lack of focus, fidgeting (Note: Body language varies by culture.)

Edition: 2008

NOT READY FOR DIET/LIFESTYLE CHANGE (NB-1.3)

Food/Nutrition History	
	Reports or observations of:
	▪ Denial of need for food- and nutrition-related changes
	▪ Inability to understand required changes
	▪ Failure to keep appointments/schedule follow-up appointments or engage in counseling
	▪ Previous failures to effectively change target behavior
	▪ Defensiveness, hostility or resistance to change
	▪ Lack of efficacy to make change or to overcome barriers to change
Client History	

References

1. Crawford S. Promoting dietary change. *Can J Cardiol.* 1995;11:14A-15A.
2. Greene GW, Rossi SR, Rossi JS, Velicer WF, Fava JS, Prochaska JO. Dietary applications of the Stages of Change Model. *J Am Diet Assoc.* 1999; 99:673-678.
3. Kumanyika SK, Van Horn L, Bowen D, Perri MG, Rolls BJ, Czajkowski SM, Schron E. Maintenance of dietary behavior change. *Health Psychol.* 2000;19:S42-S56.
4. Prochaska JO, Velicer W F. The Transtheoretical Model of behavior change. *Am J Health Promotion.* 1997;12:38-48.
5. Position of the American Dietetic Association: Total diet approach to communicating food and nutrition information. *J Am Diet Assoc.* 2007;107(in press).
6. Position of the American Dietetic Association: The role of dietetics professionals in health promotion and disease prevention. *J Am Diet Assoc.* 2006;106:1875-1884.
7. Resnicow K, Jackson A, Wang T, De A, McCarty F, Dudley W, Baronowski T. A motivational interviewing intervention to increase fruit and vegetable intake through black churches: Results of the Eat for Life trial. *Am J Public Health.* 2001; 91:1686-1693.
8. Shepherd R. Resistance to changes in diet. *Proc Nutr Soc.* 2002;61:267-272.
9. U.S. Preventive Services Task Force. Behavioral counseling in primary care to promote a healthy diet. *Am J Prev Med.* 2003;24:93-100.

Updated: 2008 Edition

Behavioral

145

BEHAVIORAL-ENVIRONMENTAL DOMAIN • Knowledge and Beliefs

SELF-MONITORING DEFICIT (NB-1.4)

Definition

Lack of data recording to track personal progress.

Etiology (*Cause/Contributing Risk Factors*)

Factors gathered during the nutrition assessment process that contribute to the existence or the maintenance of pathophysiological, psychosocial, situational, developmental, cultural, and/or environmental problems:

- Food- and nutrition-related knowledge deficit
- Lack of social support for implementing changes
- Lack of value for behavior change or competing values
- Perception that lack of resources (e.g., time, financial, or social support) prevent self-monitoring
- Cultural barrier impacting ability to track personal progress
- Learning disability, neurological, or sensory impairment
- Prior exposure to incompatible information
- Not ready for diet/lifestyle change
- Unwilling or uninterested in tracking progress
- Lack of focus and attention to detail, difficulty with time management and/or organization

Signs/Symptoms (*Defining Characteristics*)

A typical cluster of subjective and objective signs and symptoms gathered during the nutrition assessment process that provide evidence that a problem exists; quantify the problem and describe its severity.

Nutrition Assessment Category	Potential Indicators of this Nutrition Diagnosis (one or more must be present)
Biochemical Data, Medical Tests and Procedures	▪ Recorded data inconsistent with biochemical data, e.g., dietary intake is not consistent with biochemical data
Anthropometric Measurements	
Physical Exam Findings	

Edition: 2008

SELF-MONITORING DEFICIT (NB-1.4)

Food/Nutrition History	Reports or observations of:
	▪ Incomplete self-monitoring records, e.g., glucose, food, fluid intake, weight, physical activity, ostomy output records
	▪ Food intake data inconsistent with weight status or growth pattern data
	▪ Embarrassment or anger regarding need for self-monitoring
	▪ Uncertainty of how to complete monitoring records
	▪ Uncertainty regarding changes that could/should be made in response to data in self-monitoring records
	▪ No self-management equipment, e.g., no blood glucose monitor, pedometer
Client History	▪ Diagnoses associated with self-monitoring, e.g., diabetes mellitus, obesity, new ostomy
	▪ New medical diagnosis or change in existing diagnosis or condition

References

1. American Diabetes Association. Tests of glycemia in diabetes. *Diabetes Care.* 2004;27:S91-S93.
2. Baker RC, Kirschenbaum DS. Weight control during the holidays: highly consistent self-monitoring as a potentially useful coping mechanism. *Health Psychol.* 1998;17:367-370.
3. Berkowitz RI, Wadden TA, Tershakovec AM. Behavior therapy and sibutramine for treatment of adolescent obesity. *JAMA.* 2003;289:1805-1812.
4. Crawford S. Promoting dietary change. *Can J Cardiol.* 1995;11(suppl A):14A-15A.
5. Jeffery R, Drewnowski A, Epstein L, Stunkard A, Wilson G, Wing R. Long-term maintenance of weight loss: current status. *Health Psychol.* 2000;19:5-16.
6. Kumanyika SK, Van Horn L, Bowen D, Perri MG, Rolls BJ, Czajkowski SM, Schron E. Maintenance of dietary behavior change. *Health Psychol.* 2000;19(1 suppl):S42-S56.
7. Lichtman SW, Pisarska K, Berman ER, Pestone M, Dowling H, Offenbacher E, Weisel H, Heshka S, Matthews DE, Heymsfield SB. Discrepancy between self-reported and actual caloric intake and exercise in obese subjects. *N Engl J Med.* 1992;327:1893-1898.
8. Wadden, TA. Characteristics of successful weight loss maintainers. In: Allison DB, Pi-Sunyer FX, eds. *Obesity Treatment: Establishing Goals, Improving Outcomes, and Reviewing the Research Agenda.* New York: Plenum Press; 1995:103-111.

BEHAVIORAL-ENVIRONMENTAL DOMAIN • Knowledge and Beliefs

DISORDERED EATING PATTERN (NB-1.5)

Definition

Beliefs, attitudes, thoughts, and behaviors related to food, eating, and weight management, including classic eating disorders as well as less severe, similar conditions that negatively impact health.

Etiology (Cause/Contributing Risk Factors)

Factors gathered during the nutrition assessment process that contribute to the existence or the maintenance of pathophysiological, psychosocial, situational, developmental, cultural, and/or environmental problems:

- Familial, societal, biological/genetic, and/or environmental related obsessive desire to be thin
- Weight regulation/preoccupation significantly influences self-esteem

Signs/Symptoms (Defining Characteristics)

A typical cluster of subjective and objective signs and symptoms gathered during the nutrition assessment process that provide evidence that a problem exists; quantify the problem and describe its severity.

Nutrition Assessment Category	Potential Indicators of this Nutrition Diagnosis (one or more must be present)
Biochemical Data, Medical Tests and Procedures	▪ Decreased cholesterol, abnormal lipid profiles, hypoglycemia, hypokalemia [anorexia nervosa (AN)] ▪ Hypokalemia and hypochloremic alkalosis [bulimia nervosa (BN)] ▪ Hyponatremia, hypothyroid, leukopenia, elevated BUN (AN) ▪ Urine positive for ketones (AN)
Anthropometric Measurements	▪ BMI < 17.5, arrested growth and development, failure to gain weight during period of expected growth, weight less than 85% of expected (AN) ▪ BMI > 29 [eating disorder not otherwise specified (EDNOS)] ▪ Significant weight fluctuation (BN)

DISORDERED EATING PATTERN (NB-1.5)

Physical Exam Findings	• Severely depleted adipose and somatic protein stores (AN)
	• Lanugo hair formation on face and trunk, brittle listless hair, cyanosis of hands and feet, and dry skin (AN)
	• Normal or excess adipose and normal somatic protein stores (BN, EDNOS)
	• Damaged tooth enamel (BN)
	• Enlarged parotid glands (BN)
	• Peripheral edema (BN)
	• Skeletal muscle loss (AN)
	• Cardiac arrhythmias, bradycardia (AN, BN)
	• Hypotension, low body temperature
	• Inability to concentrate (AN)
	• Positive Russell's Sign (BN) callous on back of hand from self-induced vomiting
	• Bradycardia (heart rate < 60 beats/min), hypotension (systolic < 90 mm HG), and orthostatic hypotension (AN)
Food/Nutrition History	Reports or observations of:
	• Avoidance of food or calorie-containing beverages (AN, BN)
	• Fear of foods or dysfunctional thoughts regarding food or food experiences (AN, BN)
	• Denial of hunger (AN)
	• Food and weight preoccupation (AN, BN)
	• Knowledgeable about current diet fad (AN, BN, EDNOS)
	• Fasting (AN, BN)
	• Intake of larger quantity of food in a defined time period, a sense of lack of control over eating (BN, EDNOS)
	• Excessive physical activity (AN, BN, EDNOS)
	• Eating much more rapidly than normal, until feeling uncomfortably full, consuming large amounts of food when not feeling physically hungry; eating alone because of embarrassment, feeling very guilty after overeating (EDNOS)
	• Eats in private (AN, BN)
	• Irrational thoughts about food's affect on the body (AN, BN, EDNOS)
	• Pattern of chronic dieting

Behavioral

149

BEHAVIORAL-ENVIRONMENTAL DOMAIN • Knowledge and Beliefs

DISORDERED EATING PATTERN (NB-1.5)

Food/Nutrition History cont'd	▪ Excessive reliance on nutrition terming and preoccupation with nutrient content of foods
	▪ Inflexibility with food selection
Client History	▪ Self-induced vomiting, diarrhea, bloating, constipation, and flatulence (BN); always cold (AN)
	▪ Misuse of laxatives, enemas, diuretics, stimulants, and/or metabolic enhancers (AN,BN)
	▪ Muscle weakness, fatigue, cardiac arrhythmias, dehydration, and electrolyte imbalance (AN, BN)
	▪ Diagnosis, e.g., anorexia nervosa, bulimia nervosa, binge eating, eating disorder not otherwise specified, amenorrhea,
	▪ History of mood and anxiety disorders (e.g., depression, obsessive/compulsive disorder [OCD]), personality disorders, substance abuse disorders
	▪ Family history of ED, depression, OCD, anxiety disorders (AN, BN)
	▪ Irritability, depression (AN, BN)
	▪ Anemia
	▪ Avoidance of social events at which food is served

References

1. Anderson GH, Kennedy SH, eds. *The Biology of Feast and Famine.* New York: Academic Press; 1992.
2. American Psychiatric Association. *Diagnostic and statistical manual for mental disorders (fourth edition, text revision).* APA Press: Washington DC; 2000.
3. American Psychiatric Association. Practice guidelines for the treatment of patients with eating disorders. *Am J Psychiatry.* 2000;157 (suppl):1-39.
4. Cooke RA, Chambers JB. Anorexia nervosa and the heart. *Br J Hosp Med.* 1995;54:313-317.
5. Fisher M. Medical complications of anorexia and bulimia nervosa. *Adol Med Stat of the Art Reviews.* 1992;3:481-502.
6. Gralen SJ, Levin MP, Smolak L, Murnen SK. Dieting and disordered eating during early and middle adolescents: Do the influences remain the same? *Int J Eating Disorder.* 1990;9:501-512.
7. Harris JP, Kriepe RE, Rossback CN. QT prolongation by isoproterenol in anorexia nervosa. *J Adol Health.* 1993;14:390-393.
8. Kaplan AS, Garfunkel PE, eds. *Medical Issues and the Eating Disorders: The Interface.* New York: Brunner/Manzel Publishers; 1993.
9. Keys A, Brozek J, Henschel A, Mickelson O, Taylor HL. *The Biology of Human Starvation, 2nd vol.* Minneapolis, MN: University of Minnesota Press; 1950.
10. Kirkley BG. Bulimia: clinical characteristics, development, and etiology. *J Am Diet Assoc.* 1986;86:468-475.
11. Kreipe RE, Uphoff M. Treatment and outcome of adolescents with anorexia nervosa. *Adolesc Med.*1992;16:519-540.
12. Kreipe RE, Birndorf DO. Eating disorders in adolescents and young adults. *Medical Clinics of North America.* 2000;84:1027-1049.
13. Mordasini R, Klose G, Greter H. Secondary type II hyperlipoproteinemia in patients with anorexia nervosa. *Metabolism.* 1978;27:71-79.
14. Position of the American Dietetic Association: Nutrition intervention in the treatment of anorexia nervosa, bulimia nervosa, and eating disorder not otherwise specified (EDNOS). *J Am Diet Assoc.* 2006;106:2073-2082.
15. Rock C, Yager J. Nutrition and eating disorders: a primer for clinicians. *Int J Eat Disord.* 1987;6:267-280.
16. Rock, CL. Nutritional and medical assessment and management of eating disorders. *Nutr Clin Care.* 1999;2:332-343.
17. Schebendach J, Reichert-Anderson P. Nutrition in Eating Disorders. In: *Kraus's Nutrition and Diet Therapy.* Mahan K, Escott-Stump S (eds). McGraw- Hill: New York, NY; 2000.
18. Silber T. Anorexia nervosa: Morbidity and mortality. *Pediar Ann.* 1984; 13:851-859.
19. Swenne I. Heart risk associated with weight loss in anorexia nervosa and eating disorders: electrocardiographic changes during the early phase of refeeding. *Acta Paediatr.* 2000;89:447-452.
20. Turner JM, Bulsara MK, McDermott BM, Byrne GC, Prince RL, Forbes DA. Predictors of low bone density in young adolescent females with anorexia nervosa and other dieting disorders. *Int J Eat Disord.* 2001;30:245-251.

LIMITED ADHERENCE TO NUTRITION-RELATED RECOMMENDATIONS (NB-1.6)

Definition

Lack of nutrition-related changes as per intervention agreed on by client or population.

Etiology (*Cause/Contributing Risk Factors*)

Factors gathered during the nutrition assessment process that contribute to the existence or the maintenance of pathophysiological, psychosocial, situational, developmental, cultural, and/or environmental problems:

- Lack of social support for implementing changes
- Lack of value for behavior change or competing values
- Perception that time or financial constraints prevent changes
- Previous lack of success in making health-related changes
- Poor understanding of how and why to make the changes
- Unwilling or uninterested in applying information

Signs/Symptoms (*Defining Characteristics*)

A typical cluster of subjective and objective signs and symptoms gathered during the nutrition assessment process that provide evidence that a problem exists; quantify the problem and describe its severity.

Nutrition Assessment Category	Potential Indicators of this Nutrition Diagnosis (one or more must be present)
Biochemical Data, Medical Tests and Procedures	▪ Expected laboratory outcomes are not achieved
Anthropometric Measurements	▪ Expected anthropometric outcomes are not achieved
Physical Exam Findings	▪ Negative body language, e.g., frowning, lack of eye contact, fidgeting (Note: body language varies by culture)

151

BEHAVIORAL-ENVIRONMENTAL DOMAIN • Knowledge and Beliefs

LIMITED ADHERENCE TO NUTRITION-RELATED RECOMMENDATIONS (NB-1.6)

Food/Nutrition History	Reports or observations of:
	▪ Expected food/nutrition-related outcomes are not achieved
	▪ Inability to recall agreed on changes
	▪ Failure to complete any agreed on homework
	▪ Lack of compliance or inconsistent compliance with plan
	▪ Failure to keep appointments or schedule follow-up appointments
	▪ Lack of appreciation of the importance of making recommended nutrition-related changes
	▪ Uncertainty as to how to consistently apply food/nutrition information
Client History	

References

1. Crawford S. Promoting dietary change. *Can J Cardiol.* 1995;11(suppl A):14A-15A.
2. Kumanyika SK, Van Horn L, Bowen D, Perri MG, Rolls BJ, Czajkowski SM, Schron E. Maintenance of dietary behavior change. *Health Psychol.* 2000;19(1 suppl):S42-S56.
3. Position of the American Dietetic Association: Total diet approach to communicating food and nutrition information. *J Am Diet Assoc.* 2007;107(in press).
4. Shepherd R. Resistance to changes in diet. *Proc Nutr Soc.* 2002;61:267-272.
5. U.S. Preventive Services Task Force. Behavioral counseling in primary care to promote a healthy diet. *Am J Prev Med.* 2003;24:93-100.

Edition: 2008

UNDESIRABLE FOOD CHOICES (NB-1.7)

Definition

Food and/or beverage choices that are inconsistent with Dietary Reference Intakes (DRIs), US Dietary Guidelines, or My Pyramid, or with targets defined in the nutrition prescription or nutrition care process.

Etiology (*Cause/Contributing Risk Factors*)

Factors gathered during the nutrition assessment process that contribute to the existence or the maintenance of pathophysiological, psychosocial, situational, developmental, cultural, and/or environmental problems:

- Lack of prior exposure to or misunderstanding of information
- Language, religious, or cultural barrier impacting ability to apply information
- Learning disabilities, neurological or sensory impairment
- High level of fatigue or other side effect of medical, surgical or radiological therapy
- Inadequate access to recommended foods
- Perception that financial constraints prevent selection of food choices consistent with recommendations
- Food allergies and aversions impeding food choices consistent with guidelines
- Lacks motivation and or readiness to apply or support systems change
- Unwilling or uninterested in learning information
- Psychological limitations

Signs/Symptoms (*Defining Characteristics*)

A typical cluster of subjective and objective signs and symptoms gathered during the nutrition assessment process that provide evidence that a problem exists; quantify the problem and describe its severity.

Nutrition Assessment Category	Potential Indicators of this Nutrition Diagnosis (one or more must be present)
Biochemical Data, Medical Tests and Procedures	▪ Elevated lipid panel
Anthropometric Measurements	
Physical Exam Findings	▪ Findings consistent with vitamin/mineral deficiency or excess

153

BEHAVIORAL-ENVIRONMENTAL DOMAIN • Knowledge and Beliefs

UNDESIRABLE FOOD CHOICES (NB-1.7)

Food/Nutrition History	Reports or observations of:
	• Intake inconsistent with DRIs, US Dietary Guidelines, MyPyramid, or other methods of measuring diet quality, such as, the Healthy Eating Index (e.g., omission of entire nutrient groups, disproportionate intake [e.g., juice for young children])
	• Inaccurate or incomplete understanding of the guidelines
	• Inability to apply guideline information
	• Inability to select (e.g., access), or unwillingness, or disinterest in selecting, food consistent with the guidelines
Client History	• Conditions associated with a diagnosis or treatment, e.g., mental illness

References

1. Birch LL, Fisher JA. Appetite and eating behavior in children. *Pediatr Clin North Am.* 1995;42:931-953.
2. Butte N, Cobb K, Dwyer J, Graney L, Heird W, Richard K. The start healthy feeding guidelines for infants and toddlers. *J Am Diet Assoc.* 2004:104:3:442-454.
3. Position of the American Dietetic Association: Weight management. *J Am Diet Assoc.* 2002;102:1145-1155.
4. Dolecek TA, Stamlee J, Caggiula AW, Tillotson JL, Buzzard IM. Methods of dietary and nutritional assessment and intervention and other methods in the multiple risk factor intervention trial. *Am J Clin Nutr.* 1997;65(suppl):196S-210S.
5. Epstein LH, Gordy CC, Raynor HA, Beddome M, Kilanowski CK, Paluch R. Increasing fruit and vegetable intake and decreasing fat and sugar intake in families at risk for childhood obesity. *Obesity Res.* 2001;9:171-178.
6. Freeland-Graves J, Nitzke S. Total diet approach to communicating food and nutrition information. *J Am Diet Assoc.* 2002;102:100-108.
7. French SA. Pricing effects on food choices. *J Nutr.* 2003;133:S841-S843.
8. Glens K, Basil M, Mariachi E, Goldberg J, Snyder D. Why Americans eat what they do: taste, nutrition, cost, convenience and weight control concerns as influences on food consumption. *J Am Diet Assoc.* 1998;98:1118-1126.
9. Hampl JS, Anderson JV, Mullis R. The role of dietetics professionals in health promotion and disease prevention. *J Am Diet Assoc.* 2002;102:1680-1687.
10. Lin SH, Guthrie J, Frazao E. American children's' diets are not making the grade. *Food Review.* 2001;24: 8-17.
11. Satter E. Feeding dynamics: helping children to eat well. *J Pediatr Health Care.* 1995;9:178-184.
12. Story M, Holt K, Sofka D, eds. *Bright futures in practice: Nutrition, 2nd Ed.* Arlington, VA: National Center for Education in Maternal Child Health; 2002.
13. Pelto GH, Levitt E, Thairu L. Improving feeding practices, current patterns, common constraints and the design of interventions. *Food Nutr Bull.* 2003;24:45-82.

Updated: 2008 Edition

Edition: 2008

154

PHYSICAL INACTIVITY (NB-2.1)

Definition

Low level of activity/sedentary behavior to the extent that it reduces energy expenditure and impacts health.

Etiology (*Cause/Contributing Risk Factors*)

Factors gathered during the nutrition assessment process that contribute to the existence or the maintenance of pathophysiological, psychosocial, situational, developmental, cultural, and/or environmental problems:

- Harmful beliefs/attitudes about physical activity
- Injury, lifestyle change, condition (e.g., advanced stages of cardiovascular disease, obesity, kidney disease), physical disability or limitation that reduces physical activity or activities of daily living
- Lack of knowledge about the health benefits of physical activity
- Lack of prior exposure regarding need for physical activity or how to incorporate exercise, e.g., physical disability, arthritis
- Lack of role models, e.g., for children
- Lack of social support and/or environmental space or equipment
- Lack of safe environment for physical activity
- Lack of value for behavior change or competing values
- Time constraints
- Financial constraints that may prevent sufficient level of activity (e.g., to address cost of equipment or shoes or club membership to gain access)

Signs/Symptoms (*Defining Characteristics*)

A typical cluster of subjective and objective signs and symptoms gathered during the nutrition assessment process that provide evidence that a problem exists; quantify the problem and describe its severity.

Nutrition Assessment Category	Potential Indicators of this Nutrition Diagnosis (one or more must be present)
Biochemical Data, Medical Tests and Procedures	
Anthropometric Measurements	▪ Obesity—BMI > 30 (adults), BMI >95th percentile (pediatrics > 3 years)
Physical Exam Findings	▪ Excessive subcutaneous fat and low muscle mass

Behavioral

155

Edition: 2008

BEHAVIORAL-ENVIRONMENTAL DOMAIN • Physical Activity and Function

PHYSICAL INACTIVITY (NB-2.1)

Food/Nutrition History	Reports or observations of: ▪ Infrequent, low duration and/or low intensity physical activity ▪ Large amounts of sedentary activities, e.g., TV watching, reading, computer use in both leisure and work/school ▪ Low level of NEAT (non-exercise activity thermogenesis) expended by physical activities other than planned exercise, e.g., sitting, standing, walking, fidgeting
Client History	▪ Low cardiorespiratory fitness and/or low muscle strength ▪ Medical diagnoses that may be associated with or result in decreased activity, e.g., arthritis, chronic fatigue syndrome, morbid obesity, knee surgery ▪ Medications that cause somnolence and decreased cognition ▪ Psychological diagnosis, e.g., depression, anxiety disorders

References

1 Position of the American Dietetic Association: Weight management. *J Am Diet Assoc.* 2002;102:1145-1155.

2 Position of the American Dietetic Association: Total diet approach to communicating food and nutrition information. *J Am Diet Assoc* 2007;107(in press).

3 Position of the American Dietetic Association: The role of dietetics professionals in health promotion and disease prevention. *J Am Diet Assoc.* 2006;106:1875-1884.

4 Levine JA, Lanninghav-Foster LM, McCrady SK, Krizan AC, Olson LR, Kane PH, Jensen MD, Clark MM. Interindividual variation in posture allocation: Possible role in human obesity. *Science.* 2005;307:584-586.

Updated: 2008 Edition

EXCESSIVE EXERCISE (NB-2.2)

Definition

An amount of exercise that exceeds that which is necessary to improve health and/or athletic performance.

Etiology (Cause/Contributing Risk Factors)

Factors gathered during the nutrition assessment process that contribute to the existence or the maintenance of pathophysiological, psychosocial, situational, developmental, cultural, and/or environmental problems:

- Disordered eating
- Irrational beliefs/attitudes about food, nutrition, and fitness
- "Addictive" behaviors/personality

Signs/Symptoms (Defining Characteristics)

A typical cluster of subjective and objective signs and symptoms gathered during the nutrition assessment process that provide evidence that a problem exists; quantify the problem and describe its severity.

Nutrition Assessment Category	Potential Indicators of this Nutrition Diagnosis (one or more must be present)
Biochemical Data, Medical Tests and Procedures	▪ Elevated liver enzymes, e.g., LDH, AST
	▪ Altered micronutrient status, e.g., decreased serum ferritin, zinc, and insulin-like growth factor-binding protein
	▪ Increased hematocrit
	▪ Suppressed immune function
	▪ Possibly elevated cortisol levels
Anthropometric Measurements	▪ Weight loss, arrested growth and development, failure to gain weight during period of expected growth (related usually to disordered eating)
Physical Exam Findings	▪ Depleted adipose and somatic protein stores (related usually to disordered eating)
	▪ Frequent and/or prolonged injuries and/or illnesses
	▪ Chronic muscle soreness

157

BEHAVIORAL-ENVIRONMENTAL DOMAIN • Physical Activity and Function

EXCESSIVE EXERCISE (NB-2.2)

Food/Nutrition History	Reports or observations of:
	▪ Continued/repeated high levels of exercise exceeding levels necessary to improve health and/or athletic performance
	▪ Exercise daily without rest/rehabilitation days
	▪ Exercise while injured/sick
	▪ Forsaking family, job, social responsibilities to exercise
	▪ Overtraining
Client History	▪ Conditions associated with a diagnosis or treatment, e.g., anorexia nervosa, bulimia nervosa, binge eating, eating disorder not otherwise specified, amenorrhea, stress fractures
	▪ Chronic fatigue
	▪ Evidence of addictive, obsessive, or compulsive tendencies

References

1. Aissa-Benhaddad A, Bouix D, Khaled S, Micallef JP, Mercier J, Bringer I, Brun JF. Early hemorheologic aspects of overtraining in elite athletes. *Clin Hemorheol Microcirc.* 1999;20:117-125.
2. American Psychiatric Association. *Diagnostic and Statistical Manual of Mental Disorders. 4th Ed.* Washington, DC: American Psychiatric Association; 1994.
3. Davis C, Brewer H, Ratusny D. Behavioral frequency and psychological commitment: necessary concepts in the study of excessive exercising. *J Behav Med.* 1993;16:611-628.
4. Davis C, Claridge G. The eating disorder as addiction: a psychobiological perspective. *Addict Behav.* 1998;23:463-475.
5. Davis C, Kennedy SH, Ravelski E, Dionne M. The role of physical activity in the development and maintenance of eating disorders. *Psychol Med.* 1994;24:957-967.
6. Klein DA, Bennett AS, Schebendach J, Foltin RW, Devlin MJ, Walsh BT. Exercise "addiction" in anorexia nervosa: model development and pilot data. *CNS Spectr.* 2004;9:531-537.
7. Lakier-Smith L. Overtraining, excessive exercise, and altered immunity: is this a helper-1 vs helper-2 lymphocyte response? *Sports Med.* 2003;33:347-364.
8. Position of the American Dietetic Association: Nutrition intervention in the treatment of anorexia nervosa, bulimia nervosa, and eating disorder not otherwise specified (EDNOS). *J Am Diet Assoc.* 2006;106:2073-2082.
9. Shephard RJ, Shek PN. Acute and chronic over-exertion: do depressed immune responses provide useful markers? *Int J Sports Med.* 1998;19:159-171.
10. Smith LL. Tissue trauma: the underlying cause of overtraining syndrome? *J Strength Cond Res.* 2004;18:185-193.
11. Urhausen A, Kindermann W. Diagnosis of overtraining: what tools do we have. *Sports Med.* 2002;32:95-102.

Updated: 2008 Edition

INABILITY OR LACK OF DESIRE TO MANAGE SELF-CARE (NB-2.3)

Definition

Lack of capacity or unwillingness to implement methods to support healthful food- and nutrition-related behavior.

Etiology (Cause/Contributing Risk Factors)

Factors gathered during the nutrition assessment process that contribute to the existence or the maintenance of pathophysiological, psychosocial, situational, developmental, cultural, and/or environmental problems:

- Food- and nutrition-related knowledge deficit
- Lack of caretaker or social support for implementing changes
- Lack of developmental readiness to perform self-management tasks, e.g., pediatrics
- Lack of value for behavior change or competing values
- Perception that lack of resources (time, financial, support persons) prevent self-care
- Cultural beliefs and practices
- Learning disability, neurological or sensory impairment
- Prior exposure to incompatible information
- Not ready for diet/lifestyle change
- Unwilling or uninterested in learning/applying information
- No self-management tools or decision guides

Signs/Symptoms (Defining Characteristics)

A typical cluster of subjective and objective signs and symptoms gathered during the nutrition assessment process that provide evidence that a problem exists; quantify the problem and describe its severity.

Nutrition Assessment Category	Potential Indicators of this Nutrition Diagnosis (one or more must be present)		
Biochemical Data, Medical Tests and Procedures			
Anthropometric Measurements			
Physical Exam Findings			

Behavioral

159

BEHAVIORAL-ENVIRONMENTAL DOMAIN • Physical Activity and Function

INABILITY OR LACK OF DESIRE TO MANAGE SELF-CARE (NB-2.3)

Food/Nutrition History	Reports or observations of:
	▪ Inability to interpret data or self-management tools
	▪ Embarrassment or anger regarding need for self-monitoring
	▪ Uncertainty regarding changes could/should be made in response to data in self-monitoring records
Client History	▪ Diagnoses that are associated with self-management, e.g., diabetes mellitus, obesity, cardiovascular disease, renal or liver disease
	▪ Conditions associated with a diagnosis or treatment, e.g., cognitive or emotional impairment
	▪ New medical diagnosis or change in existing diagnosis or condition

References

1. Position of the American Dietetic Association: Providing nutrition services for infants, children, and adults with developmental disabilities and special health care needs. *J Am Diet Assoc.* 2004;104:97-107.
2. Crawford S. Promoting dietary change. *Can J Cardiol.* 1995;11(suppl A):14A-15A.
3. Falk LW, Bisogni CA, Sobal J. Diet change processes of participants in an intensive heart program. *J Nutr Educ.* 2000;32:240-250.
4. Glasgow RE, Hampson SE, Strycker LA, Ruggiero L. Personal-model beliefs and social-environmental barriers related to diabetes self-management. *Diabetes Care.* 1997;20:556-561.
5. Keenan DP, AbuSabha R, Sigman-Grant M. Achterberg C. Ruffing J. Factors perceived to influence dietary fat reduction behaviors. *J Nutr Educ.*1999;31:134-144.
6. Kumanyika SK, Van Horn L, Bowen D, Perri MG, Rolls BJ, Czajkowski SM, Schron E. Maintenance of dietary behavior change. *Health Psychol.* 2000;19(1 suppl):S42-S56.
7. Sporny, LA, Contento, Isobel R. Stages of change in dietary fat reduction: . *J Nutr Educ.* 1995;27:191.

Edition: 2008

IMPAIRED ABILITY TO PREPARE FOODS/MEALS (NB-2.4)

Definition

Cognitive or physical impairment that prevents preparation of foods/meals.

Etiology (Cause/Contributing Risk Factors)

Factors gathered during the nutrition assessment process that contribute to the existence or the maintenance of pathophysiological, psychosocial, situational, developmental, cultural, and/or environmental problems:

- Learning disability, neurological or sensory impairment
- Loss of mental or cognitive ability, e.g., dementia
- Physical disability
- High level of fatigue or other side effect of therapy

Signs/Symptoms (Defining Characteristics)

A typical cluster of subjective and objective signs and symptoms gathered during the nutrition assessment process that provide evidence that a problem exists; quantify the problem and describe its severity.

Nutrition Assessment Category	Potential Indicators of this Nutrition Diagnosis (one or more must be present)
Biochemical Data, Medical Tests and Procedures	
Anthropometric Measurements	
Physical Exam Findings	
Food/Nutrition History	Reports or observations of: ■ Decreased overall intake ■ Excessive consumption of convenience foods, pre-prepared meals, and foods prepared away from home resulting in an inability to adhere to nutrition prescription ■ Uncertainty regarding appropriate foods to prepare based on nutrition prescription ■ Inability to purchase and transport foods to one's home

161

BEHAVIORAL-ENVIRONMENTAL DOMAIN • Physical Activity and Function

IMPAIRED ABILITY TO PREPARE FOODS/MEALS (NB-2.4)

Client History
▪ Conditions associated with a diagnosis or treatment, e.g., cognitive impairment, cerebral palsy, paraplegia, vision problems, rigorous therapy regimen, recent surgery

References

1. Andren E, Grimby G. Activity limitations in personal, domestic and vocational tasks: a study of adults with inborn and early acquired mobility disorders. *Disabil Rehabil.* 2004;26:262-271.
2. Andren E, Grimby G. Dependence in daily activities and life satisfaction in adult subjects with cerebral palsy or spina bifida: a follow-up study. *Disabil Rehabil.* 2004;26:528-536.
3. Fortin S, Godbout L, Braun CM. Cognitive structure of executive deficits in frontally lesioned head trauma patients performing activities of daily living. *Cortex.* 2003;39:273-291.
4. Godbout L, Doucet C, Fiola M. The scripting of activities of daily living in normal aging: anticipation and shifting deficits with preservation of sequencing. *Brain Cogn.* 2000;43:220-224.
5. Position of the American Dietetic Association: Providing nutrition services for infants, children, and adults with developmental disabilities and special health care needs. *J Am Diet Assoc.* 2004;104:97-107.
6. Position of the American Dietetic Association: Food insecurity and hunger in the United States. *J Am Diet Assoc.* 2006;106:446-458.
7. Position of the American Dietetic Association: Addressing world hunger, malnutrition, and food insecurity. *J Am Diet Assoc.* 2003;103:1046-1057.
8. Sandstrom K, Alinder J, Oberg B. Descriptions of functioning and health and relations to a gross motor classification in adults with cerebral palsy. *Disabil Rehabil.* 2004;26:1023-1031.

POOR NUTRITION QUALITY OF LIFE (NQOL) (NB-2.5)

Definition

Diminished patient/client perception of quality of life in response to nutrition problems and recommendations.

Etiology (*Cause/Contributing Risk Factors*)

Factors gathered during the nutrition assessment process that contribute to the existence or the maintenance of pathophysiological, psychosocial, situational, developmental, cultural, and/or environmental problems:

- Food and nutrition knowledge–related deficit
- Not ready for diet/lifestyle change
- Negative impact of current or previous medical nutrition therapy (MNT)
- Food or activity behavior-related difficulty
- Poor self-efficacy
- Altered body image
- Food insecurity
- Lack of social support for implementing changes

Signs/Symptoms (*Defining Characteristics*)

A typical cluster of subjective and objective signs and symptoms gathered during the nutrition assessment process that provide evidence that a problem exists; quantify the problem and describe its severity.

Nutrition Assessment Category	Potential Indicators of this Nutrition Diagnosis (one or more must be present)
Biochemical Data, Medical Tests and Procedures	
Anthropometric Measurements	
Physical Exam Findings	

Behavioral

163

BEHAVIORAL-ENVIRONMENTAL DOMAIN • Physical Activity and Function

POOR NUTRITION QUALITY OF LIFE (NQOL) (NB-2.5)

Food/Nutrition History	Reports or observations of:
	▪ Unfavorable NQOL rating
	▪ Unfavorable ratings on measure of QOL, such as, SF36 (multi-purpose health survey form with 36 questions) or EORTC QLQ-C30 (quality of life tool developed for patient/clients with cancer)
	▪ Food insecurity/unwillingness to use community services that are available
	▪ Frustration or dissatisfaction with MNT recommendations
	▪ Frustration over lack of control
	▪ Inaccurate or incomplete information related to MNT recommendations
	▪ Inability to change food- or activity-related behavior
	▪ Concerns about previous attempts to learn information
	▪ MNT recommendations effecting socialization
	▪ Unwillingness or disinterest in learning information
	▪ Lack of social and familial support
	▪ Ethnic and cultural related issues
Client History	▪ New medical diagnosis or change in existing diagnosis or condition
	▪ Recent other lifestyle or life changes, e.g., quit smoking, initiated exercise, work change, home relocation

References

1. Barr JT, Schumacher GE. The need for a nutrition-related quality-of-life measure. *J Am Diet Assoc.* 2003;103:177-180.
2. Barr JT, Schumacher GE. Using focus groups to determine what constitutes quality of life in clients receiving medical nutrition therapy: First steps in the development of a nutrition quality-of-life survey. *J Am Diet Assoc.* 2003;103:844-851.
3. NQOL instrument and annotated bibliography. Available at: http://www.bouve.neu.edu (key word search: quality of life). Accessed January 29, 2007.
4. Ware JE. *SF-36 Health Survey: Manual and Interpretation Guide.* Lincoln, RI: Quality Metric Inc; 2003

Updated: 2008 Edition

SELF-FEEDING DIFFICULTY (NB-2.6)

Definition

Impaired actions to place food or beverages in mouth.

Etiology (*Cause/Contributing Risk Factors*)

Factors gathered during the nutrition assessment process that contribute to the existence or the maintenance of pathophysiological, psychosocial, situational, developmental, cultural, and/or environmental problems:

- Inability to grasp cups and utensils for self-feeding
- Inability to support and/or control head and neck
- Lack of coordination of hand to mouth
- Limited physical strength or range of motion
- Inability to bend elbow or wrist
- Inability to sit with hips square and back straight
- Limited access to foods and/or adaptive eating devices conducive for self-feeding
- Limited vision and/or impaired cognitive ability
- Reluctance or avoidance of self-feeding

Signs/Symptoms (*Defining Characteristics*)

A typical cluster of subjective and objective signs and symptoms gathered during the nutrition assessment process that provide evidence that a problem exists; quantify the problem and describe its severity.

Nutrition Assessment Category	Potential Indicators of this Nutrition Diagnosis (one or more must be present)
Biochemical Data, Medical Tests and Procedures	
Anthropometric Measurements	• Weight loss
Physical Exam Findings	• Dry mucous membranes, hoarse or wet voice, tongue extrusion

Edition: 2008

BEHAVIORAL-ENVIRONMENTAL DOMAIN • Physical Activity and Function

SELF-FEEDING DIFFICULTY (NB-2.6)

Food/Nutrition History	Reports or observations of: ▪ Being provided with foods that may not be conducive to self-feeding, e.g., peas, broth-type soups ▪ Poor lip closure, drooling ▪ Dropping of cups, utensils ▪ Emotional distress, anxiety, or frustration surrounding mealtimes ▪ Failure to recognize foods ▪ Forgets to eat ▪ Inappropriate use of food ▪ Refusal to eat or chew ▪ Dropping of food from utensil (splashing and spilling of food) on repeated attempts to feed ▪ Lack of strength or stamina to lift utensils and/or cup ▪ Utensil biting
Client History	▪ Conditions associated with a diagnosis or treatment of, e.g., neurological disorders, Parkinson's, Alzheimer's, Tardive dyskinesia, multiple sclerosis, stroke, paralysis, developmental delay ▪ Physical limitations, e.g., fractured arms, traction, contractures ▪ Surgery requiring recumbent position ▪ Dementia/organic brain syndrome ▪ Dysphagia ▪ Shortness of breath ▪ Tremors

References

1. Consultant Dietitians in Healthcare Facilities. *Dining Skills Supplement: Practical Interventions for Caregivers of Eating Disabled Older Adults.* Pensacola, FL: American Dietetic Association; 1992.
2. Morley JE. Anorexia of aging: physiological and pathologic. *Am J Clin Nutr.* 1997; 66:760-773.
3. Position of the American Dietetic Association: Providing nutrition services for infants, children, and adults with developmental disabilities and special health care needs. *J Am Diet Assoc.* 2004:104:97-107.
4. Sandman P, Norberg A, Adolfsson R, Eriksson S, Nystrom L. Prevalence and characteristics of persons with dependency on feeding at institutions. *Scand J Caring Sci.* 1990;4:121-127.
5. Siebens H, Trupe E, Siebens A, Cooke F, Anshen S, Hanauer R, Oster G. Correlates and consequences of feeding dependency. *J Am Geriatr Soc.* 1986;34:192-198.
6. Vellas B, Fitten LJ, eds. *Research and Practice in Alzheimer's Disease.* New York, NY: Springer Publishing Company; 1998.

Updated: 2008 Edition

Edition: 2008

INTAKE OF UNSAFE FOOD (NB-3.1)

Definition

Intake of food and/or fluids intentionally or unintentionally contaminated with toxins, poisonous products, infectious agents, microbial agents, additives, allergens, and/or agents of bioterrorism.

Etiology (Cause/Contributing Risk Factors)

Factors gathered during the nutrition assessment process that contribute to the existence or the maintenance of pathophysiological, psychosocial, situational, developmental, cultural, and/or environmental problems:

- Lack of knowledge about potentially unsafe food
- Lack of knowledge about proper food/feeding, (infant and enteral formula, breast milk) storage and preparation
- Exposure to contaminated water or food, e.g., community outbreak of illness documented by surveillance and/or response agency
- Mental illness, confusion, or altered awareness
- Inadequate food storage equipment/facilities, e.g., refrigerator
- Inadequate safe food supply, e.g., inadequate markets with safe, uncontaminated food

Signs/Symptoms (Defining Characteristics)

A typical cluster of subjective and objective signs and symptoms gathered during the nutrition assessment process that provide evidence that a problem exists; quantify the problem and describe its severity.

Nutrition Assessment Category	Potential Indicators of this Nutrition Diagnosis (one or more must be present)
Biochemical Data, Medical Tests and Procedures	• Positive stool culture for infectious causes, such as listeria, salmonella, hepatitis A, E. coli, cyclospora
	• Toxicology reports for drugs, medicinals, poisons in blood or food samples
Anthropometric Measurements	
Physical Examination Findings	• Evidence of dehydration, e.g., dry mucous membranes, damaged tissues

167

BEHAVIORAL-ENVIRONMENTAL DOMAIN • Food Safety and Access

INTAKE OF UNSAFE FOOD (NB-3.1)

Food/Nutrition History	Reports or observations of intake of potential unsafe foods:
	▪ Mercury content of fish, non-food items (pregnant and lactating women)
	▪ Raw eggs, unpasteurized milk products, soft cheeses, undercooked meats (infants, children, immunocompromised persons, pregnant and lactating women, and elderly)
	▪ Wild plants, berries, mushrooms
	▪ Unsafe food/feeding storage and preparation practices (enteral and infant formula, breast milk)
Client History	▪ Conditions associated with a diagnosis or treatment, e.g., foodborne illness, such as, bacterial, viral, and parasitic infection, mental illness, dementia
	▪ Poisoning by drugs, medicinals, and biological substances
	▪ Poisoning from poisonous food stuffs and poisonous plants
	▪ Diarrhea, cramping, bloating, fever, nausea, vomiting, vision problems, chills, dizziness, headache
	▪ Cardiac, neurologic, respiratory changes

References

1. Centers for Disease Control and Prevention. Diagnosis and Management of Foodborne Illnesses: A Primer for Physicians and Other Health Care Professionals. Available at: www.cdc.gov/mmwr/preview/mmwrhtml/rr5304a1.htm. Accessed July 2, 2004.

2. Food Safety and Inspection Service. The Fight BAC Survey Tool and Data Entry Tool. Available at: www.fsis.usda.gov/OA/fses/bac_datatool.htm. Accessed July 2, 2004.

3. Gerald BL, Perkin JE. Food and water safety. *J Am Diet Assoc.* 2003;103:1203-1218.

4. Partnership for Food Safety Education. Four steps. Available at: http://www.fightbac.org/foursteps.cfm?section=4. Accessed July 2, 2004.

LIMITED ACCESS TO FOOD (NB-3.2)

Definition

Diminished ability to acquire a sufficient quantity and variety of healthful food based upon the U.S. Dietary Guidelines or MyPyramid. Limitation to food because of concerns about weight or aging.

Etiology (*Cause/Contributing Risk Factors*)

Factors gathered during the nutrition assessment process that contribute to the existence or the maintenance of pathophysiological, psychosocial, situational, developmental, cultural, and/or environmental problems:

- Caregiver intentionally or unintentionally not providing access to food, e.g., unmet needs for food or eating assistance, excess of poor nutritional quality food, abuse/neglect

- Community and geographical constraints for shopping and transportation

- Food and nutrition-related knowledge deficit

- Lack of financial resources or lack of access to financial resources to purchase a sufficient quantity or variety of culturally appropriate healthful foods

- Lack of food planning, purchasing, and preparation skills

- Limited, absent, or failure to participate in community supplemental food programs, e.g., food pantries, emergency kitchens, or shelters, with a sufficient variety of culturally appropriate healthful foods

- Failure to participate in federal food programs such as WIC, National School Breakfast/Lunch Program, food stamps

- Schools lacking nutrition/wellness policies or application of policies ensuring convenient, appetizing, competitively priced culturally appropriate healthful foods at meals, snacks, and school sponsored activities.

- Physical or psychological limitations that diminish ability to shop, e.g., walking, sight, mental/emotional health

Signs/Symptoms (*Defining Characteristics*)

A typical cluster of subjective and objective signs and symptoms gathered during the nutrition assessment process that provide evidence that a problem exists; quantify the problem and describe its severity.

Nutrition Assessment Category	Potential Indicators of this Nutrition Diagnosis (one or more must be present)
Biochemical Data, Medical Tests and Procedures	▪ Indicators of macronutrient or vitamin/mineral status as indicated by physical findings, food/nutrition, and client history

Behavioral

169

BEHAVIORAL-ENVIRONMENTAL DOMAIN • Food Safety and Access

LIMITED ACCESS TO FOOD (NB-3.2)

Anthropometric Measurements	▪ Growth failure, based on National Center for Health Statistics (NCHS) growth standards
	▪ Underweight (BMI <18.5)
Physical Exam Findings	▪ Findings consistent with vitamin/mineral deficiency
Food/Nutrition History	Reports or observations of:
	▪ Food faddism or harmful beliefs and attitudes of parent or caregiver
	▪ Belief that aging can be slowed by dietary limitations and extreme exercise
	▪ Hunger
	▪ Inadequate intake of food and/or specific nutrients
	▪ Limited supply of food in home
	▪ Limited variety of foods
Client History	▪ Malnutrition, vitamin/mineral deficiency
	▪ Illness or physical disability
	▪ Conditions associated with a diagnosis or treatment, e.g., mental illness, dementia
	▪ Lack of suitable support systems

References

1. Position of the American Dietetic Association: Food insecurity and hunger in thei United States. *J Am Diet Assoc.* 2006;106:446-458.
2. Position of the American Dietetic Association: Addressing world hunger, malnutrition, and food insecurity. *J Am Diet Assoc.* 2003;103:1046-1057.

Updated: 2008 Edition

170

SNAPshot
NCP Step 3. Nutrition Intervention

What is the purpose of a nutrition intervention? The purpose is to resolve or improve the identified nutrition problem by planning and implementing appropriate nutrition interventions that are tailored to the patient/client's* needs.

How does a dietetics practitioner determine a nutrition intervention? The selection of nutrition interventions is driven by the nutrition diagnosis and its etiology. Nutrition intervention strategies are purposefully selected to change nutritional intake, nutrition-related knowledge or behavior, environmental condition, or access to supportive care and services. Nutrition intervention goals provide the basis for monitoring progress and measuring outcomes.

How are the Nutrition Intervention strategies organized? In four categories:

Food and/or Nutrient Delivery	**Nutrition Education**	**Nutrition Counseling**	**Coordination of Nutrition Care**
An individualized approach for food/nutrient provision, including meals and snacks, enteral and parenteral feeding, and supplements	*A formal process to instruct or train a patient/client in a skill or to impart knowledge to help patients/clients voluntarily manage or modify food choices and eating behavior to maintain or improve health*	*A supportive process, characterized by a collaborative counselor-patient relationship, to set priorities, establish goals and create individualized action plans that acknowledge and foster responsibility for self-care to treat an existing condition and promote health*	*Consultation with, referral to, or coordination of nutrition care with other health care providers, institutions, or agencies that can assist in treating or managing nutrition-related problems*

Intervention

What does Nutrition Intervention involve? Nutrition intervention entails two distinct and interrelated components—planning and implementing. Planning the nutrition intervention involves: a) prioritizing nutrition diagnoses, b) consulting ADA's *MNT Evidence-Based Guides for Practice* and other practice guides, c) determining patient-focused expected outcomes for each nutrition diagnosis, d) conferring with patient/client/ caregivers, e) defining a nutrition intervention plan and strategies, f) defining time and frequency of care, and g) identifying resources needed. Implementation is the action phase and involves: a) communication of the nutrition care plan, b) carrying out the plan.

Critical thinking skills required during this step...
- Setting goals and prioritizing
- Defining the nutrition prescription or basic plan
- Making interdisciplinary connections
- Initiating behavioral and other nutrition interventions
- Matching nutrition intervention strategies with client needs, nutrition diagnosis, and values
- Choosing from among alternatives to determine a course of action
- Specifying the time and frequency of care

Are dietetics practitioners limited to the Nutrition Interventions listed in this reference?
Nutrition intervention terminology includes commonly used strategies and emphasizes the application of evidence-based strategies matched to appropriate circumstances. Evaluation of the nutrition intervention terminology is ongoing and will guide future modifications. Dietetics practitioners can propose additions or revisions using the Procedure for Nutrition Controlled Vocabulary/Terminology Maintenance/Review available from ADA.

Detailed information about this step can be found in the International Dietetics and Nutrition Terminology (IDNT) Reference Manual: Standardized Language for the Nutrition Care Process, First Edition, American Dietetic Association.

*Patient/client refers to individuals, groups, family members, and/or caregivers.

Edition: 2008

Nutrition Care Process Step 3. Nutrition Intervention

INTRODUCTION

Nutrition intervention is the third step in the Nutrition Care Process, preceded by nutrition assessment and nutrition diagnosis. Nutrition intervention is defined as purposefully planned actions designed with the intent of changing a nutrition-related behavior, environmental condition, or aspect of health status for an individual (and his/her family or caregivers), target group, or the community at large. A dietetics practitioner works in conjunction with the patient/client(s) and other health care providers, programs, or agencies during the nutrition intervention phase.

While nutrition intervention is one step in the process, it consists of two interrelated components—planning and implementation. Planning involves prioritizing the nutrition diagnoses, conferring with the patient/client and/or others, reviewing practice guides and policies, and setting goals and defining the specific nutrition intervention strategy. Implementation of the nutrition intervention is the action phase that includes carrying out and communicating the plan of care, continuing data collection, and revising the nutrition intervention strategy, as warranted, based on the patient/client response.

When drafting the specific nutrition intervention terms, the Standardized Language Task Force endeavored to include the type of information necessary for medical record documentation, billing, and the description of nutrition interventions for research. Further, it is intentional that the nutrition intervention terminology distinguishes between two distinct nutrition interventions, such as nutrition education and nutrition counseling. The plan can include more that one nutrition intervention that may be implemented simultaneously during the actual interaction with the patient/client.

The nutrition intervention terminology is organized into four domains—Food and/or Nutrient Delivery, Nutrition Education, Nutrition Counseling, and Coordination of Nutrition Care. Each domain is defined with classes of nutrition interventions. Reference sheets for each nutrition intervention term define the nutrition intervention terms, list typical details for the nutrition intervention, and illustrate the potential connection to the nutrition diagnoses.

The nature of a single nutrition intervention encounter with a patient/client can be described in many ways. It could include face-to-face contact with the patient/client or an encounter via electronic mail (e-mail) or telephone. The encounter may involve an individual or group and may be described in varying increments of contact time. Throughout the course of nutrition care, the dietetics practitioner and patient/client might engage in several encounters (i.e., interactions, visits, contacts) aimed at helping the patient/client implement the nutrition intervention(s). Nutrition interventions in the Food and/or Nutrient Delivery class and Coordination of Nutrition Care class may occur without direct patient/client contact (e.g., change in enteral formula).

At all levels of practice, dietetics practitioners are competent to provide many types of nutrition interventions. However, dietetics practitioners' roles and responsibilities vary with experience, education, training, practice setting, employer expectations, and local standards of care. Responsible dietetics practitioners ensure that they are competent to practice by participating in continuing education activities and obtaining necessary education, training, and credentials related to their area of practice. The Scope of Dietetics Practice and Framework documents (available at www.eatright.org in the Practice section) provide guidance to the dietetics practitioner in identifying activities within and outside the Scope of Practice. The ADA Code of Ethics, Dietetic Practice Groups, and specialty groups also have documents that help identify appropriate dietetics practitioner roles and responsibilities.

Individualized nutrition interventions, based on a patient/client's needs identified through nutrition assessment and nutrition diagnosis, are the product of this step of the nutrition care process. Using a standardized terminology for describing the nutrition interventions extends the ability of the dietetics practitioner to document, communicate, and research the impact of nutrition care on health and disease.

What is New in this Edition Related to Nutrition Intervention?

This edition modified one nutrition education reference sheet and expanded the nutrition counseling component of nutrition intervention. Changes include:

Comprehensive Nutrition Education (E-2)
- Skill development was added to this reference sheet as an element of Comprehensive Nutrition Education.

Nutrition Counseling

Theoretical Basis/Approach (C-1) is the new title of the first reference sheet.
- This aspect of nutrition counseling was retitled from *Theory or Approach* to communicate that theory is not something a dietetics practitioner does, but influences the approach he/she takes with a patient/client. A reference sheet was developed to reflect theoretical basis/approach, defining four theories commonly used in planning nutrition interventions.
- Behavioral Theory was eliminated, because it is rarely, if ever, done without a cognitive component.
- Health Belief Model was added because it helps explain a patient/client's motivation for change.

Strategies (C-2) is a second reference sheet added describing commonly used strategies.
- The strategy *rewards/reinforcement* was relabeled *rewards/contingency management* based on the literature.
- The strategy *stimulus control/contingency management* was shortened to *stimulus control*.
- *Relapse prevention* was added as a strategy, because this is a valuable strategy used in the maintenance phase of the change process.
- *Phases of counseling* were deleted because they were not generally recognized.

Dietetics practitioners engaging in nutrition counseling are asked to indicate for each encounter both the theoretical basis or approach they are using (may be multiple) and the strategy or strategies they are using within a particular encounter.

Nutrition Intervention Components

Planning and implementation are the two components of nutrition intervention. These components are interrelated, and the dietetics practitioner will make decisions about the nutrition intervention when both planning and implementation are feasible.

Planning the Nutrition Intervention

As a dietetics practitioner plans the nutrition intervention, he/she prioritizes the nutrition diagnoses, based on the severity of the problem, safety, patient/client need, likelihood that the nutrition intervention will impact the problem, and the patient/client perception of importance.

To determine which nutrition diagnosis can be positively impacted, a dietetics practitioner needs to examine the relationship between the pieces of the nutrition diagnosis and the nutrition intervention. It has been previously established that the nutrition diagnosis defines the problem, etiology, and the signs and symptoms based on data from the nutrition assessment.

Intervention

Edition: 2008

Relationships

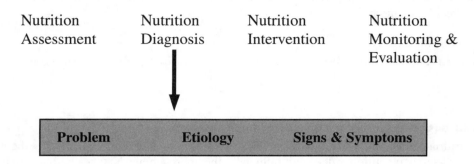

The nutrition intervention is directed, whenever possible, at the etiology or cause of the problem identified in the PES (i.e., problem, etiology, and signs/symptoms) statements. In some cases, it is not possible to direct the nutrition intervention at the etiology if the etiology cannot be changed by a dietetics practitioner. For example, if Excessive Energy Intake (NI-1.5) is caused by depression, the nutrition intervention is aimed at reducing the impact of the signs and symptoms of the problem, e.g., weight gain due to energy intake more than estimated needs.

Relationships

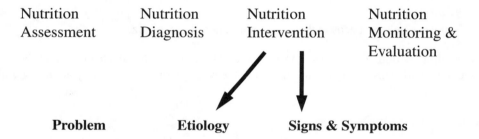

Follow-up monitoring of the signs and symptoms is used to determine the impact of the nutrition intervention on the etiology of the problem.

Relationships

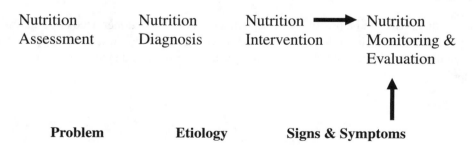

Another aspect of planning the nutrition intervention is referring to evidence-based guidelines, institutional policies and procedures, care maps, and other resources for recommended nutrition interventions, medical nutrition therapy goals, behavior changes, and/or expected outcomes. *ADA's MNT Evidence-Based Guides for Practice* provides science-based recommendations for nutrition interventions. Dietetics practitioners should carefully examine resources to determine if the recommendations are evidence-based.

An essential part of planning the nutrition intervention is detailing the Nutrition Prescription. The nutrition prescription concisely states the patient/client's individualized recommended dietary intake of energy and/or selected foods or nutrients based on current reference standards and dietary guidelines and the patient/client's health condition and nutrition diagnosis. It is determined using the assessment data, the nutrition diagnostic statement (PES), current evidence, policies and procedures, and patient/client values and preferences. The nutrition prescription either drives the nutrition intervention selection or is the context within which the nutrition intervention should be implemented. With the nutrition prescription defined, the dietetics practitioner identifies the specific nutrition intervention strategies and establishes the patient/client-focused goals to be accomplished.

Goal Setting

This is the time to establish clear patient/client goals that are measurable, achievable, and time-defined. In many cases, the goals are jointly set with the patient/client; however, this is not always possible in the case of patients/clients receiving enteral or parenteral nutrition, for example. In goal setting, the individual(s) responsible for the associated actions to achieve the goals is/are clearly identified.

These steps are essential because it is impossible to assess the impact of the nutrition intervention without quantifying or qualifying the goals so they can be measured. If the goals are not achievable, even the most appropriate nutrition intervention could be judged as unsuccessful. Additionally, the time for achieving the individual goals should be delineated into short-term (next visit) and long-term goals (over the course of the nutrition intervention).

The parties responsible for establishing the goals and the associated actions—such as joint development with patient/client and/or family or solely provider-directed (e.g., patient/client unable to participate in interaction and family/other not available)—need to be documented.

Planning Summary:
- Prioritize the nutrition diagnoses, based on problem severity, safety, patient/client need, likelihood that the nutrition intervention will impact the problem, and patient/client perception of importance
- Consult *ADA's MNT Evidence-Based Guides for Practice* and other practice guides/policies
- Confer with patient/client and other caregivers, or refer to policies throughout planning step
- Detail the nutrition prescription and identify the specific nutrition intervention strategies
- Determine patient/client-focused goals/expected outcomes
- Define time and frequency of care

Implementing the Nutrition Intervention

Implementation is the action portion of the nutrition intervention in which dietetics practitioners carry out and communicate the plan of care to all relevant parties, continue the data collection that was initiated with the nutrition assessment, and revise the nutrition intervention based on the patient/client response.

Once a dietetics practitioner has verified that the nutrition intervention is occurring, the data collected will also provide evidence of the response(s) and potentially lead to revision of the nutrition intervention.

Implementation Summary:
- Action phase
  - o Communicate the plan of care
  - o Carry out the plan
  - o Continue data collection
- Other aspects
  - o Individualize nutrition intervention
  - o Collaborate with other colleagues
  - o Follow-up and verify that nutrition intervention is occurring
  - o Adjust intervention strategies, if needed, as response occurs

NUTRITION INTERVENTION TERMS

The Standardized Language Task Force identified four domains of nutrition interventions—Food and/or Nutrient Delivery, Nutrition Education, Nutrition Counseling, and Coordination of Care—and defined classes within them. These domains and classes are intended to be used by all dietetics practitioners in all nutrition intervention settings (e.g., community, public health, home care, long-term care, private practice, and pediatric and adult acute care). Currently, the nutrition intervention terms are being tested for usability and validity in clinical settings. The specific nutrition intervention domains and classes are:

Food and/or Nutrient Delivery (ND) refers to an individualized approach for food/ nutrient provision.

Meal and Snacks (ND-1)—meals are regular eating events that include a variety of foods consisting of grains and/or starches, meat and/or meat alternatives, fruits and vegetables, and milk or milk products. A snack is defined as food served between regular meals.

Enteral and Parenteral Nutrition (ND-2)—nutrition provided through the gastrointestinal tract via tube, catheter, or stoma that delivers nutrients distal to the oral cavity (enteral) or the administration of nutrients intravenously (centrally or peripherally) (parenteral).

Supplements (ND-3)—foods or nutrients that are not intended as a sole item or a meal or diet, but that are intended to provide additional nutrients.

Medical Food Supplement (ND-3.1)—commercial or prepared foods or beverages intended to supplement the nutrient intake in energy, protein, carbohydrate, fiber, and/or fat, which may also contribute to vitamin and mineral intake.

Vitamin and Mineral Supplement (ND-3.2)—a product that is intended to supplement vitamin or mineral intake.

Bioactive Substance Supplement (ND-3.3)—a product that is intended to supplement bioactive substances (e.g., plant stanol and sterol esters, psyllium).

Feeding Assistance (ND-4)—accommodation or assistance in eating designed to restore the patient/ client's ability to eat independently, support adequate nutrient intake, and reduce the incidence of unplanned weight loss and dehydration.

Feeding Environment (ND-5)—adjustment of the physical environment, temperature, convenience, and attractiveness of the location where food is served that impacts food consumption.

Nutrition-Related Medication Management (ND-6)—modification of a drug or herbal to optimize patient/client nutritional or health status.

Nutrition Education (E) is a formal process to instruct or train a patient/client in a skill or to impart knowledge to help patients/clients voluntarily manage or modify food choices and eating behavior to maintain or improve health.

Initial/Brief Nutrition Education (E-1)—instruction or training intended to build or reinforce basic nutrition-related knowledge, or to provide essential nutrition-related information until patient/client returns.

Comprehensive Nutrition Education (E-2)—instruction or training intended to lead to in-depth nutrition-related knowledge and/or skills in given topics.

Nutrition Counseling (C) is a supportive process, characterized by a collaborative counselor-patient/client relationship, to set priorities, establish goals, and create individualized action plans that acknowledge and foster responsibility for self-care to treat an existing condition and promote health.

Theoretical basis/approach (C-1)--the theories or models used to design and implement an intervention. Theories and theoretical models consist of principles, constructs and variables, which offer systematic explanations of the human behavior change process. Behavior change theories and models provide a research-based rational for designing and tailoring nutrition interventions to achieve the desired effect. A theoretical framework for curriculum and treatment protocols, it guides determination of: 1) what information patients/clients need at different points in the behavior change process, 2) what tools and strategies may be best applied to facilitate behavior change, and 3) outcome measures to assess effectiveness in interventions or components of interventions.

Strategies (C-2)--An evidence-based method or plan of action designed to achieve a particular goal. Application of behavior change theories in nutrition practice has provided practitioners with a collection of evidence-based strategies to promote behavior change. Some strategies target change in motivation and intention to change, and others target behavior change. Dietetics practitioners selectively apply strategies based upon patient/client goals and objectives, and their personal counseling philosophy and skill.

Dietetics practitioners engaging in nutrition counseling are asked to indicate for each encounter both the theoretical basis or approach they are using (may be multiple) and the strategy or strategies they are using within a particular encounter.

Coordination of Nutrition Care (RC) is consultation with, referral to, or coordination of nutrition care with other health care providers, institutions, or agencies that can assist in treating or managing nutrition-related problems.

Coordination of Other Care During Nutrition Care (RC-1)—facilitating services or interventions with other professionals, institutions, or agencies on behalf of the patient/client prior to discharge from nutrition care.

Discharge and Transfer of Nutrition Care to New Setting or Provider (RC-2)—discharge planning and transfer of nutrition care from one level or location of care to another.

Nutrition Education vs. Nutrition Counseling

As mentioned earlier, it is intentional to *separate* nutrition education from nutrition counseling even though a dietetics practitioner may use both of these nutrition interventions at one time.

Nutrition education involves the transfer of knowledge, tailored to the specific knowledge deficit identified in the PES statement. *Nutrition counseling* involves behavior and attitude change, focused on the underlying behavioral and environmental etiologies identified in the nutrition assessment and documented in the PES statement. The etiologies leading to the two interventions differ. Knowledge deficit or no previous exposure to information would lead to nutrition education. Etiologies reflecting attitudinal issues (e.g., readiness to change, lack of willingness to change) would lead to counseling. In these cases, the patient/client knows what to do but has been unable to make or sustain a behavioral change. Therefore, these nutrition interventions are *separated* to highlight the difference between them and to show the true nature of the interaction(s) between dietetics practitioner and patient/client. This will assist a practitioner in thinking about providing distinct education and counseling approaches, while moving seamlessly between these two activities.

Uses of Nutrition Interventions Based on Practice Setting

The typical uses of the nutrition interventions may vary by practice setting, but are not limited based upon the practice setting.

- Food and/or Nutrient Delivery nutrition interventions will commonly be used by dietetics practitioners in institutional settings (e.g., hospitals, long-term care) and home care.
- Nutrition Education interventions—Initial/Brief Education (E-1) and Comprehensive Education (E-2)—Initial/Brief Education will be utilized more often in institutionalized settings and Comprehensive Education will be utilized more often in outpatient/noninstitutionalized settings (e.g., outpatient offices, private practice, community).
- Nutrition Counseling will likely be used more by dietetics practitioners in outpatient/noninstitutionalized settings (e.g., outpatient offices, private practice, community) due to the nature of the nutrition intervention and the practice setting.
- Coordination of Nutrition Care interventions will be used by dietetics practitioners from a variety of practice settings.

It is important to reiterate that these are *typical* uses of specific nutrition interventions. Dietetics practitioners in any practice setting can use the complete array of nutrition interventions as needed.

NUTRITION INTERVENTION REFERENCE SHEETS

A reference sheet for each nutrition intervention has been developed that includes the nutrition intervention label and its definition, descriptive details of the nutrition intervention, and the nutrition diagnoses with which the nutrition intervention might typically be used. Additional considerations pertinent to the nutrition intervention are also included. A partial example of a nutrition intervention reference sheet follows here:

> *Example*
>
> #### Feeding Assistance (ND-4)
>
> **Defined as** accommodation or assistance in eating designed to restore the patient/client's ability to eat independently, support adequate nutrient intake, and reduce the incidence of unplanned weight loss and dehydration.
>
> **Details of Nutrition Intervention**: A typical nutrition intervention might be further described with the following details:
> - Recommends, implements, or orders adaptive equipment, feeding position, feeding cues, meal set-up, or mouth care to facilitate eating
> - Recommends, designs, or implements a restorative dining program
> - Recommends, designs, or implements a feeding assistance training program
> - Recommends, designs, or implements menu selections that foster, promote, and maintain independent eating

These reference sheets are designed to assist dietetics practitioners with consistent and correct utilization of the nutrition interventions and are available beginning on page 186.

ENCOUNTER DETAILS

A single nutrition intervention encounter (i.e., interactions, visits, contacts, sessions) includes time spent reviewing the medical record or patient/client information and direct (i.e., face-to-face) or indirect (e.g., electronic, phone) contact with the patient/client and his/her family or caregiver. With the expanded use of electronic communication has come the growth of nutrition interventions via methods like e-mail and webinars (seminars on the Internet), along with phone and teleconference encounters.

Encounters may involve an individual or group where:
- An individual is one person with his/her family or caregiver
- A group is intended to meet more than one individual's needs

A typical method to indicate contact time in ambulatory care is in increments of 15 minutes (one unit = 15 minutes). Naturally, throughout a course of nutrition care, the dietetics practitioner and patient/client might engage in several encounters.

Roles and Responsibilities

Dietetics practice is such that practitioners differ in their need, desire, opportunity, experience, or credentials to perform various nutrition interventions. Generalist dietetics practitioners may maintain competence in a wide variety of nutrition interventions, while specialty dietetics practitioners may develop in-depth expertise with a few nutrition interventions. Some of the nutrition interventions described in the reference sheets (e.g., nutrition counseling, enteral and parenteral nutrition, or nutrition-related medication management) may require specialty or advanced education and/or training.

Practice roles and responsibilities may vary according to employer expectations or institutional tradition. Regulations, in certain practice settings, may be interpreted as restricting intervention to that authorized by order of a physician or others. Protocols may be used to allow interventions to be implemented or modified. Clinical privileges allow dietetics practitioners to autonomously intervene according to a specified scope of practice. Obtaining clinical privileges or being granted authority to make independent changes to a patient/ client's nutrition prescription or nutrition intervention may be needed. In some situations, such as private practice or community settings, a dietetics practitioner may have complete autonomy. Further, depending on the setting, the dietetics practitioner may assume various levels of autonomy for different nutrition interventions. Examples are provided below:

- *Implements the specified nutrition intervention; recommends initiating, modifying, or discontinuing a nutrition intervention as appropriate.* On completion of a nutrition assessment, the dietetics practitioner may recommend (verbally or by writing) refinements, modifications, or alternative nutrition interventions that require affirmation before they can be implemented.

    Example: The dietetics practitioner assesses a patient/client on a general diet and notices elevated serum cholesterol and triglyceride levels. The dietetics practitioner recommends a modification of the nutrition prescription to the physician or nurse practitioner, and modifies the nutrition prescription on affirmation of the recommendation.

- *Implements, within the parameters of an approved protocol or algorithm, initiation, modification, or discontinuance of a nutrition intervention.* On completion of a nutrition assessment, the dietetics practitioner modifies the original nutrition intervention within preapproved parameters.

    Example: The dietetics practitioner assesses a patient/client with a general nutrition prescription and notices elevated serum cholesterol, triglyceride, and blood glucose levels. According to an approved treatment algorithm, the dietetics practitioner can implement a "heart healthy" nutrition prescription for any patient/client with a serum cholesterol level more than 200 mg/dL. The dietetics practitioner changes the nutrition prescription to "heart healthy," initiates patient/client nutrition education, and documents the change and other details of the nutrition intervention in the medical record. Because the algorithm does not specify the nutrition intervention for hyperglycemia, the dietetics practitioner must provide (verbally or in writing) recommendations for an additional carbohydrate restriction or management in the nutrition prescription, then await affirmation for implementation.

Intervention

Edition: 2008

- *Independently orders initiation, modification, or discontinuance of a nutrition intervention based on a scope of practice. Authority may be specified in an approved clinical privileging document or inherent in the setting.* On completion of the nutrition assessment, the dietetics practitioner is able to initiate, modify, or discontinue a nutrition intervention based on independent clinical judgment.

    Example: The dietetics practitioner assesses a patient/client with a general nutrition prescription, and notices elevated serum cholesterol, triglyceride levels, and blood glucose levels. In this setting, a dietetics practitioner has the autonomy to order, change, and implement nutrition prescriptions designed to manage disorders of lipid, carbohydrate, protein, and energy metabolism. The dietetics practitioner changes the nutrition prescription to "heart healthy" with consistent carbohydrate intake and initiates patient/client nutrition education and other details of the nutrition intervention as appropriate.

The table provides examples of the common level of autonomy in a few practice settings:

Setting	Common Triggers	Common Levels of Autonomy
Inpatient	Physician or advanced practice nurse **orders** a diet or **requests** a consultation or the patient is **identified** at risk by screening criteria	• Implements the specified nutrition intervention; recommends initiating, modifying, or discontinuing a nutrition intervention. • Implements, within the parameters of an approved protocol or algorithm, initiation, modification, or discontinuance of a nutrition intervention. • Independently orders initiation, modification, or discontinuance of a nutrition intervention based on a scope of practice. Authority is usually specified in an approved clinical privileging document.
Outpatient	Physician or advanced practice nurse **refers** the patient/client or the patient/client is **self-referred**	• Implements the specified nutrition intervention; recommends initiating, modifying, or discontinuing a nutrition intervention. • Implements, within the parameters of an approved protocol or algorithm, initiation, modification, or discontinuance of a nutrition intervention. • Independently orders initiation, modification, or discontinuance of a nutrition intervention based on a scope of practice. Authority may be specified in an approved clinical privileging document or inherent in practice setting.
Private Practice	Physician or advanced practice nurse **refers** the patient/client or the patient/client is **self- referred**	• Independently orders initiation, modification, or discontinuance of a nutrition intervention based on scope of practice.
Community	Client is **self-referred** or is identified at risk by screening criteria	• Independently orders initiation, modification, or discontinuance of a nutrition intervention based on scope of practice.

As mentioned earlier, the Scope of Dietetics Practice and Framework documents provide guidance to the dietetics practitioner in identifying activities within and outside the Scope of Dietetics Practice. All Scope of Dietetics Practice documents are available on the ADA Web site, www.eatright.org, in the Practice section. Dietetic Practice Groups and specialty organizations have documents that help identify appropriate practitioner roles and responsibilities and dietetics practitioners should refer to these reports for guidance.

SUMMARY

Using a defined nutrition intervention terminology will assist the profession in communicating within and among a variety of providers. It will also be instrumental in documenting and researching the impact the profession has on specific diagnoses and/or etiologies in all patient/client populations. The nutrition intervention reference sheets are a tool that dietetics practitioners can use to select strategies and implement this aspect of the nutrition care process. Finally, evaluation of the nutrition intervention terminology is planned and will guide possible future modifications.

REFERENCES

1. Davis AM, Baker SS, Leary RA. Advancing clinical privileges for support practitioners: the dietitian as a model. *Nutr Clin Pract.* 1995;10:98-103.

2. Hager M. Hospital therapeutic diet orders and the Centers for Medicare & Medicaid Services: Steering through regulations to provide quality nutrition care and avoid survey citations. *J Am Diet Assoc.* 2006;106:198-204.

3. Kieselhorst KJ, Skates J, Pritchett E. American Dietetic Association: Standards of practice in nutrition care and updated standards of professional performance. *J Am Diet Assoc.* 2005;105:641-645.

4. Kulkarni K, Boucher J, Daly A, Shwide-Slavin C, Silvers B, Maillet JO, Pritchett E. American Dietetic Association: Standards of practice and standards of professional performance for registered dietitians (generalist, specialty, and advanced) in diabetes care. *J Am Diet Assoc.* 2005;105:819-824.

5. Lacey K, Pritchett E. Nutrition care process and model: ADA adopts road map to quality care and outcomes management. *J Am Diet Assoc.* 2003;103:1061-1072.

6. Mahan L, Escott-Stump S. *Krause's Food, Nutrition, & Diet Therapy. 11ᵗʰ ed.* Philadelphia, PA: Saunders; 2000.

7. Miller R, Rollnick S. *Motivational Interviewing: Preparing People for Change, 2ⁿᵈ ed.* New York, NY: Guilford Press; 2002.

8. Moreland K, Gotfried M, Vaughn L. Development and implementation of the clinical privileges for dietitian nutrition order writing program at a long-term acute-care hospital. *J Am Diet Assoc.* 2002;102:72-74.

9. Myers EF, Barnhill G, Bryk J. Clinical privileges: missing piece of the puzzle for clinical standards that elevate responsibilities and salaries for registered dietitians. *J Am Diet Assoc.* 2002;102:123-132.

10. O'Sullivan Maillet J, Skates J, Pritchett E. American Dietetic Association: Scope of dietetics practice framework. *J Am Diet Assoc.* 2005;105:634-640.

11. Silver H, Wellman N. Nutrition diagnosing and order writing: value for practitioners, quality for clients. *J Am Diet Assoc.* 2003;103:1470-1472.

Intervention

Edition: 2008

NUTRITION INTERVENTION TERMINOLOGY

Problem _____

Etiology _____

Signs/Symptoms _____

Nutrition Prescription
The patient's/client's individualized recommended dietary intake of energy and/or selected foods or nutrients based on current reference standards and dietary guidelines and the patient's/client's health condition and nutrition diagnosis. (*specify*)

_____

_____

_____

Intervention #1 _____

Goal (s) _____

_____

Intervention #2 _____

Goal (s) _____

_____

Intervention #3 _____

Goal (s) _____

_____

FOOD AND/OR NUTRIENT DELIVERY   ND

Meal and Snacks (1)
Regular eating event (meal); food served between regular meals (snack).
- ❑ General/healthful diet   ND-1.1
- ❑ Modify distribution, type,   ND-1.2
  or amount of food and nutrients
  within meals or at specified time
- ❑ Specific foods/beverages   ND-1.3
  or groups
- ❑ Other   ND-1.4
  (specify)

Enteral and Parenteral Nutrition (2)
Nutrition provided through the GI tract via tube, catheter, or stoma (enteral) or intravenously (centrally or peripherally) (parenteral).
- ❑ Initiate EN or PN   ND-2.1
- ❑ Modify rate, concentration,   ND-2.2
  composition or schedule
- ❑ Discontinue EN or PN   ND-2.3
- ❑ Insert enteral feeding tube   ND-2.4
- ❑ Site care   ND-2.5
- ❑ Other   ND-2.6
  (specify)

Supplements (3)
Medical Food Supplements (3.1)
Commercial or prepared foods or beverages that supplement energy, protein, carbohydrate, fiber, fat intake.
  Type
- ❑ Commercial beverage   ND-3.1.1
- ❑ Commercial food   ND-3.1.2
- ❑ Modified beverage   ND-3.1.3
- ❑ Modified food   ND-3.1.4
- ❑ Purpose   ND-3.1.5
  (specify)

Vitamin and Mineral Supplements (3.2)
Supplemental vitamins or minerals.
- ❑ Multivitamin/mineral   ND-3.2.1
- ❑ Multi-trace elements   ND-3.2.2
- ❑ Vitamin   ND-3.2.3
  - ❑ A   ❑ Riboflavin
  - ❑ C   ❑ Niacin
  - ❑ D   ❑ Folate
  - ❑ E   ❑ B6
  - ❑ K   ❑ B12
  - ❑ Thiamin
  - ❑ Other (specify) _____
- ❑ Mineral   ND-3.2.4
  - ❑ Calcium   ❑ Phosphorus
  - ❑ Iron   ❑ Potassium
  - ❑ Magnesium   ❑ Zinc
  - ❑ Other (specify) _____

Bioactive Substance Supplement (3.3)
Supplemental bioactive substances.
- ❑ Initiate   ND-3.3.1
- ❑ Dose change   ND-3.3.2
- ❑ Form change   ND-3.3.3
- ❑ Route change   ND-3.3.4
- ❑ Administration schedule   ND-3.3.5
- ❑ Discontinue   ND-3.3.6
  (specify)

Feeding Assistance (4)
Accommodation or assistance in eating.
- ❑ Adaptive equipment   ND-4.1
- ❑ Feeding position   ND-4.2
- ❑ Meal set-up   ND-4.3
- ❑ Mouth care   ND-4.4
- ❑ Other   ND-4.5
  (specify)

Feeding Environment (5)
Adjustment of the factors where food is served that impact food consumption.
- ❑ Lighting   ND-5.1
- ❑ Odors   ND-5.2
- ❑ Distractions   ND-5.3
- ❑ Table height   ND-5.4
- ❑ Table service/set up   ND-5.5
- ❑ Room temperature   ND-5.6
- ❑ Other   ND-5.7
  (specify)

Nutrition-Related Medication Management (6)
Modification of a drug or herbal to optimize patient/client nutritional or health status.
- ❑ Initiate   ND-6.1
- ❑ Dose change   ND-6.2
- ❑ Form change   ND-6.3
- ❑ Route change   ND-6.4
- ❑ Administration schedule   ND-6.5
- ❑ Discontinue   ND-6.6
  (specify)

NUTRITION EDUCATION   E

Initial/Brief Nutrition Education (1)
Build or reinforce basic or essential nutrition-related knowledge.
- ❑ Purpose of the nutrition education   E-1.1
- ❑ Priority modifications   E-1.2
- ❑ Survival information   E-1.3
- ❑ Other   E-1.4
  (specify)

Comprehensive Nutrition Education (2)
Instruction or training leading to in-depth nutrition-related knowledge or skills.
- ❑ Purpose of the nutrition education   E-2.1
- ❑ Recommended modifications   E-2.2
- ❑ Advanced or related topics   E-2.3

Comprehensive Nutrition Education (2) *cont'd*
- ❑ Result interpretation   E-2.4
- ❑ Skill development   E-2.5
- ❑ Other   E-2.6
  (specify)

NUTRITION COUNSELING   C

Theoretical Basis/Approach (1)
The theories or models used to design and implement an intervention.
- ❑ Cognitive-Behavioral Theory   C-1.2
- ❑ Health Belief Model   C-1.3
- ❑ Social Learning Theory   C-1.4
- ❑ Transtheoretical Model/   C-1.5
  Stages of Change
- ❑ Other   C-1.6
  (specify)

Strategies (2)
Selectively applied evidence-based methods or plans of action designed to achieve a particular goal.
- ❑ Motivational interviewing   C-2.1
- ❑ Goal setting   C-2.2
- ❑ Self-monitoring   C-2.3
- ❑ Problem solving   C-2.4
- ❑ Social support   C-2.5
- ❑ Stress management   C-2.6
- ❑ Stimulus control   C-2.7
- ❑ Cognitive restructuring   C-2.8
- ❑ Relapse prevention   C-2.9
- ❑ Rewards/contingency management   C-2.10
- ❑ Other
  (specify)

COORDINATION OF NUTRITION CARE   RC

Coordination of Other Care During Nutrition Care (1)
Facilitating services with other professionals, institutions, or agencies during nutrition care.
- ❑ Team meeting   RC-1.1
- ❑ Referral to RD with different   RC-1.2
  expertise
- ❑ Collaboration/referral to other   RC-1.3
  providers
- ❑ Referral to community agencies/   RC-1.4
  programs
  (specify)

Discharge and Transfer of Nutrition Care to New Setting or Provider (2)
Discharge planning and transfer of nutrition care from one level or location of care to another.
- ❑ Collaboration/referral to other   RC-2.1
  providers
- ❑ Referral to community   RC-2.2
  agencies/programs
  (specify)

NUTRITION INTERVENTION TERMS AND DEFINITIONS

Nutrition Intervention Term	Term Number	Definition	Reference Sheet Page Numbers
DOMAIN: FOOD AND/OR NUTRIENT DELIVERY	ND	**Individualized approach for food/nutrient provision.**	
Meals and Snacks	ND-1	Meals are defined as regular eating events that include a variety of foods consisting of grains and/or starches, meat and/or meat alternatives, fruits and vegetables, and milk or milk products. A snack is defined as food served between regular meals.	186-187
Enteral and Parenteral Nutrition	ND-2	Enteral nutrition is defined as nutrition provided through the gastrointestinal (GI) tract via tube, catheter, or stoma that delivers nutrients distal to the oral cavity. Parenteral nutrition is defined as the administration of nutrients intravenously, centrally (delivered into a large-diameter vein, usually the superior vena cava adjacent to the right atrium) or peripherally (delivered into a peripheral vein, usually of the hand or forearm).	188-189
Supplements	ND-3	Foods or nutrients that are not intended as a sole item or a meal or diet, but that are intended to provide additional nutrients.	
Medical Food Supplements	ND-3.1	Commercial or prepared foods or beverages intended to supplement energy, protein, carbohydrate, fiber, and/or fat intake that may also contribute to vitamin and mineral intake.	190-191
Vitamin and Mineral Supplements	ND-3.2	A product that is intended to supplement vitamin or mineral intake.	192-193
Bioactive Substance Supplement	ND-3.3	A product that is intended to supplement bioactive substances (e.g., plant stanol and sterol esters, psyllium).	194
Feeding Assistance	ND-4	Accommodation or assistance in eating designed to restore the patient's/client's ability to eat independently, support nutrient intake, and reduce the incidence of unplanned weight loss and dehydration.	195-196
Feeding Environment	ND-5	Adjustment of the physical environment, temperature, convenience, and attractiveness of the location where food is served that impacts food consumption.	197-197
Nutrition-Related Medication Management	ND-6	Modification of a drug or herbal to optimize patient/client nutritional or health status.	199-200

183

Intervention

NUTRITION INTERVENTION TERMS AND DEFINITIONS

Nutrition Intervention Term	Term Number	Definition	Reference Sheet Page Numbers
DOMAIN: NUTRITION EDUCATION	E	**Formal process to instruct or train a patient/client in a skill or to impart knowledge to help patients/clients voluntarily manage or modify food choices and eating behavior to maintain or improve health.**	
Initial/Brief Nutrition Education	E-1	Instruction or training intended to build or reinforce basic nutrition-related knowledge, or to provide essential nutrition-related information until patient/client returns.	201-202
Comprehensive Nutrition Education	E-2	Instruction or training intended to lead to in-depth nutrition-related knowledge and/or skills in given topics.	203-204
DOMAIN: NUTRITION COUNSELING	C	**A supportive process, characterized by a collaborative counselor-patient/client relationship, to set priorities, establish goals, and create individualized action plans that acknowledge and foster responsibility for self-care to treat an existing condition and promote health.**	
Theoretical basis/approach	C-1	The theories or models used to design and implement an intervention. Theories and theoretical models consist of principles, constructs and variables, which offer systematic explanations of the human behavior change process. Behavior change theories and models provide a research-based rational for designing and tailoring nutrition interventions to achieve the desired effect. A theoretical framework for curriculum and treatment protocols, it guides determination of: 1) what information patients/clients need at different points in the behavior change process, 2) what tools and strategies may be best applied to facilitate behavior change, and 3) outcome measures to assess effectiveness in interventions or components of interventions.	205-216
Strategies	C-2	An evidence-based method or plan of action designed to achieve a particular goal. Application of behavior change theories in nutrition practice has provided practitioners with a collection of evidence-based strategies to promote behavior change. Some strategies target change in motivation and intention to change, and others target behavior change. Dietetics practitioners selectively apply strategies based upon patient/client goals and objectives, and their personal counseling philosophy and skill.	217-224

Edition: 2008

NUTRITION INTERVENTION TERMS AND DEFINITIONS

Nutrition Intervention Term	Term Number	Definition	Reference Sheet Page Numbers
DOMAIN: COORDINATION OF NUTRITION CARE	RC	**Consultation with, referral to, or coordination of nutrition care with other providers, institutions, or agencies that can assist in treating or managing nutrition-related problems.**	
Coordination of Other Care During Nutrition Care	RC-1	Facilitating services or interventions with other professionals, institutions, or agencies on behalf of the patient/client prior to discharge from nutrition care.	225-227
Discharge and Transfer of Nutrition Care to New Setting or Provider	RC-2	Discharge planning and transfer of nutrition care from one level or location of care to another.	228-229

185

Intervention

Edition: 2008

FOOD AND/OR NUTRIENT DELIVERY DOMAIN

Food & Nutrient

MEALS AND SNACKS (ND-1)

Definition

Meals are defined as regular eating events that include a variety of foods consisting of grains and/or starches, meat and/or meat alternatives, fruits and vegetables, and milk or milk products. A snack is defined as food served between regular meals.

Details of Intervention

A typical intervention might be further described with the following details:

- Recommend, implement, or order an appropriate distribution of type or quantity of food and nutrients within meals or at specified times
- Identify specific food/beverage(s) or groups for meals and snacks

Typically used with the following

Nutrition Diagnostic Terminology Used in PES Statements	Common Examples (Not intended to be inclusive)
Nutrition Diagnoses	▪ Increased energy expenditure (NI-1.2) ▪ Excessive fat intake (NI-5.6.2) ▪ Excessive carbohydrate intake (NI-5.8.2) ▪ Inconsistent carbohydrate intake (NI-5.8.4)
Etiology	▪ Lack of access to healthful food choices, e.g., food provided by caregiver ▪ Physiologic causes, e.g., increased energy needs due to increased activity level or metabolic change, malabsorption ▪ Psychological causes, e.g., disordered eating ▪ Difficulty chewing, swallowing, extreme weakness

Edition: 2008

MEALS AND SNACKS (ND-1)

| Signs and Symptoms | Biochemical Data, Medical Tests and Procedures
  ▪ Serum cholesterol level > 200 mg/dL
  ▪ Hemoglobin A1C > 6%
Physical Assessment
  ▪ Weight change
  ▪ Dental caries
  ▪ Diarrhea in response to carbohydrate feeding
Food/Nutrition History
  ▪ Cultural or religious practices that do not support modified food/nutrition intake
  ▪ Changes in physical activity
  ▪ Intake of inappropriate foods
Client History
  ▪ Conditions associated with diagnosis or treatment, e.g., surgery, trauma, sepsis, diabetes mellitus, inborn errors of metabolism, digestive enzyme deficiency, obesity
  ▪ Chronic use of medications that increase or decrease nutrient requirements or impair nutrient metabolism |

Other considerations (*e.g., patient/client negotiation, patient/client needs and desires, and readiness to change*)

- Compliance skills and abilities
- Economic concerns with purchasing special food items
- Willingness/ability to change behavior to comply with diet
- Availability/access to a qualified practitioner for follow-up and monitoring

References

1. Lacey K, Pritchett E. Nutrition Care Process and Model: ADA adopts road map to quality care and outcomes management. *J Am Diet Assoc.* 2003;103:1061-1071.

Food & Nutrient

Edition: 2008

FOOD AND/OR NUTRIENT DELIVERY DOMAIN

ENTERAL AND PARENTERAL NUTRITION (ND-2)

Definition

Enteral nutrition is defined as nutrition provided through the gastrointestinal (GI) tract via tube, catheter, or stoma that delivers nutrients distal to the oral cavity. Parenteral nutrition is defined as the administration of nutrients intravenously, centrally (delivered into a large-diameter vein, usually the superior vena cava adjacent to the right atrium) or peripherally (delivered into a peripheral vein, usually of the hand or forearm).

Details of Intervention

A typical intervention might be further described with the following details:

- Recommend, implement, or order changes in the rate, composition, schedule, and/or duration of feeding
- Recommend, implement, or order the initiation, route, and discontinuation of enteral nutrition
- Insert the feeding tube, provide tube site care; administer feedings
- Change dressings and provide line care
- Review changes in the intervention with the patient/client(s) and/or caregivers

Typically used with the following

Nutrition Diagnostic Terminology Used in PES Statements	Common Examples (Not intended to be inclusive)
Nutrition Diagnoses	▪ Swallowing difficulties (NC-1.1) ▪ Altered GI function (NC-1.4) ▪ Inadequate oral food/beverage intake (NI-2.1) ▪ Inadequate intake from enteral/parenteral nutrition infusion (NI-2.3) ▪ Excessive intake from parenteral nutrition infusion (NI-2.4)
Etiology	▪ Altered gastrointestinal tract function, inability to absorb nutrients ▪ Inability to chew/swallow

Edition: 2008

ENTERAL AND PARENTERAL NUTRITION (ND-2)

Signs and Symptoms
Physical Assessment
▪ Weight loss > 10% in 6 months, > 5% in 1 month
▪ Obvious muscle wasting
▪ Skin turgor (tenting, edema)
▪ Growth failure
▪ Insufficient maternal weight gain
▪ BMI < 18.5
Food/Nutrition History
▪ Intake < 75% of requirements (insufficient intake)
▪ Existing or expected inadequate intake for 7-14 days
Client History
▪ Malabsorption, maldigestion
▪ Emesis
▪ Diffuse peritonitis, intestinal obstruction, paralytic ileus, intractable diarrhea or emesis, gastrointestinal ischemia, or perforated viscus, short-bowel syndrome

Other considerations *(e.g., patient/client negotiation, patient/client needs and desires, and readiness to change)*

- End-of-life issues, ethical considerations, patient/client rights and family/caregiver issues.
- Other nutrient intake (oral, parenteral, or enteral nutrition)
- Enteral formulary composition and product availability
- Availability/access to a qualified practitioner for follow-up and monitoring
- Economic constraints that limit availability of food/enteral/parenteral products

References

1. A.S.P.E.N. Board of Directors and Standards Committee. Definition of terms, style, and conventions used in A.S.P.E.N. guidelines and standards. *Nutr Clin Pract.* 2005;20:281-285.
2. A.S.P.E.N. Board of Directors and the Clinical Guidelines Task Force. Guidelines for the use of parenteral and enteral nutrition in adult and pediatric patients. *JPEN J Parenter Enteral Nutr.* 2002;26:1SA-138SA.
3. McClave SA, Lowen CC, Kleber MJ, Nicholson JF, Jimmerson SC, McConnell JW, Jung LY. Are patients fed appropriately according to their caloric requirements? *JPEN J Parenter Enteral Nutr.* 1998;22:375-381.
4. Mirtallo J, Canada T, Johnson D, Kumpf V, Petersen C, Sacks G, Seres D, Guenter P. Task force for the revision of safe practices for parenteral nutrition. *JPEN J Parenter Enteral Nutr.* 2004;28:S39-S70.

Food &
Nutrient

FOOD AND/OR NUTRIENT DELIVERY DOMAIN

MEDICAL FOOD SUPPLEMENTS (ND-3.1)

Definition

Commercial or prepared foods or beverages intended to supplement energy, protein, carbohydrate, fiber, and/or fat intake that may also contribute to vitamin and mineral intake.

Details of Intervention

A typical intervention might be further described with the following details:

- Recommend, implement, or order changes in an individualized feeding plan including the initiation, composition, type, frequency, timing, and discontinuation of oral supplements

- Describe the purpose of the supplement (e.g., to supplement energy, protein, carbohydrate, fiber, and/or fat intake)

Typically used with the following

Nutrition Diagnostic Terminology Used in PES Statements	Common Examples (Not intended to be all inclusive)
Nutrition Diagnoses	▪ Inadequate oral food/beverage intake (NI-2.1) ▪ Inadequate fluid intake (NI-3.1) ▪ Increased nutrient needs (NI-5.1)
Etiology	▪ Neurologic deficit (stroke) ▪ Difficulty chewing or swallowing ▪ Food allergies or intolerance ▪ Altered GI function ▪ Partial GI obstruction
Signs and Symptoms	Physical Examination Findings ▪ Weight loss > 10% in 6 months or > 5% in 1 month ▪ Obvious muscle wasting ▪ Poor skin turgor (tenting or edema) Food/Nutrition History ▪ Insufficient usual food/beverage intake Client History ▪ Diagnosis consistent with elevated nutrient needs ▪ Potential for repletion of nutritional status ▪ Ability to feed self ▪ Choking on foods, oral/facial trauma ▪ Insufficient vitamin-mineral intake

Edition: 2008

MEDICAL FOOD SUPPLEMENTS (ND-3.1)

Other considerations *(e.g., patient/client negotiation, patient/client needs and desires, and readiness to change)*

- Appetite sufficient to take medical food supplements
- System constraints that prevent meeting the client's preferences for specific flavors, textures, foods and the timing of feedings
- Availability of feeding assistance
- Economic concerns and product/food availability

References

1. Milne AC, Avenell A, Potter J. Meta-analysis: Protein and energy supplementation in older people. *Ann Intern Med.* 2006;144:37-48.

191

FOOD AND/OR NUTRIENT DELIVERY DOMAIN

VITAMIN OR MINERAL SUPPLEMENTS (ND-3.2)

Definition

A product that is intended to supplement vitamin or mineral intake.

Details of Intervention

A typical intervention might be further described with the following details:

- Recommend, implement, or order initiation, change in administration schedule and dose/form/route, or discontinuation of a vitamin and/or mineral supplement

Typically used with the following

Nutrition Diagnostic Terminology Used in PES Statements	Common Examples (Not intended to be inclusive)
Nutrition Diagnoses	▪ Inadequate vitamin intake (NI-5.9.1) ▪ Excessive vitamin intake (NI-5.9.2) ▪ Inadequate mineral intake (NI-5.10.1) ▪ Excessive mineral intake (NI-5.10.2) ▪ Food–medication interaction (NC-2.3) ▪ Food- and nutrition-related knowledge deficit (NB-1.1) ▪ Undesirable food choices (NB-1.7)
Etiology	▪ Poor intake of nutrient dense foods that contain vitamins and minerals ▪ Excessive use of vitamin and mineral supplements ▪ Medical diagnosis consistent with altered vitamin and mineral requirements ▪ Malabsorption of vitamins and minerals
Signs and Symptoms	Physical Examination Findings ▪ Cutaneous abnormalities consistent with vitamin and mineral deficiency of excess Food/Nutrition History ▪ Nutrient intake analysis reveals vitamin and mineral intake more or less than recommended ▪ Laboratory or radiologic indexes of vitamin-mineral depletion

Edition: 2008

192

VITAMIN OR MINERAL SUPPLEMENTS (ND-3.2)

Other considerations (*e.g., patient/client negotiation, patient/client needs and desires, and readiness to change*)

- Emerging scientific evidence to support the use of vitamin and mineral supplements in specific populations
- Availability of a qualified practitioner with additional education/training in the use of vitamin and mineral supplements in practice
- Economic considerations and product availability

References

1. Federal Food, Drug and Cosmetic Act. US Code, Title 21, Chapter 9, Subchapter II, Section 321 (ff). 2000 Edition. Available at: http://frwebgate.access.gpo.gov/cgi-bin/getdoc.cgi?dbname=browse_usc&docid=Cite:+21USC321. Accessed April 26, 2005.
2. Position of the American Dietetic Association: Fortification and nutritional supplements. *J Am Diet Assoc*. 2005;105:1300-1311.

Food & Nutrient

Edition: 2008

FOOD AND/OR NUTRIENT DELIVERY DOMAIN

BIOACTIVE SUBSTANCE SUPPLEMENT (ND-3.3)

Definition

A product that is intended to supplement bioactive substances (e.g., plant stanol and sterol esters, psyllium).

Details of Intervention

A typical intervention might be further described with the following details:

- Recommend, implement, or order initiation, changed in administration schedule or dose/form/route, or discontinuation of a bioactive substances (e.g., soluble fiber, soy protein, fish oils, plant sterol and stanol esters)

Typically used with the following

Nutrition Diagnostic Terminology Used in PES Statements	Common Examples (Not intended to be inclusive)
Nutrition Diagnoses	▪ Inadequate bioactive substance intake (NI-4.1) ▪ Excessive bioactive substance intake (NI-4.2) ▪ Excessive alcohol intake (NI-4.3) ▪ Food–medication interaction (NC-2.3) ▪ Food- and nutrition-related knowledge deficit (NB-1.1) ▪ Undesirable food choices (NB-1.7)
Etiology	▪ Poor intake of bioactive substance–containing foods ▪ Excessive use of bioactive substance supplements
Signs and Symptoms	Food/Nutrition History ▪ Nutrient intake analysis reveals bioactive substance intake more or less than recommended Client History ▪ Medical diagnosis associated with increased bioactive substance need

Other considerations *(e.g., patient/client negotiation, patient/client needs and desires, and readiness to change)*

- Emerging scientific evidence to support the use of bioactive supplements in specific populations
- Availability of a qualified practitioner with additional education/training in the use of bioactive supplements in practice

References

1. Position of the American Dietetic Association: Functional foods. *J Am Diet Assoc.* 2004;104:814-826.

Food &
Nutrient

Edition: 2008

FOOD AND/OR NUTRIENT DELIVERY DOMAIN

FEEDING ASSISTANCE (ND-4)

Definition

Accommodation or assistance in eating designed to restore the patient /client's ability to eat independently, support adequate nutrient intake, and reduce the incidence of unplanned weight loss and dehydration.

Details of Intervention

A typical intervention might be further described with the following details:

- Recommend, implement, or order adaptive equipment, feeding position, feeding cues, meal set-up, or mouth care to facilitate eating
- Recommend, design, or implement a restorative dining program
- Recommend, design, or implement a feeding assistance training program
- Recommends, designs, or implements menu selections that foster, promote, and maintain independent eating

Typically used with the following

Nutrition Diagnostic Terminology Used in PES Statements	Common Examples (Not intended to be inclusive)
Nutrition Diagnoses	• Inadequate energy intake (NI-1.4) • Inadequate oral/food beverage intake (NI-2.1) • Involuntary weight loss (NC-3.2)
Etiology	• Physical disability • Poor food/nutrient intake • Decreased memory/concentration problems
Signs and Symptoms	Physical Examination Findings • Dropping the utensils or food • Weight loss Client History • Cerebral palsy, stroke, dementia • Refusal to use prescribed adaptive eating devices, or follow prescribed positioning techniques

Food & Nutrient

195

Food & Nutrient

FOOD AND/OR NUTRIENT DELIVERY DOMAIN

FEEDING ASSISTANCE (ND-4)

Other considerations *(e.g., patient/client negotiation, patient/client needs and desires, and readiness to change)*

- Acceptance of feeding assistance/feeding devices
- Poor environment to foster adequate intake
- Lack of individual to provide assistance at meal time
- Lack of training in methods of feeding assistance
- Lack of available physical therapy, occupational therapy, or speech therapy evaluations
- Ability to understand the reasoning behind the recommendations and then want to make personal changes

References

1. Consultant Dietitians in Health Care Facilities. *Eating Matters: A training Manual for Feeding Assistants.* Chicago, IL: Consultant Dietitians in Health Care Facilities, American Dietetic Association; 2003.
2. Niedert K, Dorner B, eds. *Nutrition Care of the Older Adult, 2nd edition.* Chicago, IL: Consultant Dietitians in Health Care Facilities, American Dietetic Association; 2004.
3. Position of the American Dietetic Association: Liberalization of the diet prescription improves quality of life for older adults in long-term care. *J Am Diet Assoc.* 2005;105:1955-1965.
4. Position of the American Dietetic Association: Providing nutrition services for infants, children, and adults with developmental disabilities and special health care needs. *J Am Diet Assoc.* 2004;104:97-107.
5. Robinson GE, Leif B, eds. *Nutrition Management and Restorative Dining for Older Adults: Practical Interventions for Caregivers.* Chicago, IL: Consultant Dietitians in Health Care Facilities, American Dietetic Association; 2001.
6. Russell C, ed. *Dining Skills: Practical Interventions for the Caregivers of Older Adults with Eating Problems.* Consultant Dietitians in Health Care Facilities. Chicago, IL: American Dietetic Association; 2001.
7. Simmons SF, Osterweil D, and Schnelle JF. Improving food intake in nursing home residents with feeding assistance. *J Gerontol A Biol Sci Med Sci.* 2001;56:M790-M794.
8. Simmons SF, Schnelle JF. Individualized feeding assistance care for nursing home residents: Staffing requirements to implement two interventions. *J Gerontol A Biol Sci Med Sci.* 2004;59:M966-M973.

FOOD AND/OR NUTRIENT DELIVERY DOMAIN

FEEDING ENVIRONMENT (ND-5)

Definition

Adjustment of the physical environment, temperature, convenience, and attractiveness of the location where food is served that impacts food consumption.

Details of Intervention

A typical intervention might be further described with the following details:

- Recommend, implement, or order changes in table service/colors/set up/height, room temperature and lighting, meal schedule, menu choice, appetite enhancers, proper positioning, and minimize distractions and odors
- Recommend, implement, or order seating arrangements considering groupings that inspire social interactions

Typically used with the following:

Nutrition Diagnostic Terminology Used in PES Statements	Common Examples (Not intended to be inclusive)
Nutrition Diagnoses	▪ Inadequate oral food/beverage intake (NI-2.1) ▪ Disordered eating pattern (NB-1.5) ▪ Self-feeding difficulty (NB-2.6)
Etiology	▪ Dementia ▪ Inability to stick to task/easily distracted by others
Signs and Symptoms	Food/Nutrition History ▪ Changes in appetite attributed to mealtime surroundings ▪ Easily distracted from eating ▪ Food sanitation and safety issues ▪ Available foods not of the patient's choosing ▪ Decline in patient/client ability to eat independently Client History ▪ Pacing, wandering, changes in affect

Other considerations (*e.g., patient/client negotiation, patient/client needs and desires, and readiness to change*)

- Resources available to improve/modify the feeding environment

Food &
Nutrient

197

Food &
Nutrient

FOOD AND/OR NUTRIENT DELIVERY DOMAIN

FEEDING ENVIRONMENT (ND-5)

References

1. Niedert K, Dorner B, eds. *Nutrition Care of the Older Adult, 2nd edition.* Chicago, IL: Consultant Dietitians in Health Care Facilities, American Dietetic Association; 2004.
2. Position of the American Dietetic Association: Liberalization of the diet prescription improves quality of life for older adults in long-term care. *J Am Diet Assoc.* 2005;105:1955-1965.
3. Position of the American Dietetic Association: Providing nutrition services for infants, children, and adults with developmental disabilities and special health care needs. *J Am Diet Assoc.* 2004;104:97-107.
4. Robinson GE, Leif B, eds. *Nutrition Management and Restorative Dining for Older Adults: Practical Interventions for Caregivers.* Chicago, IL: Consultant Dietitians in Health Care Facilities, American Dietetic Association; 2001.
5. Russell C, ed. *Dining Skills: Practical Interventions for the Caregivers of Older Adults with Eating Problems.* Consultant Dietitians in Health Care Facilities. Chicago, IL: American Dietetic Association; 2001.

Edition: 2008

FOOD AND/OR NUTRIENT DELIVERY DOMAIN

NUTRITION-RELATED MEDICATION MANAGEMENT (ND-6)

Definition
Modification of a drug or herbal to optimize patient/client nutritional or health status.

Details of Intervention
A typical intervention might be further described with the following details:

- Recommend, implement, order initiation, changes in dose/form/route, change in administration schedule, or discontinuance of medications or herbals including insulin, appetite stimulants, digestive enzymes, or probiotics

Typically used with the following

Nutrition Diagnostic Terminology Used in PES Statements	Common Examples (Not intended to be inclusive)
Nutrition Diagnoses	▪ Altered GI function (NC-1.4) ▪ Impaired nutrient utilization (NC-2.1) ▪ Food–medication interaction (NC-2.3)
Etiology	▪ Appetite insufficient resulting in adequate nutrient intake ▪ Frequent hypo- or hyperglycemia ▪ Pancreatic insufficiency ▪ Malabsorption of fat, protein, lactose, or other carbohydrates ▪ Polypharmacy and medication abuse ▪ Drug toxicity
Signs and Symptoms	Physical Examination Findings ▪ Thin, wasted appearance Food/Nutrition History ▪ Sufficient oral intake ▪ Report of herbal use Client History ▪ Diabetes with poorly controlled blood sugar

Food & Nutrient

199

FOOD AND/OR NUTRIENT DELIVERY DOMAIN

NUTRITION-RELATED MEDICATION MANAGEMENT (ND-6)

Other considerations *(e.g., patient/client negotiation, patient/client needs and desires, and readiness to change)*

- Availability/access to a clinical pharmacist
- Availability of a qualified practitioner with appropriate pharmacology training and/or education

References

1. Position of the American Dietetic Association: Integration of medical nutrition therapy and pharmacotherapy. *J Am Diet Assoc.* 2003;103:1363-1370.
2. Kris-Etherton P, Pearson T. Over-the-counter statin medications: Emerging opportunities for RDs. *J Am Diet Assoc.* 2000;100:1126-1130.
3. Moyers B. Medications as adjunct therapy for weight loss: Approved and off-label agents in use. *J Am Diet Assoc.* 2005;105:948-959.

Food & Nutrient

INITIAL/BRIEF NUTRITION EDUCATION (E-1)

Definition

Instruction or training intended to build or reinforce basic nutrition-related knowledge, or to provide essential nutrition-related information until patient/client returns.

Details of Intervention

A typical intervention might be further described related the following details:

- Discuss the purpose of the nutrition education intervention
- Communicate relationship between nutrition and specific disease/health issue
- Begin instruction of nutrition issue of most concern to patient/client's health and well-being
- Provide basic nutrition-related educational information until client is able to return for comprehensive education

Typically used with the following

Nutrition Diagnostic Terminology Used in PES Statements	Common Examples (Not intended to be inclusive)
Nutrition Diagnoses	▪ Food–medication interaction (NC-2.3) ▪ Food- and nutrition-related knowledge deficit (NB-1.1) ▪ Harmful beliefs/attitudes about food- or nutrition-related topics (NB-1.2) ▪ Self-monitoring deficit (NB-1.4) ▪ Other: Any diagnoses related to inadequate, excessive, inappropriate, or inconsistent intake
Etiology	▪ Capacity for learning ▪ Knowledge deficit related to newly diagnosed medical condition ▪ Interest and/or motivation ▪ Medical or surgical procedure requiring modified diet ▪ Unable to distinguish legitimate from false information
Signs and Symptoms	Food/Nutrition History ▪ Unable to explain purpose of the nutrition prescription or rationale for nutrition prescription in relationship to disease/health ▪ Expresses need for additional information or clarification of education or additional time to learn information ▪ Unable to select appropriate foods or supplements ▪ Unable to choose appropriate timing, volume, or preparation/handling of foods

Education

Edition: 2008

NUTRITION EDUCATION DOMAIN

INITIAL/BRIEF NUTRITION EDUCATION (E-1)

Other considerations *(e.g., patient/client negotiation, patient/client needs and desires, and readiness to change)*

- Met with several providers in one day and is unable or unwilling to receive more nutrition education at this time
- Profile reflects complicated situation warranting additional education/instruction
- Being discharged from the hospital
- Caregiver unavailable at time of nutrition education
- Baseline knowledge
- Learning style
- Other education and learning needs, e.g., new medication or other treatment administration

References

1. Position of the American Dietetic Association: Total diet approach to communicating food and nutrition information. *J Am Diet Assoc* 2007;107(in press).
2. Holli BB, Calabrese RJ, O'Sullivan-Maillet J. *Communication and education skills for dietetics professionals. 4th ed.* New York, NY: Lipincott Williams and Wilkins; 2003.
3. Sahyoun NR, Pratt CA, Anderson A. Evaluation of nutrition education interventions for older adults: A proposed framework. *J Am Diet Assoc.* 2004;104:58-69.
4. Contento I. The effectiveness of nutrition education and implications for nutrition education policy, programs, and research: a review of research. *J Nutr Ed.* 1995;27: 279-283.
5. Medeiros LC, Butkus SN, Chipman H, Cox RH, Jones L, Little D. A logic model framework for community nutrition education. *J Nutr Educ Behav.* 2002;37: 197-202.

Edition: 2008

COMPREHENSIVE NUTRITION EDUCATION (E-2)

Definition

Instruction or training intended to lead to in-depth nutrition-related knowledge and/or skills in given topics.

Details of Intervention

A typical intervention might be further described with the following details:

- Provide information related to purpose of the nutrition prescription
- Initiate thorough instruction of relationship between nutrition and disease/health
- Explain detailed or multiple nutrition prescription modifications recommended given patient/client situation
- Introduce more advanced nutrition topics related to patient/condition (e.g., saturated and *trans* fatty acid intake vs. total fat intake, menu planning, food purchasing)
- Support skill development (e.g., glucometer use, home tube feeding and feeding pump training, cooking skills/preparation)
- Commence training on interpreting medical or other results to modify nutrition prescription (e.g., distribution of carbohydrates throughout the day based on blood glucose monitoring results)

Typically used with the following

Nutrition Diagnostic Terminology Used in PES Statements	Common Examples (Not intended to be inclusive)
Nutrition Diagnoses	▪ Food–medication interaction (NC-2.3) ▪ Food- and nutrition-related knowledge deficit (NB-1.1) ▪ Harmful beliefs/attitudes about food- or nutrition-related topics (NB-1.2) ▪ Self-monitoring deficit (NB-1.4) ▪ Other: Any diagnoses related to inadequate or excessive, inappropriate, or inconsistent intake
Etiology	▪ Deficient understanding of relevant nutrition-related topics ▪ Exposure to incorrect food and nutrition information ▪ Lack of skill in self management techniques
Signs and Symptoms	Food/Nutrition History ▪ Expresses desire for knowledge/information ▪ Food and nutrient intake assessment indicates food choice incompatible with recommendations

NUTRITION EDUCATION DOMAIN

COMPREHENSIVE NUTRITION EDUCATION (E-2)

Other considerations (*e.g., patient/client negotiation, patient/client needs and desires, and readiness to change*)

- Profile reflects complicated situation warranting additional education/instruction
- Increased capacity and willingness to learn information
- Quality of life may be enhanced with in-depth nutrition education and understanding
- Baseline knowledge
- Lifestyle factors
- Education approaches that enhance knowledge/skill transfer

References

1. Position of the American Dietetic Association: Total diet approach to communicating food and nutrition information. *J Am Diet Assoc.* 2007;107(in press).
2. Carmona RH. Improving health literacy: Preventing obesity with education. *J Am Diet Assoc.* 2005;105:S9-S10.
3. Contento I. The effectiveness of nutrition education and implications for nutrition education policy, programs, and research: a review of research. *J Nutr Educ.* 1995;27: 279-283.
4. Holli BB, Calabrese RJ, O'Sullivan-Maillet J. *Communication and education skills for dietetics professionals. 4th ed.* New York, NY: Lipincott Williams and Wilkins; 2003.
5. Holmes AL, Sanderson B, Maisiak R, Brown R, Bittner V. Dietitian services are associated with improved patient outcomes and the MEDFICTS dietary assessment questionnaire is a suitable outcome measure in cardiac rehabilitation. *J Am Diet Assoc.* 2005;105:1533-1540.
6. Medeiros LC, Butkus SN, Chipman H, Cox RH, Jones L, Little D. A logic model framework for community nutrition education. *J Nutr Educ Behav.* 2005;37:197-202.
7. Sahyoun NR, Pratt CA, Anderson A. Evaluation of nutrition education interventions for older adults: A proposed framework. *J Am Diet Assoc.* 2004;104:58-69.

THEORETICAL BASIS/APPROACH (C-1)

Definition

The theories or models used to design and implement an intervention. Theories and theoretical models consist of principles, constructs and variables, which offer systematic explanations of the human behavior change process. Behavior change theories and models provide a research-based rationale for designing and tailoring nutrition interventions to achieve the desired effect. A theoretical framework for curriculum and treatment protocols, it guides determination of: 1) what information patients/clients need at different points in the behavior change process, 2) what tools and strategies may be best applied to facilitate behavior change, and 3) outcome measures to assess effectiveness in interventions or components of interventions.

Application Guidance

One or more of the following theories or theoretical models may influence a practitioner's counseling style or approach. Practitioners are asked to identify those theories (C-1) that most influence the intervention being documented. An intervention might also incorporate tools and strategies derived from a variety of behavior change theories and models. The practitioner is also asked to indicate which strategies (C-2) they used in a particular intervention session.

Details of Intervention

A typical intervention might be further described with the following details:

The following theories and models have proven valuable in providing a theoretical framework for evidence-based individual and interpersonal level nutrition interventions. Other theories may be useful for community level interventions (e.g., Community Organization, Diffusion of Innovations, Communication Theory).

- Cognitive-Behavioral Theory
- Health Belief Model
- Social Learning Theory
- Transtheoretical Model/Stages of Change

Additional information regarding each of the above theories and models can be found within this reference sheet.

205

Counseling

NUTRITION COUNSELING DOMAIN

THEORETICAL BASIS/APPROACH (C-1)

Typically used with the following

Nutrition Diagnostic Terminology Used in PES Statements	Common Examples (Not intended to be inclusive)
Nutrition Diagnoses	▪ Overweight/obesity (NC-3.3) ▪ Harmful beliefs/attitudes about food or nutrition-related topics (NB-1.2) ▪ Not ready for diet/lifestyle change (NB-1.3) ▪ Self-monitoring deficit (NB-1.4) ▪ Disordered eating pattern (NB-1.5) ▪ Limited adherence to nutrition-related recommendations (NB-1.6) ▪ Undesirable food choices (NB-1.7) ▪ Physical inactivity (NB-2.1) ▪ Excessive exercise (NB-2.2) ▪ Inability or lack of desire to manage self care (NB 2.3) ▪ Poor nutrition quality of life (NB-2.5) ▪ Other: Any diagnoses related to inadequate, excessive, inappropriate, or inconsistent intake
Etiology	▪ New medical diagnosis ▪ Harmful beliefs/attitudes about food, nutrition, and nutrition-related topics ▪ Lack of value for behavior change, competing values ▪ Cultural/religious practices that interfere with implementation of the nutrition prescription ▪ Lack of efficacy to make changes or to overcome barriers to change ▪ Lack of focus/attention to detail, difficulty with time management and/or organization ▪ Perception that time, interpersonal, or financial constraints prevent change ▪ Prior exposure to incorrect or incompatible information ▪ Not ready for diet/lifestyle change ▪ Lack of caretaker or social support for implementing changes ▪ High level of fatigue or other side effect of medical condition
Signs and Symptoms (Defining Characteristics)	Food/Nutrition History ▪ Frustration with MNT recommendations ▪ Previous failures to effectively change target behavior ▪ Defensiveness, hostility, or resistance to change ▪ Sense of lack of control of eating ▪ Inability to apply food- and nutrition-related information/guidelines ▪ Inability to change food- and nutrition-related behavior ▪ Absent or incomplete self-monitoring records ▪ Inability to problem-solve/self manage ▪ Irrational thoughts about self and effects of food intake ▪ Unrealistic expectations ▪ Inflexibility with food selection ▪ Evidence of excessive, inadequate, inappropriate, or inconsistent intake related to needs

Counseling

206

Edition: 2008

NUTRITION COUNSELING DOMAIN

THEORETICAL BASIS/APPROACH (C-1)

Other considerations (*e.g., patient/client negotiation, patient/client needs and desires, and readiness to change*)

- Lifestyle factors
- Language barrier
- Educational level
- Culture
- Socioeconomic status

References

1. Glanz K. Current theoretical bases for nutrition intervention and their uses. In Coulston AM, Rock CL, Monsen E. *Nutrition in the Prevention and Treatment of Disease.* San Diego, CA: Academy Press; 2001:83-93.
2. U.S. Department of Health and Human Services, National Institutes of Health, National Cancer Institute. Theory at a Glance: A Guide for Health Promotion Practice, Spring 2005. Available at: http://www.cancer.gov/PDF/481f5d53-63df-41bc-bfaf-5aa48ee1da4d/TAAG3.pdf, Accessed on January 22, 2007.
3. Powers MA, Carstensen K, Colon K, Rickheim P, Bergenstal RM. Diabetes BASICS: education, innovation, revolution. *Diabetes Spectrum.* 2006;19:90-98.
4. Glanz K, Rimer BK, Lewis FM. *Health Behavior and Health Education: Theory Research and Practice, 3rd ed.* San Francisco, CA:Jossey-Bass Publishers; 2002.

Edition: 2008

NUTRITION COUNSELING DOMAIN

THEORETICAL BASIS/APPROACH (C-1)
Cognitive-Behavioral Theory

Description

Cognitive-behavioral theory (CBT) is based on the assumption that all behavior is learned and is directly related to internal factors (e.g., thoughts and thinking patterns) and external factors (e.g., environmental stimulus and reinforcement) that are related to the problem behaviors. Application involves use of both cognitive and behavioral change strategies to effect behavior change.

Implication for Counseling Interventions

CBT, derived from an educational model, is based upon the assumption that most emotional and behavioral reactions are learned and can be unlearned. The goal of CBT is to facilitate client identification of cognitions and behaviors that lead to inappropriate eating or exercise habits and replace these with more rational thoughts and actions.

The process is:

- Goal directed
- Process oriented
- Facilitated through a variety of problem solving tools

Behavioral and cognitive techniques to modify eating and exercise habits are taught for continuous application by the patient/client. Practitioners implement Cognitive-Behavioral Theory by partnering with clients to study their current environment to:

- Identify determinants or antecedents to behavior that contribute to inappropriate eating/exercise
- Identify resultant inappropriate behavior (e.g., overeating, vomiting)
- Analyze consequences of this behavior (cognitions, positive and negative reinforcers and punishments, e.g., decreased anxiety, feeling over full, losing or gaining weight)
- Make specific goals to modify the environment/cognitions to reduce target behaviors

Cognitive and behavioral strategies used to promote change in diet and physical activity may include:

- Goal setting
- Self-monitoring
- Problem solving
- Social support
- Stress management
- Stimulus control
- Cognitive restructuring
- Relapse prevention
- Rewards/contingency management

Edition: 2008

THEORETICAL BASIS/APPROACH (C-1)

References

1. Fabricatore AN. Behavior therapy and cognitive-behavioral therapy of obesity: Is there a difference? *J Am Diet Assoc.* 2007;107:92-99.
2. Brownell KD, Cohen LR. Adherence to Dietary Regimens 2: Components of effective interventions. *Behav Med.* 1995;20:155–163.
3. Kiy AM. Cognitive-behavioral and psychoeducational counseling and therapy. In: Helm KK, Klawitter B. *Nutrition Therapy: Advanced Counseling Skills.* Lake Dallas, TX: Helms Seminars; 1995:135-154.
4. Foster GD. Clinical implications for the treatment of obesity. *Obesity.* 2006;14:182S-185S.
5. Berkel LA, Poston WS 2d, Reeves RS, Foreyt JP. Behavioral interventions for obesity. *J Am Diet Assoc.* 2005;105:S35-S43.

Edition: 2008

NUTRITION COUNSELING DOMAIN

THEORETICAL BASIS/APPROACH (C-1)

Health Belief Model

Description

The Health Belief Model is a psychological model, which focuses on an individual's attitudes and beliefs to attempt to explain and predict health behaviors. The HBM is based on the assumption that an individual will be motivated to take health-related action if that person 1) feels that a negative health condition (e.g., diabetes) can be avoided or managed, 2) has a positive expectation that by taking a recommended action, he/she will avoid negative health consequences (e.g., good blood glucose control will preserve eye sight), and believes he/she can successfully perform a recommended health action (e.g., I can use carbohydrate counting and control my diet).

Implication for Counseling Interventions

The Health Belief Model is particularly helpful to practitioners planning interventions targeted to individuals with clinical nutrition-related risk factors, such as diabetes, high blood cholesterol and/or hypertension. The six major constructs of the model have been found to be important in impacting an individual's motivation to take health-related action. The following table provides definitions and application guidance for the key constructs of the theory. Motivational interviewing strategies may be appropriate to address perceived susceptibility, severity, benefits and barriers. Behavioral strategies are most appropriate once the patient/client begins to take action to modify his/her diet.

These six constructs are useful components in designing behavior change programs. It is important for the practitioner to understand the patient's perception of the health threat and potential benefits of treatment. According to the HBM, an asymptomatic diabetic may not be compliant with his/her treatment regiment if he/she does not:

- believe he or she has diabetes (susceptibility)
- believe diabetes will seriously impact his/her life (perceived seriousness)
- believe following the diabetic diet will decrease the negative effects of diabetes (perceived benefits)
- believe the effort to follow the diet is worth the benefit to be gained (perceived barriers)
- have stimulus to initiate action (cue to action)
- have confidence in their ability to achieve success (self-efficacy)

210

NUTRITION COUNSELING DOMAIN

THEORETICAL BASIS/APPROACH (C-1)

Construct	Definition	Strategies
Perceived susceptibility	Client's belief or opinion of the personal threat a health condition represents for them; client opinion regarding whether they have the condition (e.g., diabetes or hypertension) or their chance of getting the disease or condition	▪ Educate on disease/condition risk factors ▪ Tailor information to the client ▪ Ask client if they think they are at risk or have the disease/condition ▪ Guided discussions ▪ Motivational interviewing (express empathy, open-ended questions, reflective listening, affirming, summarizing, and eliciting self-motivation statements)
Perceived severity	Client's belief about the impact a particular health threat will have on them and their lifestyle	▪ Educate on consequences of the disease/condition; show graphs, statistics ▪ Elicit client response ▪ Discuss potential impact on client's lifestyle ▪ Motivational interviewing
Perceived benefits and barriers	Client's belief regarding benefits they will derive from taking nutrition-related action; perceived benefits versus barriers--client's perception of whether benefits will outweigh the sacrifices and efforts involved in behavior change	▪ Clearly define benefits of nutrition therapy ▪ Role models, testimonials ▪ Explore ambivalence and barriers ▪ Imagine the future ▪ Explore successes ▪ Summarize and affirm the positive
Cues to action	Internal or external triggers that motivate or stimulate action	▪ How-to education ▪ Incentive programs ▪ Link current symptoms to disease/condition ▪ Discuss media information ▪ Reminder phone calls/mailings ▪ Social support
Self-efficacy	Client confidence in their ability to successfully accomplish the necessary action	▪ Skill training/demonstration ▪ Introduce alternatives and choices ▪ Behavior contracting; small, incremental goals ▪ Coaching, verbal reinforcement

References
1. Glanz K. Current theoretical bases for nutrition intervention and their uses. In Coulston AM, Rock CL, Monsen E. *Nutrition in the Prevention and Treatment of Disease*. San Diego, Ca: Academy Press; 2001:83-93.
2. U.S. Department of Health and Human Services, National Institutes of Health, National Cancer Institute. Theory at a Glance: A Guide for Health Promotion Practice, Spring 2005. Available at: http://www.cancer.gov/PDF/481f5d53-63df-41bc-bfaf-5aa48ee1da4d/TAAG3.pdf, Accessed on January 22, 2007.
3. Powers MA, Carstensen K, Colon K, Rickheim P, Bergenstal RM. Diabetes BASICS: education, innovation, revolution. *Diabetes Spectrum*. 2006;19:90-98.

Edition: 2008

NUTRITION COUNSELING DOMAIN

Counseling

THEORETICAL BASIS/APPROACH (C-1)

Social Learning Theory

Description

Social learning theory, also known as Social Cognitive Theory, provides a framework for understanding, predicting, and changing behavior. The theory identifies a dynamic, reciprocal relationship between environment, the person, and behavior. The person can be both an agent for change and a responder to change. It emphasizes the importance of observing and modeling behaviors, attitudes and emotional reactions of others. Determinants of behavior include goals, outcome expectations and self-efficacy. Reinforcements increase or decrease the likelihood that the behavior will be repeated.[1]

Implication for Counseling Interventions

Social Learning Theory is rich in concepts applicable to nutrition counseling. The following table provides definitions and application guidance for the key concepts of the theory.

212

NUTRITION COUNSELING DOMAIN

THEORETICAL BASIS/APPROACH (C-1)

Concept	Definition	Strategies
Reciprocal Determinism	A person's ability to change a behavior is influenced by characteristics within the person (e.g., beliefs), the environment, and the behavior itself (e.g., difficulty doing the behavior). All three interact to influence if the behavior change will happen.	Consider multiple behavior change strategies targeting motivation, action, the individual and the environment: • Motivational interviewing • Social support • Stimulus control • Demonstration • Skill development training/coaching
Behavioral Capability	The knowledge and skills that are needed for a person to change behavior	• Comprehensive education • Demonstration • Skill development training/coaching
Expectations	For a person to do a behavior, they must believe that the behavior will result in outcomes important to them	• Motivational interviewing • Model positive outcomes of diet/exercise
Self-Efficacy	Confidence in ability to take action and persist in action	• Break task down to component parts • Demonstration/modeling • Skill development training/coaching • Reinforcement • Small, incremental goals/behavioral contracting
Observational Learning	When a person learns how to do a behavior by watching credible others do the same behavior	• Demonstrations • Role modeling • Group problem-solving sessions
Reinforcement	Response to a behavior that will either increase or decrease the likelihood that the behavior will be repeated	• Affirm accomplishments • Encourage self reward/self-reinforcement • Incentives for process components of change (e.g., keeping a food diary)

References

1. Glanz K. Current theoretical bases for nutrition intervention and their uses. In Coulston AM, Rock CL, Monsen E. *Nutrition in the Prevention and Treatment of Disease.* San Diego, Ca: Academy Press; 2001:83-93.
2. U.S. Department of Health and Human Services, National Institutes of Health, National Cancer Institute. Theory at a Glance: A Guide for Health Promotion Practice, Spring 2005. Available at: http://www.cancer.gov/PDF/481f5d53-63df-41bc-bfaf-5aa48ee1da4d/TAAG3.pdf. Accessed on January 22, 2007.
3. Bandru A. *Social Foundations of Thought and Action: A Social Cognitive Theory.* Englewood Cliffs, NJ: Prentice-Hall; 1986.
4. Bandra A. Self-Efficacy: *The Exercise of Control.* New York, NY: W.H. Freeman; 1997.
5. Glanz K, Rimer BK, Lewis FM. Health Behavior and Health Education: Theory Research and Practice, 3ed. San Francisco, Ca:Jossey-Bass Publishers, 2002.

Edition: 2008

NUTRITION COUNSELING DOMAIN

THEORETICAL BASIS/APPROACH (C-1)

Transtheoretical Model/Stages of Change

Definition

A theoretical model of intentional health behavior change that describes a sequence of cognitive (attitudes and intentions) and behavioral steps people take in successful behavior change. The model, developed by Prochaska and DiClemente, is composed of a core concept known as Stages of Change, a series of independent variables, the Processes of Change, and outcome measures including decision balance and self-efficacy. The model has been used to guide development of effective interventions for a variety of health behaviors.

Implication for Counseling Interventions

One of the defining characteristics of this model is that it describes behavior change not as a discrete event (e.g., today I am going to stop overeating), but as something that occurs in stages, over time. The five stages reflect an individual's attitudes, intentions and behavior related to change of a specific behavior and include the following:

- Precontemplation – no recognition of need for change; no intention to take action within the next 6 months
- Contemplation – recognition of need to change; intends to take action within the next 6 months
- Preparation – intends to take action in the next 30 days and has taken some behavioral steps in that direction
- Action – has made changes in target behavior for less than 6 months
- Maintenance – has changed target behavior for more than 6 months

Determination of a patient/client stage of change is relatively simple, involving a few questions regarding intentions and current diet. One of the appealing aspects of the theory is that the Process of Change construct describes cognitive and behavioral activities or strategies, which may be applied at various stages to move a person forward through the stages of change. This movement is not always linear, and patients can cycle in and out of various stages. The model has been used to effectively tailor interventions to the needs of clients at various stages. Knowing a patient/client's stage of change can help a practitioner determine:

- Whether intervention now is appropriate
- The type and content of intervention to use (motivational versus action oriented)
- Appropriate and timely questions about past efforts, pros and cons of change, obstacles, challenges and potential strategies
- The amount of time to spend with the patient

The following table provides guidance for applying stages and processes of change to the adoption of healthy diets.

THEORETICAL BASIS/APPROACH (C-1)

Table 3
General guidelines for applying stages and processes of change to adoption of healthful diets

State of readiness	Key strategies for moving to next stage	Treatment do's at this stage	Treatment don'ts at this stage
Precontemplation	Increased information and awareness, emotional acceptance	■ Provide personalized information. ■ Allow client to express emotions about his or her disease or about the need to make dietary changes.	■ Do not assume client has knowledge or expect that providing information will automatically lead to behavior change. ■ Do not ignore client's emotional adjustment to the need for dietary change, which could override ability to process relevant information.
Contemplation	Increased confidence in one's ability to adopt recommended behaviors	■ Discuss and resolve barriers to dietary change. ■ Encourage support networks. ■ Give positive feedback about a client's abilities. ■ Help to clarify ambivalence about adopting behavior and emphasize expected benefits.	■ Do not ignore the potential impact of family members, and others, on client's ability to comply. ■ Do not be alarmed or critical of a client's ambivalence.
Preparation	Resolution of ambivalence, firm commitment, and specific action plan	■ Encourage client to set specific, achievable goals (eg, use 1% milk instead of whole milk). ■ Reinforce small changes that client may have already achieved.	■ Do not recommend general behavior changes (eg, "Eat less fat"). ■ Do not refer to small changes as "not good enough."
Action	Behavioral skill training and social support	■ Refer to education program for self-management skills. ■ Provide self-help materials.	■ Do not refer clients to information-only classes.
Maintenance	Problem-solving skills and social and environmental support	■ Encourage client to anticipate and plan for potential difficulties (eg, maintaining dietary changes on vacation). ■ Collect information about local resources (eg, support groups, shopping guides). ■ Encourage client to "recycle" if he or she has a lapse or relapse. ■ Recommended more challenging dietary changes if client is motivated.	■ Do not assume that initial action means permanent change. ■ Do not be discouraged or judgmental about a lapse or relapse.

Source: Kristal AR, Glanz K, Curry S, Patterson RE. How can stages of change be best used in dietary interventions? *J Am Diet Assoc.* 1999;99:683.

215

Counseling

NUTRITION COUNSELING DOMAIN

THEORETICAL BASIS/APPROACH (C-1)

Prochaska recommends the following strategies, which target motivation, be used in the early stages of change: consciousness raising, dramatic relief (e.g., emotional arousal via role playing or personal testimonials), environmental reevaluation (e.g., empathy training and family interactions), social liberation (e.g., advocacy, empowerment) and self-reevaluation (e.g., value clarification, healthy role models and imagery). These strategies are very consistent with motivational interviewing techniques. In the later stages of change, behavioral strategies are most appropriate.

References

1   Kristal AR, Glanz K, Curry S, Patterson RE. How can stages of change be best used in dietary interventions? *J Am Diet Assoc.* 1999;99:679-684.

2.   Nothwehr F, Snetselaar L, Yang J, Wu H. Stage of change for healthful eating and use of behavioral strategies. *J Am Diet Assoc.* 2006;106:1035-1041.

3.   Green GW, Rossi SR, Rossi JS, Velicer WF, Fava JL, Prochaska JO. Dietary applications of the stages of change model. *J Am Diet Assoc.* 1999;99:673-678.

4.   Glanz K. Current theoretical bases for nutrition intervention and their uses. In Coulston AM, Rock CL, Monsen E. *Nutrition in the Prevention and Treatment of Disease.* San Diego, CA: Academy Press; 2001:83-93.

5.   Prochaska JO, Norcross JC, DiClemente V. *Changing for Good: A Revolutionary Six-Stage Program for Overcoming Bad Habits and Moving Your Life Positively Forward.* New York, NY: Avon Books Inc; 1994

Edition: 2008

STRATEGIES (C-2)

Definition

An evidence-based method or plan of action designed to achieve a particular goal. Application of behavior change theories in nutrition practice has provided practitioners with a collection of evidence-based strategies to promote behavior change. Some strategies target change in motivation and intention to change, and others target behavior change. Practitioners selectively apply strategies based upon patient/client goals and objectives, and their personal counseling philosophy and skill.

Application Guidance

An intervention typically incorporate tools and strategies derived from a variety of behavior change theories and models. The practitioner is asked to indicate which strategies (C-2) he/she used in a particular intervention session along with the theories (C-1), which most influence the intervention being documented.

Details of Intervention

A typical intervention might be further described with the following details:

The following strategies have proven valuable in providing effecting nutrition-related behavior change.

- Motivational interviewing
- Goal setting
- Self-monitoring
- Problem solving
- Social support

- Stress management
- Stimulus control
- Cognitive restructuring
- Relapse prevention
- Rewards/contingency management

Additional information regarding each of the above strategies can be found within this reference sheet.

Edition: 2008

NUTRITION COUNSELING DOMAIN

STRATEGIES (C-2)

Typically used with the following:

Nutrition Diagnostic Terminology Used in PES Statements	Common Examples (Not intended to be inclusive)
Nutrition Diagnoses	▪ Overweight/obesity (NC-3.3) ▪ Harmful beliefs/attitudes about food or nutrition-related topics (NB-1.2) ▪ Not ready for diet/lifestyle change (NB-1.3) ▪ Self-monitoring deficit (NB-1.4) ▪ Disordered eating pattern (NB-1.5) ▪ Limited adherence to nutrition-related recommendations (NB-1.6) ▪ Undesirable food choices (NB-1.7) ▪ Physical inactivity (NB-2.1) ▪ Excessive exercise (NB-2.2) ▪ Inability or lack of desire to manage self care (NB 2.3) ▪ Poor nutrition quality of life (NB-2.5) ▪ Other: Any diagnoses related to inadequate, excessive, inappropriate, or inconsistent intake
Etiology	▪ New medical diagnosis ▪ Harmful beliefs/attitudes about food, nutrition, and nutrition-related topics ▪ Lack of value for behavior change, competing values ▪ Cultural/religious practices that interfere with implementation of the nutrition prescription ▪ Lack of efficacy to make changes or to overcome barriers to change ▪ Lack of focus/attention to detail, difficulty with time management and/or organization ▪ Perception that time, interpersonal, or financial constraints prevent change ▪ Prior exposure to incorrect or incompatible information ▪ Not ready for diet/lifestyle change ▪ Lack of caretaker or social support for implementing changes ▪ High level of fatigue or other side effect of medical condition
Signs and Symptoms (Defining Characteristics)	Food/Nutrition History ▪ Frustration with MNT recommendations ▪ Previous failures to effectively change target behavior ▪ Defensiveness, hostility, or resistance to change ▪ Sense of lack of control of eating ▪ Inability to apply food- and nutrition-related information/guidelines ▪ Inability to change food- and nutrition-related behavior ▪ Absent or incomplete self-monitoring records ▪ Inability to problem-solve/self manage ▪ Irrational thoughts about self and effects of food intake ▪ Unrealistic expectations ▪ Inflexibility with food selection ▪ Evidence of excessive, inadequate, inappropriate, or inconsistent intake related to needs

Counseling

218

Edition: 2008

NUTRITION COUNSELING DOMAIN

STRATEGIES (C-2)

Other considerations *(e.g., patient/client negotiation, patient/client needs and desires, and readiness to change)*

- Lifestyle factors
- Language barrier
- Educational level
- Culture
- Socioeconomic status

References

1. Glanz K. Current theoretical bases for nutrition intervention and their uses. In Coulston AM, Rock CL, Monsen E. *Nutrition in the Prevention and Treatment of Disease*. San Diego, CA: Academy Press; 2001:83-93.

2. U.S. Department of Health and Human Services, National Institutes of Health, National Cancer Institute. Theory at a Glance: A Guide for Health Promotion Practice, Spring 2005. Available at: http://www.cancer.gov/PDF/481f5d53-63df-41bc-bfaf-5aa48ee1da4d/TAAG3.pdf. Accessed on January 22, 2007.

3. Powers MA, Carstensen K, Colon K, Rickheim P, Bergenstal RM. Diabetes BASICS: education, innovation, revolution. *Diabetes Spectrum*. 2006;19:90-98.

4. Glanz K, Rimer BK, Lewis FM. *Health Behavior and Health Education: Theory Research and Practice, 3ed*. San Francisco, CA: Jossey-Bass Publishers, 2002.

Edition: 2008

NUTRITION COUNSELING DOMAIN

STRATEGIES (C-2)

Strategy descriptions and application guidance

Strategy	Description	Implementation Tips
Motivational interviewing	A directive, client-centered counseling style for eliciting behavior change by helping clients to explore and resolve ambivalence.[1]	Tone of counseling:
	The approach involves selective response to client speech in a way that helps the client resolve ambivalence and move toward change.	▪ Partnership ▪ Nonjudgmental ▪ Empathetic/supportive/encouraging
	The four guiding principles that underlie this counseling approach include:	▪ Nonconfrontational ▪ Quiet and eliciting
	▪ Express empathy ▪ Develop discrepancy ▪ Roll with resistance ▪ Support self-efficacy.	The client does most of the talking and the counselor guides the client to explore and resolve ambivalence by:
	The following specific practitioner behaviors are characteristic of the MI style:[2]	▪ Asking open ended questions ▪ Listening reflectively ▪ Summarizing ▪ Affirming
	▪ Expressing acceptance and affirmation ▪ Eliciting and selectively reinforcing the client's own self motivational statements, expressions of problem recognition, concern, desire, intention to change, and ability to change ▪ Monitoring the client's degree of readiness to change, and ensuring that jumping ahead of the client does not generate resistance ▪ Affirming the client's freedom of choice and self-direction	▪ Eliciting self-motivational statements ▪ Shared agenda setting/decision making ▪ Allowing clients to interpret information ▪ Rolling with resistance, rather than confronting ▪ Building discrepancy ▪ Eliciting "change talk" ▪ Negotiating a change plan
	The source of motivation is presumed to reside within the client and the counselor encourages the client to explore ambivalence, motivation and possibilities to change, so it is the client who chooses what to change, determines the change plan and strategy.	Motivational interviewing is best applied in situations when a patient is not ready, is unwilling or ambivalent about changing their diet or lifestyle.
	MI is an evidence-based counseling strategy which builds on Carl Roger's client-centered counseling model, Prochaska and DiClemente's transtheoretical model of change, Milton Rokeach's human values theory and Daryl Bern's theory of self-perception.	MI integrates well with the readiness to change model to move individuals from the early stages to the action stage of change.
		MI is a major paradigm change from the problem solving oriented counseling frequently employed by practitioners.
		MI is not a set of techniques that can be learned quickly, but a style or approach to counseling.

STRATEGIES (C-2)

Goal setting	A collaborative activity between the client and the practitioner in which the client decides from all potential activity recommendations what changes he/she will expend effort to implement.	▪ Appropriate for patients ready to make dietary changes ▪ Coach on goal setting skills ▪ Document and track progress toward short-term and long-term goals ▪ Probe client about pros and cons of proposed goals ▪ Assist client in gaining the knowledge and skills necessary to succeed ▪ Encourage strategies to build confidence (discuss realistic steps and start with easily achievable goals) ▪ Aid clients in building a supportive environment ▪ Celebrate successes
Self-monitoring	A technique that involves keeping a detailed record of behaviors that influence diet and/or weight and may include: ▪ What, when, how much eaten ▪ Activities during eating ▪ Emotions and cognitions related to meals/snacks ▪ Frequency, duration and intensity of exercise ▪ Target nutrient content of foods consumed (i.e., calories, fat, fiber) ▪ Event, thoughts about event, emotional response, behavioral response ▪ Negative self-talk, replacement thoughts ▪ Blood glucose, blood pressure Self-monitoring is associated with improved treatment outcomes.	▪ Provide rationale and instructions for self-monitoring ▪ Review and identify patterns ▪ Assist with problem solving and goal setting ▪ Celebrate successes ▪ The amount of feedback required, typically diminishes as patient/client skill improves
Problem solving	Techniques that are taught to assist clients in identifying barriers to achieving goals, identifying and implementing solutions and evaluating the effectiveness of the solutions.[2]	Work collaboratively with client to: ▪ Define the problem ▪ Brainstorm solutions ▪ Weigh pros/cons of potential solutions ▪ Select/implement strategy ▪ Evaluate outcomes ▪ Adjust strategy

221

Counseling

STRATEGIES (C-2)

Counseling

Social support	Increased availability of social support for dietary behavior change. Social support may be generated among an individual's family, church, school, co-workers, health club or community.	A dietetics practitioner may assist a client by: ▪ Establishing a collaborative relationship ▪ Identifying family/community support ▪ Assisting clients in developing assertiveness skills. ▪ Utilize modeling, skill training, respondent and operant conditioning ▪ Conducting education in a group ▪ Encourage family involvement
Stress management	Reaction to stress can cause some clients to loss their appetite and others to overeat. Dietetics practitioners are particularly interested in management of stressful situations, which result in inappropriate eating behaviors.	Two approaches may be used to manage stress, one focuses on changing the environment, and the other focuses on modifying the client's response to stress. Environmental-focused strategies may include: ▪ Guidance on planning ahead ▪ Use of time-management skills ▪ Developing a support system ▪ Building skills to prepare quick and healthful meals ▪ Guidance on eating on the run Emotion-focused strategies may include: ▪ Use of positive self-talk ▪ Building assertiveness in expressing eating desires ▪ Setting realistic goals ▪ Learning to deal appropriately with emotion-driven eating cravings ▪ Relaxation exercises

STRATEGIES (C-2)

Stimulus control	Identifying and modifying social or environmental cues or triggers to act, which encourage undesirable behaviors relevant to diet and exercise. In accordance with operant conditioning principles, attention is given to reinforcement and rewards.	▪ Review of self-monitoring records with clients may help to identify triggers for undesirable eating
		▪ Assist client in identifying ways to modify the environment to eliminate triggers. This may include things such as:
		  □ Keeping food out of sight
		  □ Removing high sugar/high fat snacks from the house
		  □ Bringing lunch to work
		  □ Establishing a rule – no eating in the car
		▪ Help client establish criteria for rewards for desirable behavior
		▪ Ensure reward (reinforcement) received only if criteria met

Cognitive restructuring	Techniques used to increase client awareness of their perceptions of themselves and their beliefs related to diet, weight and weight loss expectations.	▪ Self-monitoring and techniques such as the ABC Technique of Irrational Beliefs may help clients to become more aware of thoughts that interfere in their ability to meet behavioral goals
		▪ Help clients replace dysfunctional thoughts with more rationale ones
		  □ Challenge shoulds, oughts, musts
		  □ Decatastrophize expected outcomes
		  □ Confront faulty self-perceptions
		  □ Decenter by envisioning other perspectives
		▪ Coach clients on replacing negative self-talk with more positive, empowering and affirming statements

Relapse prevention	Techniques used to help clients prepare to address high-risk situations for relapse with appropriate strategies and thinking. Incorporates both cognitive and behavioral strategies to enhance long-term behavior change outcomes.	Assist clients: ▪ Assess if external circumstances are contributing to lapse e.g., loss of job or support system ▪ Identify high-risk situations for slips ▪ Analyze reactions to slips ▪ Acquire knowledge and skills necessary to address high-risk situations ▪ Gain confidence in their ability to succeed in high-risk situations

223

Counseling

NUTRITION COUNSELING DOMAIN

STRATEGIES (C-2)

Rewards/contingency management	A systematic process by which behaviors can be changed through the use of rewards for specific actions. Rewards may be derived from the client or the provider.	▪ Provide rewards for desired behaviors e.g., attendance, diet progress, consistent self-monitoring ▪ Rewards can be monetary, prizes, parking space, gift certificates ▪ Assist clients in determining rewards for achievement ▪ Ensure rewards are not received if progress is not made

References

1. Miller WR, Rollnick S. *Motivational Interviewing: Preparing People for Change.* 2nd ed., New York: Guilford Press; 2002
2. Miller WR, Rollnick. S Motivational Interviewing: resources for clinicians, researchers and trainers. Available at: http://www.motivationalinterview.org/clinical/. Accessed January 12, 2007
3. Berg-Smith SM, Stevens VJ, Brown KM, Van Horn L, Gernhofer N, Peters E, Greenberg R, Snetselaar L, Ahrens L, Smith K for the Dietary Intervention Study in Children (DISC) Research Group. A brief motivational intervention to improve dietary adherence in adolescents. *Health Educ Res.* 1999; 14:399-410.
4. Snetselaar L. Counseling for change. In: Mahan LK, Escott-Stump S, eds. *Krause's Food, Nutrition, & Diet Therapy.* 10th ed. Philadelphia: Saunders; 2000.
5. Brug J, Spikmans F, Aartsen C, Breedveld B, Bes R, Fereira I. Training dietitians in basic motivational interviewing skills results in changes in their counseling style and in lower saturated fat intakes in their patients. *J Nutr Ed Behav.* 2007;39:8-12.
6. DiLillo V, Siegfried NJ, West DS. Incorporating motivational interviewing into behavioral obesity training. *Cogn Behav Prac.* 2003;10:120-130
7. National Heart, Lung, and Blood Institute, National Institute of Diabetes and Digestive and Kidney Diseases. Clinical Guidelines on the Identification, Evaluation, and Treatment of Overweight and Obesity in Adults: The Evidence Report. Washington, DC: U.S. Government Printing Office. 1998. Guidelines available at http://www.nhlbi.nih.gov/guidelines/obesity/ob_gdlns.htm.
8. Estabrooks P, Nelson C, Xu S, King D, Bayliss E, Gaglio B, Nutting P, Glasgow R. the frequency and behavioral outcomes of goal choices in the self-management of diabetes. *Diabetes Educ.* 2005;31(3):391-400.
9. Boutelle KN, Kirschenbaum DS. Further support for consistent self-monitoring as a vital component of successful weight control. *Obes Res.* 1998;52:219-224.
10. Foster GD. Clinical implications for the treatment of obesity. *Obesity.* 2006;14:182S-185S.
11. Brownell KD, Cohen LR. Adherence to Dietary Regimens 2: components of effective interventions. *Behav Med.* 1995; 20: 155–163.
12. D'Zurilla TJ, Goldfried MR. Problem solving and behavior modification. *J Abnorm Psychol.* 1971;78:107-126.
13. Barrere M, Toobert D, Angell K, Glasgow R, Mackinnon D. Social support and social-ecological resources as mediators of lifestyle intervention effects for type 2 diabetes. *J Health Psychol.* 2006;11:483-495.
14. Berkel LA, Poston WS 2d, Reeves RS, Foreyt JP. Behavioral Interventions for Obesity. *J Am Diet Assoc.* 2005;105: S35-S43.
15. Snetselaar L. *Nutritional Counseling for Lifestyle Change.* New York:Taylor & Francis Group; 2007: 117-119.
16. Snetselaar LG. *Nutrition Counseling Skills for Medical Nutrition Therapy.* 2nd ed. Gaithersburg, MD: Aspen Press; 2007
17. Fabricatore AN. Behavior therapy and cognitive-behavioral therapy of obesity: Is there a difference? *J Am Diet Assoc.* 2007:107:92-99.
18. Kiy AM. Cognitive-behavioral and psychoeducational counseling and therapy. In: Helm KK, Klawitter B. *Nutrition Therapy: Advanced Counseling Skills.* Lake Dallas, TX: Helms Seminars: 1995:135-154.
19. Irvin JE, Bowers CA, Dunn ME, Wang MC. Efficacy of relapse prevention: A meta-analytic review. *J Consult Clin Psychol.* 1999;67:563-570.
20. Prochaska JO, Norcross JC, DiClemente V. *Changing for Good: A Revolutionary Six-Stage Program for Overcoming Bad Habits and Moving Your Life Positively Forward.* New York, NY: Avon Books Inc; 1994

COORDINATION OF OTHER CARE DURING NUTRITION CARE (RC-1)

Definition

Facilitating services or interventions with other professionals, institutions, or agencies on behalf of the patient/client prior to discharge from nutrition care.

Details of Intervention

A typical intervention might be further described with the following details:

- Holding a team meeting to develop a comprehensive plan of care
- A formal referral for care by other dietetics practitioners who provide different expertise
- Collaboration with or referral to others such as the physician, dentist, physical therapist, social worker, occupational therapist, speech therapist, nurse, pharmacist, or other specialist dietitian
- Referral to an appropriate agency/program (e.g., home delivered meals, WIC, food pantry, soup kitchen, food stamps, housing assistance, shelters, rehabilitation, physical and mental disability programs, education training, and employment programs)

Typically used with the following:

Nutrition Diagnostic Terminology Used in PES Statements	Common Examples (Not intended to be inclusive)
Nutrition Diagnoses	▪ Inadequate oral food and beverage intake (NI 2.1) ▪ Involuntary weight loss (NC-3.2) ▪ Excessive alcohol intake (NI-4.3) ▪ Inappropriate intake of food fats (NI-5.6.3) ▪ Overweight/obesity (NC-3.3) ▪ Physical inactivity (NB-2.1) ▪ Food–medication interaction (NC-2.3) ▪ Self-feeding difficulty (NB-2.6) ▪ Limited access to food (NB-3.2)

225

Coordination

COORDINATION OF NUTRITION CARE DOMAIN

COORDINATION OF OTHER CARE DURING NUTRITION CARE (RC-1)

Etiology	Physical Examination Findings • Physical disability with impaired feeding ability, other impairments related to activities of daily living • Growth and development issues Food/Nutrition History • Inadequate intake • Nutrient drug interactions Psychological/Social History • Transportation issues • Food acceptance issues • Developmental issues • Economic considerations impacting food/nutrient intake	
Signs and Symptoms	Physical Examination Findings • Weight loss • Unacceptable growth rates compared to standard growth charts Food/Nutrition History • More than 10% weight loss in 6 months • Hyperglycemia and weight loss • Poor wound healing Client History • Inability to procure food • Anorexia nervosa • Lack of access to food sources • Lack of food preparation skills	

Other considerations (*e.g., patient/client negotiation, patient/client needs and desires, and readiness to change*)

- Availability of services related to patient/client need (specialty dietitians, clinical pharmacists, speech pathologists, nurse practitioners, etc.)
- Anticipated duration of health care encounter/hospital or long-term care discharge
- Resources available for care
- Medicare/Medicaid/insurance guidelines and restrictions
- Food assistance program (e.g., food stamp program) guidelines and regulations

226

Edition: 2008

COORDINATION OF OTHER CARE DURING NUTRITION CARE (RC-1)

References

1. Position of the American Dietetic Association. Nutrition, aging, and the continuum of care. *J Am Diet Assoc.* 2000;100:580-595.
2. Mclaughlin C, Tarasuk V, Kreiger N. An examination of at-home food preparation activity among low-income, food insecure women. *J Am Diet Assoc.* 2003;103:1506-1512.
3. Greger JL, Maly A, Jensen N, Kuhn J, Monson K, Stocks A. Food pantries can provide nutritionally adequate food packets but need help to become effective referral units for public assistance programs. *J Am Diet Assoc.* 2002;102:1125-1128.
4. Olson CM, Holben DH. Position of the American Dietetic Association: Domestic food and nutrition security. *J Am Diet Assoc.* 2002;102:1840-1847.
5. Millen BE, Ohls JC, Ponza M, McCool AC. The elderly nutrition program: An effective national framework for preventive nutrition interventions. *J Am Diet Assoc.* 2002;102:234-240.

227

Coordination

COORDINATION OF NUTRITION CARE DOMAIN

DISCHARGE AND TRANSFER OF NUTRITION CARE TO A NEW SETTING OR PROVIDER (RC-2)

Definition

Discharge planning and transfer of nutrition care from one level or location of care to another.

Details of Intervention

A typical intervention might be further described with the following details:

- Change in the nutrition prescription with consideration for changes in patient/client schedule, activity level, and food/nutrient availability in the new setting
- Collaboration with or referral to others such as the physician, dentist, physical therapist, social worker, occupational therapist, speech therapist, nurse, pharmacist, or other specialist dietitian
- Referral to an appropriate agency/program (e.g., home delivered meals, WIC, food pantry, soup kitchen, food stamps, housing assistance, shelters, rehabilitation, physical and mental disability programs, education, training and employment programs)

Typically used with the following

Nutrition Diagnostic Terminology Used in PES Statements	Common Examples (Not intended to be inclusive)
Nutrition Diagnoses	▪ Inadequate oral food/beverage intake (NI-2.1) ▪ Imbalance of nutrients (NI-5.5) ▪ Inappropriate intake of food fats (NI-51.3) ▪ Food-medication interaction (NC-2.3) ▪ Underweight (NC-3.1) ▪ Overweight/obesity (NC-3.3) ▪ Impaired ability to prepare foods/meals (NB-2.4) ▪ Self-feeding difficulty (NB-2.6)
Etiology	Food/Nutrition History ▪ Long-term insufficient intake mandating home enteral or parenteral nutrition ▪ Growth and development considerations requiring intervention in a new setting

228

DISCHARGE AND TRANSFER OF NUTRITION CARE TO A NEW SETTING OR PROVIDER (RC-2)

Signs and Symptoms
Biochemical Data, Medical Tests and Procedures
▪ Abnormal lab values
Anthropometric Measurements
▪ Inappropriate weight status
▪ Continuing weight gain or loss
Food/Nutrition History
▪ Inappropriate dietary practices
▪ Harmful beliefs and attitudes
Client History
▪ Treatment failure
▪ Readmission

Other considerations *(e.g., patient/client negotiation, patient/client needs and desires, and readiness to change)*

- Availability of discharge planning services, options for care
- Preferences for the level and location of care
- Resources available for care
- Medicare/Medicaid/insurance guidelines and restrictions
- Health literacy
- Ability to implement treatment at home
- Food assistance program (e.g., food stamp program) guidelines and regulations

References

1. Baker EB, Wellman NS. Nutrition concerns for discharge planning for older adults: A need for multidisciplinary collaboration. *J Am Diet Assoc.* 2005;105:603-607.
2. Position of the American Dietetic Association. Nutrition, aging, and the continuum of care. *J Am Diet Assoc.* 2000;100:580-595.

229

Coordination

Edition: 2008

SNAPshot
NCP Step 4. Nutrition Monitoring and Evaluation

What is the purpose of Nutrition Monitoring and Evaluation? The purpose is to determine the amount of progress made and if goals/expected outcomes are being met. Nutrition monitoring and evaluation identifies patient/client* outcomes relevant to the nutrition diagnosis and intervention plans and goals. Nutrition care outcomes—the desired results of nutrition care—are defined in this step. The change in specific nutrition care outcome indicators can be measured and compared to the patient/client's previous status, nutrition intervention goals, or reference standards. The aim is to promote more uniformity within the dietetics profession in assessing the effectiveness of nutrition intervention.

How does a dietetics practitioner determine what to measure for Nutrition Monitoring and Evaluation? Practitioners select nutrition care outcome indicators that will reflect a change as a result of nutrition care. In addition, dietetics practitioners will consider factors such as the nutrition diagnosis and its etiology and signs or symptoms, the nutrition intervention, medical diagnosis, health care outcome goals, quality management goals for nutrition, practice setting, patient/client population, and disease state and/or severity.

How are outcomes used in Nutrition Monitoring and Evaluation organized? In four categories.

Nutrition-Related Behavioral and Environmental Outcomes	Food and Nutrient Intake Outcomes	Nutrition-Related Physical Sign and Symptom Outcomes	Nutrition-Related Patient/Client-Centered Outcomes
Nutrition-related knowledge, behavior, access, and ability that impact food and nutrient intake	*Food and/or nutrient intake from all sources*	*Anthropometric, biochemical, and physical exam parameters*	*Perception of patient/ client's nutrition intervention and its impact*

What does Nutrition Monitoring and Evaluation involve? Practitioners do three things as part of nutrition monitoring and evaluation—monitor, measure, and evaluate the changes in nutrition care indicators to determine patient/client progress. Practitioners *monitor* by providing evidence that the nutrition intervention is or is not changing the patient/client behavior or status. They *measure* outcomes by collecting data on the appropriate nutrition outcome indicator(s). Finally, dietetics practitioners compare the current findings with previous status, nutrition intervention goals, and/or reference standards (i.e., criteria) and *evaluate* the overall impact of the nutrition intervention on the patient's health outcomes. The use of standardized indicators and criteria increases the validity and reliability outcome data are collected. All these procedures facilitate electronic charting, coding, and outcomes measurement.

Critical thinking during this step...
- Selecting appropriate indicators/measures
- Using appropriate reference standards for comparison
- Defining where patient/client is in terms of expected outcomes
- Explaining a variance from expected outcomes
- Determining factors that help or hinder progress
- Deciding between discharge and continuation of nutrition care

---

Are dietetics practitioners limited to the Nutrition Monitoring and Evaluation outcomes terms? A cascade of outcomes of nutrition care have been identified; each outcome has several possible indicators that can be measured depending on the patient/client population, practice setting, and disease state/severity. Dietetics practitioners can propose additions or revisions using the Procedure for Nutrition Controlled Vocabulary/Terminology Maintenance/Review available from ADA.

Detailed information about this step can be found in the International Dietetics and Nutrition Terminology (IDNT) Reference Manual: Standardized Language for the Nutrition Care Process, First Edition, American Dietetic Association.

Patient/client refers to individuals, groups, family members, and/or caregivers.

Monitoring & Evaluation

Nutrition Care Process Step 4. Nutrition Monitoring and Evaluation

INTRODUCTION

Since 2003, the ADA has been working to describe and research the initial three steps in the Nutrition Care Process (NCP), Nutrition Assessment, Nutrition Diagnosis, and Nutrition Intervention. These three steps, along with the fourth, Nutrition Monitoring and Evaluation, are described to enhance the ability to communicate within and outside of the profession and improve the consistency and quality of individualized patient/client care and the measurement of patient/client outcomes.

The fourth step is a critical component of the nutrition care process because it identifies important measures of change or patient/client outcomes relevant to the nutrition diagnosis and nutrition intervention and describes how best to measure and evaluate these outcomes. The aim is to promote more uniformity within the profession in evaluating the efficacy of nutrition intervention.

In defining a nutrition monitoring and evaluation taxonomy, it was clear that there is substantial overlap between nutrition assessment and nutrition monitoring and evaluation. Many data points may be the same or related; however, the data purpose and use are distinct in these two steps. The items included in the monitoring and evaluation terms are those thought to be useful in evaluating the outcomes of nutrition interventions.

> **Special Note.** The terms **patient/client** are used in association with the NCP; however, the process is also intended for use with groups. In addition, family members or caregivers are an essential asset to the patient/client and dietetics practitioner in the NCP. Therefore, groups and families and caregivers of patients/clients are implied each time a reference is made to patient/client.

While the nutrition care process steps are not necessarily linear, simply stated, a dietetics practitioner using the process completes a nutrition assessment, identifies and labels the patient/client nutrition diagnosis, and targets the nutrition intervention at the etiology of the nutrition diagnosis. Nutrition monitoring and evaluation determines if the patient/client is achieving the nutrition intervention goals or desired outcomes (1).

Nutrition care outcomes, those which dietetics practitioners are striving to measure, result directly from the nutrition care process and represent the practitioner's contribution to care. Many dietetics practitioners have been involved in tracking physician-centric or institution-centric health care outcomes, such as length of stay or reduction in health risk profile, but efforts to measure the nutrition specific contributions to patient/client care have been sporadic and uncoordinated. This section of the publication will focus on describing and defining nutrition care outcomes. Nutrition care outcomes contribute to favorable health care outcomes, however, describing and defining the profession's impact on health care outcomes is beyond the scope of this publication.

The following figure illustrates how nutrition care outcomes are categorized and are linked together in a logical cascade that flows to other health care outcomes that are of concern to other health care providers, health systems, payors, and patients/clients.

Monitoring & Evaluation

Edition: 2008

Cascade of Nutrition Care and Health Care Outcomes

	Nutrition Care Outcomes				Health Care Outcomes		
	Nutrition-Related Behavior and Environmental Outcomes	Food and Nutrient Intake Outcomes	Nutrition-Related Physical Sign and Symptom Outcomes	Nutrition-Related Patient/ Client– Centered Outcomes	Health and Disease Outcomes	Cost Outcomes	Patient Outcomes
Appropriate nutrition intervention	Changes in knowledge, behavior, access, and ability.	Improved nutrient intake.	Changes in (normalization of) anthropometric, biochemical, and physical exam indices.	Improved measures of function, nutrition quality of life, and satisfaction.	↓ Risk Improvement of disease or condition. Prevention of adverse event.	↓ Diagnostic and treatment costs. ↓ Hospital and outpatient visits.	↓ Disability. ↑ Quality of life.

The ADA has developed a language and methodology to aid in standardizing the dietetics practitioner's approach to nutrition monitoring and evaluation of the nutrition care process. The nutrition monitoring and evaluation reference sheets, at the end of this chapter, are based on scientific literature and describe how dietetics practitioners measure nutrition care indicators and evaluate them.

Dietetics practitioners are encouraged to pool or aggregate data from the nutrition monitoring and evaluation step to create an outcomes management system. Like nutrition screening, the outcome management system is not a part of the nutrition care process. The primary purpose of an outcome management system is to evaluate the efficacy and efficiency of the entire process.

NUTRITION CARE PROCESS AND NUTRITION MONITORING AND EVALUATION

Nutrition monitoring and evaluation determines if the patient/client is meeting the nutrition intervention goals or desired outcomes (1). To reach this point in the process, a nutrition assessment is needed to identify whether a nutrition-related problem exists.

If a nutrition diagnosis/problem does exist, the dietetics practitioner labels the problem and creates a PES (Problem, Etiology, Signs/Symptoms) statement.

Relationships

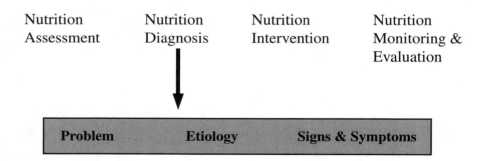

The nutrition intervention is, almost always, aimed at the etiology (E) of the nutrition diagnosis/problem identified in the PES statement. Less frequently, the nutrition intervention is directed at the signs and symptoms (S) to minimize their impact.

Relationships

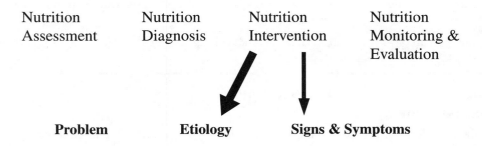

Nutrition monitoring and evaluation determines whether the patient/client is achieving the nutrition intervention goals or desired outcomes.

Relationships

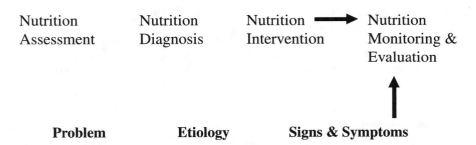

Nutrition monitoring and evaluation answers the question, "Is the nutrition intervention strategy working to resolve the nutrition diagnosis, its etiology, and/or signs and symptoms?" This step clearly defines the outcomes specific to nutrition care. For instance, a patient newly diagnosed with hyperlipidemia, may have goals related to nutrition knowledge and fat, fiber, and energy intake along with biochemical measures of total cholesterol and LDL cholesterol. The dietetics practitioner may develop an action plan to periodically monitor, evaluate and document nutrition knowledge, intake of fat and/or saturated fat, and/or lab values.

As will be described in greater detail throughout in this chapter, nutrition monitoring and evaluation assesses the patient/client's progress by comparing very specific markers or nutrition care indicators against recognized, science-based standards or baseline. Some of the terminology essential to this step is defined here. Its application to patient/client nutrition care will be covered thoroughly.

Edition: 2008

Nutrition Monitoring and Evaluation Definitions

Nutrition monitoring—pre-planned review and measurement of selected nutrition care outcome indicators of patient/client's status relevant to the defined needs, nutrition diagnosis, nutrition intervention, and outcomes.

Nutrition evaluation—the systematic comparison of current findings with the previous status, nutrition intervention goals, effectiveness of overall nutrition care, or a reference standard.

Nutrition care outcomes—the results of nutrition care that are directly related to the nutrition diagnosis and the goals of the intervention plan.

Nutrition care outcome indicators—markers that can be measured and evaluated to determine the effectiveness of the nutrition care.

NUTRITION MONITORING AND EVALUATION COMPONENTS:
Monitor, Measure, and Evaluate

In the fourth step of the nutrition care process, dietetics practitioners do the following three things—monitor progress, measure outcomes, and evaluate the outcomes against criteria to determine changes in specific indicators of nutrition care outcomes.

Monitor

Nutrition intervention typically involves activities completed with the patient/client (e.g., self-monitoring record review, education) and actions taken by the patient/client as a result of the intervention (e.g., adjusting insulin dosage based upon self-monitoring, label reading and interpretation, self-feeding with an adapted feeding device). At each encounter, the dietetics practitioner monitors some or all of the nutrition care outcome indicators to determine if nutrition goals have been achieved or if further intervention is necessary.

In many cases, nutrition monitoring and evaluation will begin with a determination of the patient/client's understanding of the nutrition intervention and how it should or if it has been implemented. Progress may be impacted if the patient/client did not or was not clear about how to implement the nutrition intervention.

Measure

Patient/client records, counseling sessions, and classes offer an abundance of potential nutrition care outcomes. The appropriate nutrition care outcome indicators are determined by the nutrition diagnosis and its etiology and signs or symptoms. In addition, the nutrition intervention, medical diagnosis and health care outcome goals, and quality management goals for nutrition may influence the nutrition care outcome indicators chosen. Other factors, such as practice setting, patient/client population, and disease state and/or severity may also impact the choice of indicator. As noted earlier, nutrition care outcomes and health care outcomes are different and distinct. Only nutrition care outcomes are discussed here.

Sometimes the measurement or data collection will occur during the initial encounter and other times it will occur at a later date during subsequent encounters. For example, you can measure knowledge change immediately but you may only be able to measure a nutrition-related physical sign and symptom such as laboratory indicator at a subsequent encounter.

Use of standardized indicators and measures will increase the likelihood that valid and reliable measures of change will be collected and facilitate electronic charting, coding, and outcomes measurement.

Evaluate

Comparing the nutrition care outcome indicators against standards shown to produce the desired effect (e.g., $\leq 30\%$ of calories from fat/day), will aid in more consistent and comparable nutrition care changes and outcomes across patient populations, practitioners, and practice settings. The criteria used for comparison may be a national, institutional, and/or regulatory standard. Fortunately, the monitoring and evaluation step is flexible. Dietetics practitioners must select the most appropriate reference standard or goal based upon the patient/client condition and patient care setting. Not all patients/clients may be able to achieve the goals established by a national standard, for example, < 2,300 mg sodium per day from the *Dietary Guidelines for Americans* (2). Mitigating circumstances may be defined and a more suitable goal established, for example, a dietetics practitioner might establish a nutrition prescription for 4,000 mg of sodium per day, and evaluate a patient/client's progress toward this nutrition prescription. A second component of the evaluation is to look at the entire picture of the nutrition care by simultaneously evaluating multiple outcome indicators and determine overall impact on the patient/client outcomes.

The following types of critical thinking skills are essential for the nutrition monitoring and evaluation step:
- Selecting appropriate indicators/measures
- Using appropriate criteria (i.e., previous status, nutrition intervention goals, or reference standards) for comparison
- Defining where patient/client is now in terms of expected outcome
- Explaining variance from expected outcomes
- Identifying factors that help or hinder progress
- Deciding between discharge or continuation of nutrition care

Following is a summary of the three components of the nutrition monitoring and evaluation step.

Nutrition Monitoring and Evaluation Components Summary

Monitor progress
- Check patient/client's understanding and compliance with nutrition intervention
- Determine if the intervention is being implemented as prescribed
- Provide evidence that the nutrition intervention is or is not changing the patient/client's behavior or status
- Identify other positive or negative outcomes
- Gather information indicating reasons for lack of progress
- Support conclusions with evidence

Measure outcomes
- Select the nutrition care outcome indicator(s) to measure the desired outcome(s)
- Use standardized nutrition care outcome indicator(s) to increase the validity and reliability of the measurements of change

Evaluate outcomes
- Compare monitoring data with the nutrition prescription/goals or reference standard to assess progress and determine future action
- Evaluate impact of the sum of all interventions on overall patient/client health outcomes

NUTRITION CARE OUTCOMES

Nutrition care should result in important changes that lead to improved behaviors and/or nutritional status. In outpatient and community settings, this might include improvement in the patient/client's understanding of the food and nutrient needs and their ability and motivation to meet those needs. In hospital settings, this might include an improvement in biochemical parameters or a basic understanding of the nutrition prescription. In long term care facilities, this might include an improvement in a patient/client's ability to feed him or herself independently and a reduction in need for supplemental enteral nutrition support.

Edition: 2008

Nutrition care outcomes are often intermediate outcomes to other broader health care outcomes (e.g., occurrence, duration or severity of acute and chronic disease, infections, wound healing, health care cost, and patient functional ability).

Nutrition care outcomes are distinguished by several characteristics. They:

- Represent results that the practitioner/nutrition care impacted independently
- Can be linked to nutrition intervention goals
- Are measurable with tools and resources available to the practitioner
- Occur in reasonable time period
- Can be attributed to the nutrition care
- Are logical and biologically or psychologically plausible stepping stones to other health care outcomes (e.g., health and disease, cost, and patient/client outcomes)

NUTRITION CARE OUTCOME CATEGORIES

Nutrition care outcomes are distinct from health care outcomes as they represent the dietetics practitioner's specific contribution to care. They are categorized into the four domains shown in the previous figure (see page 232). Within each of the four domains are classes of outcomes.

Nutrition Care Outcome Domains

Nutrition-Related Behavioral and Environmental Outcome Domain
Level or degree of understanding, behavior, access, and ability, which may impact food and nutrient intake. The following are classes of outcomes within this domain:

Class: Knowledge and belief outcomes—improved understanding of nutrition concepts and change in beliefs and attitudes that increase the probability that the patient/client will successfully implement nutrition prescription/goal.

Class: Behavioral outcomes—patient/client activities and actions necessary to achieve nutrition-related goals.

Class: Access outcomes—availability of a sufficient quantity of safe, healthful food.

Class: Physical activity and function outcomes—improved physical activity and ability to engage in specific tasks (e.g., breastfeeding).

Food and Nutrient Intake Outcome Domain
Food and/or nutrient intake, from all sources, e.g., food, beverages, supplements, and via enteral and parenteral routes.

Class: Energy intake outcomes—total energy intake.

Class: Food and beverage intake outcomes—foods and food groups and fluid intake.

Class: Enteral/parenteral nutrition intake outcomes—specialized nutrition support intake.

Class: Bioactive substance intake outcomes—alcohol, plant stanol and sterol esters, soy protein, psyllium and β-glucan, and caffeine intake.

Class: Macronutrient intake outcomes—carbohydrate, fiber, protein, and fat and cholesterol intake.

Class: Micronutrient intake outcomes—vitamins and mineral intake.

Nutrition-Related Physical Sign and Symptom Outcome Domain
Measures associated with anthropometric, biochemical, and physical exam parameters.

Class: Anthropometric outcomes—measures such as weight, body mass index (BMI) percentile/age, waist circumference, and length.

Class: Biochemical and medical test outcomes—lab values or medical tests such as glucose, lipids, electrolytes, and bone densitometry.

Class: Physical examination outcomes—physical exam parameters such as edema, nausea, vomiting, bowel function, skin integrity, and blood pressure.

Nutrition-Related Patient/Client-Centered Outcome Domain
Measures associated with a patient/client's perception of his/her nutrition intervention and its impact on life.

Class: Nutrition quality of life outcomes—perception of the impact of nutrition care on quality of life

Class: Satisfaction outcomes—satisfaction with nutrition prescription recommendations, nutrition counseling, nutrition education and/or meals and snacks or food service.

Health Care Outcomes

Health care outcomes represent outcomes of interest to health care providers, health systems and payors and are defined in other standardized languages. Health Care Outcomes often include the cumulative outcomes of all medical care—including nutrition care. They include:

- Health and Disease Outcomes—Change in severity, duration, or course of a condition or disease; changes in risk level; prevention of an adverse event; or maintenance of health.

- Cost Outcomes—Change in factors that influence the cost of health care such as hospitalization, length of stay, ICU days; number of outpatient visits; home, intermediate and long-term care; diagnostic and treatment procedures; and medication and equipment consumed.

- Patient/Client Outcomes—Changes in patient/client-centered indicators that reflect such things as level of disability, functional status, quality of life, and satisfaction with care.

Health care outcomes can be impacted with appropriate nutrition care of sufficient intensity and duration. Adoption of the nutrition care process (including assessment, diagnosis, intervention, and monitoring and evaluation) associated process improvements and practice innovations should result in positive changes in nutrition care outcomes that in turn improve other health care outcomes. This publication will focus only on nutrition care monitoring and evaluation and nutrition care outcomes. These represent the principle nutrition care contributions to global health care outcomes.

NUTRITION CARE OUTCOME INDICATORS

Nutrition care outcome indicators are clearly defined markers that can be observed and measured and are used to quantify the changes that are the result of nutrition care. Selected indicators for nutrition monitoring should be relevant to and reflect a change in the patient/client's nutrition diagnosis and its etiology and signs/symptoms. The indicators selected may also be relevant to the patient/client disease state, quality management goals for nutrition, and health care outcome goals.

Well-chosen indicators enable practitioners to monitor and evaluate progress made toward desired nutrition care outcomes. Nutrition care outcome indicators provide information about the type and magnitude of progress made, when the nutrition problem is resolved, and what aspects of nutrition intervention are working or where adjustments are needed. This is in contrast to data used for nutrition assessment. Many data points may be the same or related; however, dietetics practitioners use additional nutrition assessment data to identify and provide evidence about a nutrition-related problem or diagnosis.

Edition: 2008

Monitoring & Evaluation

While not part of the nutrition care process, nutrition care outcome indicators are ideal components of a quality improvement program, which will be discussed further at the end of this chapter. Commonly used indicators vary by practice setting.

Nutrition care outcomes and indicators include:
- Factors that dietetics practitioners can impact directly, such as food and nutrient intake; growth and body composition; food and nutrition-related knowledge, attitudes and behaviors; and food access
- Laboratory values such as HgbA1c, hematocrit, serum cholesterol
- Functional capabilities such as physical activity
- Patient perception of nutrition care and results of nutrition care such as nutrition quality of life

Nutrition monitoring and evaluation reference sheets define the nutrition care outcome and the indicators that may be appropriate for measuring and evaluating outcomes within a variety of practice settings.

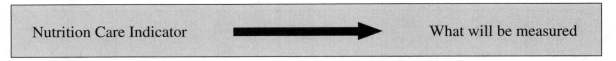

Nutrition Care Indicator ⟶ What will be measured

MEASUREMENT AND EVALUATION OF NUTRITION OUTCOME INDICATORS

Dietetics practitioners make judgments about progress toward nutrition-related outcomes by comparing the actual value of the measured indicator to a science-based criteria or individualized goal/expected outcome.

The dietetics practitioner does this based upon the *criteria* and *scale* established for the nutrition care outcome.

Criteria

Two criteria are suggested for nutrition monitoring and evaluation:
- Nutrition prescription or goal/expected outcome (e.g. a behavior change has a goal not a nutrition prescription)
- Reference standard (e.g., national, institutional, and/or regulatory standards)

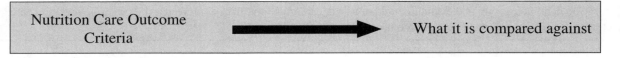

Nutrition Care Outcome Criteria ⟶ What it is compared against

The nutrition prescription is the patient/client's individualized recommended dietary intake of energy and/or selected foods or nutrients based on current reference standards or and dietary guidelines and the patient/client's health condition and nutrition diagnosis. For example, a patient of normal body weight has a serum LDL-cholesterol of 150 mg/dL. His nutrition prescription is <30% calories from fat with <10% calories from saturated fat. If a behavior change outcome is desired, the patient/client would also have a goal (e.g., take lunch to work at least three times per week and reduce high-fat fast food intake at lunch to one time per week).

For biochemical outcomes such as LDL-cholesterol, the criteria that may be used is the reference standard established by the National Heart Lung and Blood Institute of serum LDL <100 mg/dL. This could also be stated as a goal to reduce baseline LDL by a specific percentage.

Monitoring & Evaluation

Scale

Once the nutrition care indicator is selected and the criteria established, the next step is evaluating the changes using a scale. Practitioners use the scale to define the degree to which the indicator changed to meet the criteria.

Other professions, such as nursing and speech-language pathology have developed validated scales for evaluating the changes in a patient/client's status. The dietetics profession has a critical need to have reliable and valid indicators and scales to demonstrate the impact of nutrition care. This need is balanced with the desire to have these measures as soon as is practical to facilitate measuring outcomes and research and to move toward electronic medical records.

This publication contains the nutrition care outcomes and indicators, along with the references related to the criteria and sample documentation examples. A future edition will incorporate recommendations for practitioners to evaluate the degree to which the indicators meet the criteria using scales. While additional time is needed, it is believed that a staged approach would improve the likelihood of developing reliable and valid measures of nutrition care that are critical to the profession.

Selection and Interpretation of the Nutrition Care Indicators

Primary factors affecting indicator selection and interpretation

Although the nutrition monitoring and evaluation reference sheets define the nutrition care outcome and the wide variety of indicators that are appropriate for measuring and evaluating outcomes, the reference sheets do not distinguish which nutrition care outcome indicators are best for a particular situation. The dietetics practitioner makes this decision based on the individual situation.

Three primary factors will influence the selection, measurement, and interpretation of the individual nutrition care outcomes indicators:

- Practice setting (e.g., inpatient or outpatient, long-term care, community)
- Age of the patient/client (e.g., pediatrics, geriatrics)
- Disease state and severity (e.g., renal disease, diabetes, critical illness)

National reference standards are available for many outcome indicators; for example, ADA has a Critical Illness Evidence-Based Guideline which addresses glucose level (indicator) for critically ill patients/clients with hyperglycemia (3). This guideline reads: "Dietitians should promote attainment of strict glycemic control (80-110 mg/dL) to reduce time on mechanical ventilation in critically ill medical ICU patients."

Glucose is the appropriate indicator in a stressed ICU patient and the criteria have been defined. HgbA1c is not used as an indicator in this instance. It is the dietetics practitioner's responsibility to distinguish which indictor is appropriate for the given practice and patient/client situation.

Edition: 2008

Secondary factor affecting indicator selection and interpretation
The time frame over which a patient/client receives nutrition care influences the selection of the indicator. The previous example illustrates this point. HgbA1c is a measure of glucose status over a 60-90 day period and is not useful in monitoring and evaluation of the ICU patient/client with acute elevation of blood glucose. HgbA1c *is* appropriate, however, in the outpatient setting when patient/clients are observed over a period of time.

Other considerations
Interpretation of the change seen in particular nutrition care indicators may require evidence or explanation by a dietetics practitioner. For example, if a patient/client attains the goal to reduce overall body fat through nutrition intervention, one may see a negative change or increase in body mass index (BMI) due to the patient/client's increase in muscle mass. Occurrences such as these should be anticipated and appropriate evidence and explanation documented.

The considerations described, along with the examples, illustrate the importance of appropriate indictor selection and interpretation. Each situation will be different depending upon the practice setting, population, and disease state and severity, and the time interval over which the patient/client receives nutrition care. Selection of the incorrect indicator may lead to incorrect conclusions about the impact of nutrition interventions.

NUTRITION MONITORING AND EVALUATION REFERENCE SHEETS

Following this introduction to nutrition monitoring and evaluation are reference sheets for the nutrition care outcomes identified. Reference sheets contain seven distinct components: definition of the nutrition care outcome, the potential nutrition care outcome indicators, measurement method or data sources, the nutrition interventions with which the outcomes are associated, the nutrition diagnoses with which the nutrition monitoring and evaluation data are used, the criteria for evaluation, and the patient/client nutrition monitoring documentation example.

The reference sheets provide references for suggested measurement techniques and reference standards for some common patient/client populations and settings associated with the outcome. Dietetics practitioners are not limited to the references offered and are encouraged to use others pertinent to their patient/client and practice setting needs. Once measurement techniques and criteria are identified, they should be noted in the dietetics practitioner's policies and procedures or other documents for use in patient/client records, quality or performance improvement, or in formal research projects.

Following is a description of the seven components of the nutrition monitoring and evaluation reference sheet:

The **Definition** of Nutrition Care Outcome defines the specific parameters of the outcome.

The **Potential Nutrition Care Outcome Indicators** identify the indicators that can be used to measure *change* based upon nutrition intervention.

The **Measurement Method or Data Sources** for the outcome identify some of the resources dietetics practitioners use to obtain nutrition monitoring and evaluation data.

The typical **Nutrition Interventions** with which the nutrition care outcomes are associated are listed.

The typical **Nutrition Diagnoses** with which the nutrition care outcomes are associated are listed.

Two **Criteria** are identified for comparison of the nutrition care outcome indicators: 1) goal/nutrition prescription, or 2) reference standard.

The **Patient/Client Example** includes sample nutrition monitoring and evaluation documentation. It describes only *one* of the nutrition care outcome indicators associated with the nutrition care outcome. As described earlier, depending on the practice setting (e.g., inpatient or outpatient, long-term care, community), patient/client (e.g., pediatrics, geriatrics), and disease state and severity, one or multiple indicators may be followed at a time.

It is important to reiterate that while patient/client is used throughout this reference, these terms refer to individuals and groups, as well as family and caregivers. Following is an example of one nutrition monitoring and evaluation indicator that may be used with an individual or a group.

Individual Patient/Client Example

Nutrition care outcome: Nutritional anemia profile

Nutrition care outcome indicator: Serum ferritin

Criteria: Based on a reference standard: The patient/client's serum ferritin is 8 ng/mL, which is below (*above, below, or a percent of*) the reference standard for adult females.

Nutrition monitoring and evaluation documentation:

Initial encounter with patient/client	Patient/client's serum ferritin is 8 ng/mL, which is below the reference standard for adult females. Will monitor change in serum ferritin at the next appointment.
Re-assessment after nutrition intervention	Goal/reference standard achieved as patient/client's serum ferritin is 10.9 ng/mL, within normal limits.

Group Example

Nutrition care outcome: Nutritional anemia profile

Nutrition care outcome indicator: Serum ferritin

Criteria: Based on a reference standard: 20% or fewer of low-income women will have a hemoglobin level <11.0 g/dL during the third trimester of pregnancy based upon Healthy People 2010.

Nutrition monitoring and evaluation documentation:

Initial encounter with population	44% of low-income black women have a hemoglobin level of < 11.0 g/dL during the third trimester of pregnancy. Monitor change in prevalence of low hemoglobin levels among low-income women.
Re-assessment after nutrition intervention	Prevalence of anemia among low-income pregnant women is 29%. Significant progress made toward the Healthy People 2010 target, 20% or less, for prevalence of anemia.

These reference sheets will assist dietetics practitioners working in a variety of settings, with individuals and groups, when measuring and evaluating nutrition care outcome indicators.

NUTRITION MONITORING AND EVALUATION: Documentation

Several components of documentation are recommended throughout the nutrition care process. Documentation is an on-going process that supports all of the steps. Documentation that is relevant, accurate, and timely is essential, but lacking if it does not include specific statements of where the patient/client is now in terms of expected nutrition outcomes.

Edition: 2008

Quality documentation for nutrition monitoring and evaluation includes:

- Date and time
- Indicators measured, results, and the method for obtaining the measurement
- Criteria to which the indicator is compared (i.e., nutrition prescription/goal or a reference standard)
- Factors facilitating or hampering progress
- Other positive or negative outcomes
- Future plans for nutrition care, nutrition monitoring, and follow up or discharge

In an initial encounter, it may not be possible to include all of these elements because the nutrition prescription and goals have just been established, and the nutrition intervention may not have occurred. Two complete Case Studies with examples of documentation in various charting formats are available in the Nutrition Care Process and Model Resource section of the ADA Web site, www.eatright.org, in the either the Research or Practice sections. *Brief excerpts* of documentation may look like this:

Initial encounter 7/15

Nutrition assessment: Based upon a three-day food diary, patient consumes approximately 120 grams fat per day.

Nutrition diagnosis: Excessive fat intake related to frequent restaurant meals as evidence by a current average intake of 120 grams of fat per day.

Nutrition intervention: Nutrition prescription is 60 grams of fat per day. Nutrition counseling provided.

Nutrition monitoring and evaluation: Intake of fat (indicator) is currently 200% of nutrition prescription (criteria). Will monitor change in fat intake at next encounter.

Follow-up encounter 8/10

Nutrition intervention: Patient/client reports difficulty ordering low fat selections at restaurants. Provided comprehensive education to identify low fat items on restaurant menus and at a variety of fast food restaurants. Patient/client implementing self-monitoring log.

Nutrition monitoring and evaluation: Based upon three-day diet record, some progress toward nutrition prescription as intake of fat is reduced from 120 to 90 grams per day. Will monitor change in restaurant selections (using patient/client's self-monitoring log) and fat intake at next encounter.

NUTRITION MONITORING AND EVALUATION: Data Sources and Tools

To monitor and evaluate a patient/client's progress, the following tools may be used:

- Patient/client questionnaires
- Surveys
- Pre-tests and post-tests
- Patient/client/family member interview
- Anthropometric measurements
- Biochemical and medical test results
- Food and nutrition intake tools

These tools can be used when patients are seen individually or in groups, or when the encounter is conducted by phone or via computer. Pooled data can be monitored and evaluated using tracking forms and computer software programs.

The Nutrition Monitoring and Evaluation Reference Sheet is a guide developed for dietetics practitioners to use when completing this step. The reference sheet gathers together, in one resource, valuable information from the scientific literature. Since nutrition monitoring and evaluation have not been comprehensively described before now, the reference sheets break new ground as dietetics practitioners aim to accurately describe the impact of nutrition care.

NUTRITION CARE OUTCOME MANAGEMENT SYSTEM

Nutrition monitoring and evaluation applies to individual patient/clients and to groups of patients/clients. Selecting nutrition monitoring and evaluation data for an individual patient/client depends primarily upon the nutrition diagnosis and the nutrition intervention. An additional consideration when selecting the nutrition monitoring and evaluation outcome indicators for patients/clients is how data may be used when pooled to assess quality of care provided to specific groups of patients. Choosing what to monitor may also be influenced by facility strategic goals and quality improvement plans, regulatory or certifying agency requirements (e.g., American Diabetes Association Self-Management Education certification, Joint Commission).

Aggregate nutrition care outcome indicator data may be reported to administrators, payers, quality improvement organizations, and other decision makers of health care funding.

Potential benefits of the aggregate data include:
- Provides for process improvement and leads to understanding of what works and what does not
- Can be used for outcomes measurement studies and quality improvement initiatives
- Links care processes and resource utilization
- Gives an opportunity to identify and analyze causes of less than optimal performance and outcomes
- Defines information for inclusion in centralized data systems relevant to nutrition care
- Can be used to quantify the dietetics practitioner's contribution to health care

Various factors that can impact aggregate nutrition care outcome indicator data interpretation and need consideration include:
- Method for collecting the outcome, e.g., three-day diet record versus a 24-hour recall
- Data source, e.g., patient/client, family/caregiver, chart, bedside record
- Intervention components (e.g., type, duration, and intensity)
- Education and skill level of dietetics practitioner
- Nutrition program attributes

A case example integrating nutrition monitoring and evaluation data into a department quality improvement program, Case C, is available in the Nutrition Care Process and Model Resource section of the ADA Web site, www.eatright.org, in the either the Research or Practice sections.

SUMMARY

Nutrition monitoring and evaluation describes the patient/client's progress through consistent terms that are evaluated based upon carefully selected indicators and criteria. As more and more dietetics practitioners use these tools and share their progress and nutrition care outcomes, the body of literature quantifying the dietetics practitioner's contribution to improving the health of patients/clients and describing effective methods of intervention will grow.

REFERENCES
1. Lacey K, Pritchett E. Nutrition care process and model: ADA adopts road map to quality care and outcomes management. *J Am Diet Assoc.* 2003;103:1061-1072.
2. Dietary Guidelines for Americans, 2005. Available at: http://www.health.gov/dietaryguidelines/dga2005/document/html/executivesummary.htm. Accessed October 27, 2006.
3. American Dietetic Association. Critical illness evidence-based nutrition guideline, 2006. Available at: http://www.adaevidencelibrary.com/topic.cfm?cat=2809. Accessed November 1, 2006.

Monitoring & Evaluation

NUTRITION MONITORING AND EVALUATION TERMINOLOGY

During nutrition monitoring and evaluation, practitioners list the signs and symptoms from the PES statement that are the targets of the nutrition intervention. Then, practitioners list the nutrition interventions and goals/expected outcome along with the indicators and criteria to provide evidence for the nutrition monitoring and evaluation. There may be more than one indicator per goal and one indicator may be used for multiple goals.

Signs/Symptoms from PES statement(s)

_____

_____

_____

Nutrition Intervention(s) and Goal/expected outcome(s)	Indicator(s)	Criteria
Intervention _____ #1 Goal _____ #2 Goal _____	_____ _____ _____ _____	_____ _____ _____
Intervention _____ #3 Goal _____ #4 Goal _____	_____ _____ _____ _____	_____ _____ _____
Intervention _____ #5 Goal _____ #6 Goal _____	_____ _____ _____ _____	_____ _____ _____

NUTRITION-RELATED BEHAVIORAL-ENVIRONMENTAL OUTCOMES — BE

Knowledge/Beliefs (1)
Improved understanding of nutrition concepts and change in beliefs and attitudes that increase the probability that the patient/client will successfully implement nutrition prescription/goal.

Beliefs and attitudes (1.1)
- ☐ Readiness to change — BE-1.1.1
- ☐ Perceived consequence of change — BE-1.1.2
- ☐ Perceived costs versus benefits of change — BE-1.1.3
- ☐ Perceived risk — BE-1.1.4
- ☐ Outcome expectancy — BE-1.1.5
- ☐ Conflict with personal/ family value system — BE-1.1.6
- ☐ Self-efficacy — BE-1.1.7 _(breastfeeding, eating, weight loss)_

Food and nutrition knowledge (1.2)
- ☐ Level of knowledge — BE-1.2.1 _(e.g., none, limited, minimal, substantial, and extensive)_
- ☐ Areas of knowledge — BE-1.2.2 _(food/nutrient requirements, physiological functions, disease/condition, nutrition recommendations, food products, consequences of food behavior, food label understanding, self-management parameters)_

Behavior (2)
Patient/client activities and actions necessary to achieve nutrition-related goals.

Ability to plan meals/snacks (2.1)
- ☐ Meal/snack planning ability — BE-2.1.1

Ability to select healthful food/meals (2.2)
- ☐ Food/meal selection — BE-2.2.1

Ability to prepare food/meals (2.3)
- ☐ Food/meal preparation ability — BE-2.3.1

Adherence (2.4)
- ☐ Self-reported adherence — BE-2.4.1

Goal setting (2.5)
- ☐ Goal setting ability — BE-2.5.1

Portion control (2.6)
- ☐ Portion size eaten — BE-2.6.1

Self-care management (2.7)
- ☐ Self-care management ability — BE-2.7.1

Self-monitoring (2.8)
- ☐ Self-monitoring ability — BE-2.8.1

Social support (2.9)
- ☐ Ability to build and utilize social support — BE-2.9.1

Stimulus control (2.10)
- ☐ Ability to manage behavior in response to stimuli — BE-2.10.1

Access (3)
Availability of a sufficient quantity of safe, healthful food.

Access to food (3.1)
- ☐ Access to a sufficient quantity of healthful food — BE-3.1.1
- ☐ Access to safe food — BE-3.1.2

Physical Activity and Function (4)
Improved physical activity and ability to engage in specific tasks (e.g., breastfeeding).

Breastfeeding success (4.1)
- ☐ Initiation of breastfeeding — BE-4.1.1
- ☐ Duration of breastfeeding — BE-4.1.2
- ☐ Exclusive breastfeeding — BE-4.1.3
- ☐ Breastfeeding problems — BE-4.1.4

Nutrition-related ADLs and IADLs (4.2)
- ☐ Acceptance of assistance with eating — BE-4.2.1
- ☐ Ability to use adaptive eating devices — BE-4.2.2
- ☐ Time taken to eat and consume meals — BE-4.2.3
- ☐ Ability to shop for food — BE-4.2.4
- ☐ Nutrition-related ADL — BE-4.2.5
- ☐ Nutrition-related IADL — BE-4.2.6

Physical activity (4.3)
- ☐ Consistency/frequency — BE-4.3.1
- ☐ Duration — BE-4.3.2
- ☐ Intensity — BE-4.3.3
- ☐ Strength — BE-4.3.4

FOOD AND NUTRIENT INTAKE OUTCOMES — FI

Energy intake (1)
Total energy intake from all sources, e.g., food, beverages, supplements, and via enteral and parenteral routes.

Energy intake (1.1)
- ☐ Total energy intake — FI 1.1.1

Food and Beverage (2)
Foods and food groups and fluids from all sources, e.g., food, beverages, supplements.

Fluid/Beverage intake (2.1)
- ☐ Oral Fluids Amounts — FI-2.1.1 _(water, coffee/tea, juice, milk, soda)_
- ☐ Food derived fluids — FI-2.1.2
- ☐ IV Fluids — FI-2.1.3
- ☐ Liquid meal replacement — FI-2.1.4

Food intake (2.2)
- ☐ Food variety — FI-2.2.1
- ☐ Number of food group servings — FI-2.2.2 _(grains, fruits, vegetables, milk/ dairy, meat/protein substitutes)_
- ☐ Healthy Eating Index — FI-2.2.3
- ☐ Children's Diet Quality Index — FI-2.2.4
- ☐ Revised Children's Diet Quality Index — FI-2.2.5

Enteral and Parenteral (3)
Specialized nutrition support intake from all sources, e.g., enteral and parenteral routes.

Enteral/parenteral nutrition intake (3.1)
- ☐ Access — FI-3.1.1
- ☐ Formula/solution — FI-3.1.2
- ☐ Discontinuation — FI-3.1.3
- ☐ Initiation — FI-3.1.4
- ☐ Rate/schedule — FI-3.1.5

Bioactive Substances (4)
Alcohol, plant stanol and sterol esters, soy protein, psyllium and β-glucan, and caffeine intake from all sources, e.g., food, beverages, supplements, and via enteral and parenteral routes.

Alcohol intake (4.1)
- ☐ Drink size/volume — FI-4.1.1
- ☐ Frequency — FI-4.1.2

Monitoring & Evaluation

Bioactive substance intake (4.2)
- ❑ Plant sterol and stanol esters   FI-4.2.1
- ❑ Soy protein   FI-4.2.2
- ❑ Psyllium and β-glucan   FI-4.2.3

Caffeine intake (4.3)
- ❑ Total caffeine   FI-4.3.1

Macronutrients (5)
Carbohydrate, fiber, protein, and fat and cholesterol intake from all sources, e.g., food, beverages, supplements, and via enteral and parenteral routes.

Fat and cholesterol intake (5.1)
- ❑ Total fat   FI-5.1.1
- ❑ Saturated fat   FI-5.1.2
- ❑ Trans fatty acids   FI-5.1.3
- ❑ Polyunsaturated fat   FI-5.1.4
- ❑ Monounsaturated fat   FI-5.1.5
- ❑ Omega-3 fatty acids   FI-5.1.6
  (marine/plant derived, alpha-linolenic acid)
- ❑ Dietary cholesterol   FI-5.1.7

Protein intake (5.2)
- ❑ Total protein   FI-5.2.1
- ❑ High biological value protein   FI-5.2.2
- ❑ Casein   FI-5.2.3
- ❑ Whey   FI-5.2.4
- ❑ Soy protein   FI-5.2.5
- ❑ Amino acids   FI-5.2.6
- ❑ Essential amino acids   FI-5.2.7

Carbohydrate intake (5.3)
- ❑ Total carbohydrate   FI-5.3.1
- ❑ Sugar   FI-5.3.2
- ❑ Starch   FI-5.3.3
- ❑ Glycemic index   FI-5.3.4
- ❑ Glycemic load   FI-5.3.5

Fiber intake (5.4)
- ❑ Total fiber   FI-5.4.1
- ❑ Soluble fiber   FI-5.4.2
- ❑ Insoluble fiber   FI-5.4.3
  (fructo-oligosaccharides)

Micronutrients (6)
Vitamins and mineral intake from all sources, e.g., food, beverages, supplements, and via enteral and parenteral routes.

Vitamin intake (6.1)
- ❑ A   ❑ Riboflavin
- ❑ C   ❑ Niacin
- ❑ D   ❑ Folate
- ❑ E   ❑ B6
- ❑ K   ❑ B12
- ❑ Thiamin
- ❑ Other *(specify)* _____

Mineral/element intake (6.2)
- ❑ Calcium   ❑ Potassium
- ❑ Iron   ❑ Sodium
- ❑ Magnesium   ❑ Zinc
- ❑ Phosphorus
- ❑ Other *(specify)* _____

NUTRITION-RELATED PHYSICAL SIGN/ SYMPTOM OUTCOMES   S

Anthropometric (1)
Measures such as weight, body mass index (BMI) percentile/age, waist circumference, and length.

Body composition/Growth (1.1)
- ❑ Body mass index (kg/m2)   S-1.1.1
- ❑ IBW or UBW percentage   S-1.1.2
- ❑ Growth pattern   S-1.1.3
  (head circumference, length/height, weight for length/ stature, BMI percentile/age, also see Weight change)
- ❑ Weight/weight change   S-1.1.4
  (e.g. % change, weight gain/day)
- ❑ Lean body mass, fat free mass   S-1.1.5
- ❑ Mid-arm muscle circumference   S-1.1.6

- ❑ Body fat percentage   S-1.1.7
- ❑ Triceps skin fold   S-1.1.8
- ❑ Waist circumference   S-1.1.9
- ❑ Waist-hip ratio   S-1.1.10
- ❑ Bone age   S-1.1.11
- ❑ Bone mineral density   S-1.1.12

Biochemical and Medical Tests (2)
Lab values or medical tests such as glucose, lipids, electrolytes, and fecal fat test.

Acid-base balance (2.1)
- ❑ pH, serum   S-2.1.1
- ❑ Bicarbonate   S-2.1.2
- ❑ Partial pressure of carbon   S-2.1.3
  dioxide in arterial blood

Electrolyte and renal profile (2.2)
- ❑ BUN   S-2.2.1
- ❑ Creatinine   S-2.2.2
- ❑ BUN:creatinine ratio   S-2.2.3
- ❑ Glomerular filtration rate   S-2.2.4
- ❑ Sodium   S-2.2.5
- ❑ Chloride   S-2.2.6
- ❑ Potassium   S-2.2.7
- ❑ Magnesium   S-2.2.8
- ❑ Calcium   S-2.2.9
- ❑ Calcium, ionized   S-2.2.10
- ❑ Phosphorus   S-2.2.11
- ❑ Serum osmolality   S-2.2.12
- ❑ Parathyroid hormone   S-2.2.13

Essential fatty acid profile (2.3)
- ❑ Triene:Tetraene ratio   S-2.3.1

Gastrointestinal profile (2.4)
- ❑ Amylase   S-2.4.1
- ❑ Alkaline phophatase   S-2.4.2
- ❑ Alanine aminotransferase   S-2.4.3
- ❑ Aspartate aminotransferase   S-2.4.4
- ❑ Gamma glutamyl transferase   S-2.4.5
- ❑ Bilirubin, total   S-2.4.6
- ❑ Ammonia, serum   S-2.4.7
- ❑ Prothrombin time   S-2.4.8
- ❑ Partial thromboplastin time   S-2.4.9
- ❑ INR *(ratio)*   S-2.4.10
- ❑ Fecal fat   S-2.4.11

Glucose profile (2.5)
- ❑ Glucose, fasting   S-2.5.1
- ❑ Glucose, casual   S-2.5.2
- ❑ HgbA1c   S-2.5.3
- ❑ Pre-prandial capillary   S-2.5.4
  plasma glucose
- ❑ Peak postprandial capillary   S-2.5.5
  plasma glucose

Lipid profile (2.6)
- ❑ Cholesterol, serum   S-2.6.1
- ❑ Cholesterol, HDL   S-2.6.2
- ❑ Cholesterol, LDL   S-2.6.3
- ❑ Triglycerides, serum   S-2.6.4

Mineral profile (2.7)
- ❑ Copper, serum   S-2.7.1
- ❑ Iodine, urinary excretion   S-2.7.2
- ❑ Thyroid stimulating hormone   S-2.7.3
- ❑ Zinc, plasma   S-2.7.4

Nutritional anemia profile (2.8)
- ❑ Hemoglobin   S-2.8.1
- ❑ Hematocrit   S-2.8.2
- ❑ Mean corpuscular volume   S-2.8.3
- ❑ Red blood cell folate   S-2.8.4
- ❑ Red cell distribution width   S-2.8.5
- ❑ Serum B12   S-2.8.6
- ❑ Serum methylmalonic acid   S-2.8.7
- ❑ Serum folate   S-2.8.8
- ❑ Serum homocysteine   S-2.8.9
- ❑ Serum ferritin   S-2.8.10

- ❑ Serum iron   S-2.8.11
- ❑ Total iron-binding capacity   S-2.8.12
- ❑ Transferrin saturation   S-2.8.13

Protein profile (2.9)
- ❑ Albumin   S-2.9.1
- ❑ Prealbumin   S-2.9.2
- ❑ Transferrin   S-2.9.3
- ❑ Phenylalanine, plasma   S-2.9.4
- ❑ Tyrosine, plasma   S-2.9.5

Respiratory quotient (2.10)
- ❑ RQ   S-2.10.1

Urine profile (2.11)
- ❑ Urine color   S-2.11.1
- ❑ Urine osmolality   S-2.11.2
- ❑ Urine specific gravity   S-2.11.3
- ❑ Urine tests   S-2.11.4
  (e.g., ketones, sugar, protein)
- ❑ Urine volume   S-2.11.5

Vitamin profile (2.12)
- ❑ Vitamin A *(serum or*   S-2.12.1
  plasma retinol)
- ❑ Vitamin C *(plasma or serum)*   S-2.12.2
- ❑ Vitamin D *(25-hydroxy)*   S-2.12.3
- ❑ Vitamin E   S-2.12.4
  (plasma alpha-tocopherol)
- ❑ Thiamin   S-2.12.5
  (activity coefficient for erythrocyte transketolase activity)
- ❑ Riboflavin   S-2.12.6
  (activity coefficient for erythrocyte glutathione reductase activity)
- ❑ Niacin   S-2.12.7
  (urinary N'methyl-nicotinamide concentration)
- ❑ Vitamin B6   S-2.12.8
  (plasma or serum pyridoxal 5'phosphate concentration)

Physical Examination (3)
Physical exam parameters such as such as edema, nausea, vomiting, bowel function, skin integrity, and blood pressure.

Nutrition physical exam findings (3.1)
- ❑ Cardiovascular-pulmonary   S-3.1.1
  (pulmonary edema)
- ❑ Extremities, musculo-skeletal   S-3.1.2
  (e.g., nails, subcutaneous fat, muscle)
- ❑ Gastrointestinal   S-3.1.3
  (e.g., nausea, vomiting, bowel function)
- ❑ Head and neck   S-3.1.4
  (e.g. tongue, mouth, and hair changes)
- ❑ Neurological   S-3.1.5
  (e.g. confusion, fine/gross motor)
- ❑ Skin   S-3.1.6
  (e.g., appearance, turgor, integrity)
- ❑ Vital signs   S-3.1.7
  (blood pressure, respiratory rate)

**NUTRITION-RELATED
PC PATIENT/CLIENT-CENTERED
OUTCOMES**

Nutrition Quality of Life (1)
Patient/client's perception of his/her nutrition intervention and its impact on life.

Nutrition quality of life (1.1)
- ❑ Food impact   PC-1.1.1
- ❑ Physical state   PC-1.1.2
- ❑ Psychological factors   PC-1.1.3
- ❑ Self-image   PC-1.1.4
- ❑ Self-efficacy   PC-1.1.5
- ❑ Social/interpersonal factors   PC-1.1.6
- ❑ Nutrition quality of life score   PC-1.1.7

Satisfaction (2)
To be added

NUTRITION MONITORING AND EVALUATION TERMS AND DEFINITIONS

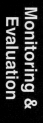

Monitoring & Evaluation

Nutrition Monitoring and Evaluation Term	Term Number	Definition	Reference Sheet Page Numbers
DOMAIN: NUTRITION-RELATED BEHAVIORAL-ENVIRONMENTAL OUTCOMES	BE	**Level or degree of understanding, behavior, access, and ability, which may impact food and nutrient intake.**	
Class: Knowledge/ Beliefs (1)			
		Improved understanding of nutrition concepts and changes in beliefs and attitudes that increase the probability that the patient/client will successfully implement the nutrition prescription	
Beliefs and attitudes	BE-1.1	Beliefs/attitudes about and/or readiness to change food, nutrition, or nutrition-related behaviors	252-254
Food and nutrition knowledge	BE-1.2	Patient/client level of knowledge about food, nutrition or nutrition-related information and guidelines	255-257
Class: Behavior (2)			
		Patient/client activities and actions necessary to achieve nutrition-related goals	
Ability to plan meals/snacks	BE-2.1	Ability level related to planning healthful meals/snacks, which are compatible with dietary goals	258-259
Ability to select healthful food/meals	BE-2.2	Ability level related to making selections at food stores and/or restaurants compatible with dietary goals	260-261
Ability to prepare food/meals	BE-2.3	Ability level related to preparing food and meals compatible with dietary goals	262-263
Adherence	BE-2.4	Level of compliance with nutrition-related recommendations or behavioral changes agreed upon by patient/client to achieve nutrition related goals	264-265
Goal setting	BE-2.5	Ability related to setting specific, realistic (in light of current skill level and beliefs), and positive goals pertinent to food and nutrition related behaviors	266-267
Portion control	BE-2.6	Ability level related to selecting and eating appropriate quantities of food (portion sizes) for a meal or snack, **compatible** with dietary goals	268-269

246

Edition: 2008

NUTRITION MONITORING AND EVALUATION TERMS AND DEFINITIONS

Nutrition Monitoring and Evaluation Term	Term Number	Definition	Reference Sheet Page Numbers
Self-care management	BE-2.7	Ability level related to making judgments and implementing action on a day-to-day basis to control a nutrition-related condition	270-271
Self-monitoring	BE-2.8	Ability level related to using techniques to observe and document feelings, behaviors, weight or blood/urine values to achieve a goal	272-273
Social support	BE-2.9	Ability level related to building and utilizing a network of family, friends, colleagues, health professionals, and community resources for encouragement, emotional support and enhancing environment to support behavior change	274-275
Stimulus control	BE-2.10	Ability level related to developing and/or implementing strategies to manage eating behavior and physical activity in response to stimuli	276-277
Class: Access (3)			
Access to food	BE-3.1	Availability of a sufficient quantity of safe, healthful food Degree to which enough healthful, safe food are available	278-279
Class: Physical Activity and Function (4)			
Breastfeeding success	BE-4.1	Amount of physical activity and ability to engage in specific tasks Degree to which breastfeeding plans and experience meet nutritional and other needs of the infant and mother	280-281
Nutrition-related instrumental activities of daily living	BE-4.2	Level of cognitive and physical ability to perform nutrition-related activities of daily living and instrumental activities of daily living by older and/or disabled persons	282-283
Physical activity	BE-4.3	Level of physical activity and/or amount of exercise performed	284-285

247

Monitoring & Evaluation

Edition: 2008

NUTRITION MONITORING AND EVALUATION TERMS AND DEFINITIONS

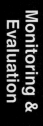

Nutrition Monitoring and Evaluation Term	Term Number	Definition	Reference Sheet Page Numbers
DOMAIN: FOOD AND NUTRIENT INTAKE OUTCOMES	**FI**	**Food and/or nutrient intake, from all sources, e.g., food, beverages, supplements, and via enteral and parenteral routes.**	
Class: Energy Intake (1)			
Energy intake	FI-1.1	Total energy intake from all sources including food, beverages, supplements and via enteral and parenteral routes	
		Amount of energy intake from all sources, e.g., food, beverages, supplements, and via enteral and parenteral routes	286-287
Class: Food and Beverage Intake (2)		Intake of foods, food groups, and fluids from all sources including food, beverages, and supplements	
Fluid/beverage intake	FI-2.1	Amount and type of fluid/beverage intake from all sources, e.g. beverages, supplements, and via enteral and parenteral routes	288-289
Food intake	FI-2.2	Amount and type of food consumed orally	290-292
Class: Enteral and Parenteral Intake (3)		Specialized nutrition support intake from all sources including enteral and parenteral routes	
Enteral/parenteral nutrition intake	FI-3.1	Amount or type of enteral and/or parenteral nutrition intake	293-294
Class: Bioactive Substances Intake (4)		Intake of bioactive substances such as caffeine, plant stanols and sterol esters, and alcohol from all sources including food, beverages, supplements and via enteral and parenteral routes	
Alcohol intake	FI-4.1	Amount and pattern of alcohol consumption	295-296
Bioactive substances intake	FI-4.2	Amount and type of bioactive substances consumed	297-298
Caffeine intake	FI-4.3	Amount of caffeine intake from all sources, e.g., food, beverages, supplements, and via enteral and parenteral routes	299-300

248

Edition: 2008

NUTRITION MONITORING AND EVALUATION TERMS AND DEFINITIONS

Nutrition Monitoring and Evaluation Term	Term Number	Definition	Reference Sheet Page Numbers
Class: Macronutrient Intake (5)		Carbohydrate, fiber, protein and fat and cholesterol intake from all sources including food, beverages, supplements, and via enteral and parenteral routes	
Fat and cholesterol intake	FI-5.1	Fat and cholesterol consumption from all sources, e.g., food, beverages, supplements, and via enteral and parenteral routes	301-303
Protein intake	FI-5.2	Protein intake from all sources, e.g., food, beverages, supplements, and via enteral and parenteral routes	304-305
Carbohydrate intake	FI-5.3	Carbohydrate consumption from all sources, e.g., food, beverages, supplements, and via enteral and parenteral routes	306-307
Fiber intake	FI-5.4	Amount and/or type of indigested carbohydrate from all sources e.g., food, beverages, supplements, and via enteral routes	308-309
Class: Micronutrient Intake (6)		Vitamin and mineral intake from all sources , e.g., foods, beverages, supplements, and enteral and/or parenteral routes	
Vitamin intake	FI-6.1	Vitamin intake from all sources, e.g., food, beverages, supplements, and via enteral and parenteral routes	310-311
Mineral/element intake	FI-6.2	Mineral/element intake from all sources, e.g., food, beverages, supplements, and via enteral and parenteral routes	312-313
DOMAIN: NUTRITION-RELATED PHYSICAL SIGN/SYMPTOM OUTCOMES	S	**Measures associated with anthropometric, biochemical, and physical exam parameters.**	
Class: Anthropometric (1)		Measures of the body such as weight, height /length, waist or head circumference, and composite indicators such as body mass index (BMI) and growth determination	
Body composition/Growth	S-1.1	The body's fat , muscle, and bone tissue, including growth	314-316

249

Monitoring & Evaluation

Edition: 2008

NUTRITION MONITORING AND EVALUATION TERMS AND DEFINITIONS

Nutrition Monitoring and Evaluation Term	Term Number	Definition	Reference Sheet Page Numbers
Class: Biochemical and Medical Tests (2)			
Acid-base balance	S-2.1	Laboratory values such as glucose, lipids, and electrolytes or medical tests such as a bone scan.	317-318
	S-2.1	Degree of acidity and alkalinity in the blood as measured by the systemic arterial pH	317-318
Electrolyte and renal profile	S-2.2	Laboratory measures associated with electrolyte balance and kidney function	319-320
Essential fatty acid profile	S-2.3	Laboratory measures of essential fatty acids	321-322
Gastrointestinal profile	S-2.4	Laboratory measures associated with function of the gastrointestinal tract and related organs	323-324
Glucose profile	S-2.5	Laboratory measures associated with glycemic control	325-326
Lipid profile	S-2.6	Laboratory measures associated with lipid disorders	327-328
Mineral profile	S-2.7	Laboratory measures associated with body mineral status	329-330
Nutritional anemia profile	S-2.8	Laboratory measures associated with nutritional anemias	331-332
Protein profile	S-2.9	Laboratory measures associated with hepatic and circulating proteins	333-334
Respiratory quotient	S-2.10	Ratio of the volume of carbon dioxide produced to the volume of oxygen consumed, which, under controlled conditions, is a reflection of net substrate utilization in the body	335-336
Urine profile	S-2.11	Physical and/or chemical properties of urine	337-338
Vitamin profile	S-2.12	Laboratory measures associated with body vitamin status	339-340

250

NUTRITION MONITORING AND EVALUATION TERMS AND DEFINITIONS

Nutrition Monitoring and Evaluation Term	Term Number	Definition	Reference Sheet Page Numbers
Class: Physical Examination (3)			
Nutrition physical exam findings	S-3.1	Parameters determined through physical exam of the patient/client such as edema, skin integrity and blood pressure	341-343
		Nutrition-related physical characteristics associated with pathophysiological states derived from observation or the medical record	
DOMAIN: NUTRITION-RELATED PATIENT/ CLIENT-CENTERED OUTCOMES	PC	**Measures associated with a patient/client's perception of his/her nutrition intervention and its impact on life.**	
Class: Nutrition Quality of Life (1)		Patient/client's perception of the impact of nutrition care on their satisfaction and quality of life	
Nutrition quality of life	PC-1.1	Extent to which the nutrition care process impacts a patient/client's physical, mental and social well-being related to food and nutrition	344-346
Class: Satisfaction (2)		Satisfaction with the nutrition prescription recommendations, nutrition counseling and nutrition education, and/or meals and snacks or food service	
To be added		To be added	

251

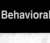

BELIEFS AND ATTITUDES (BE-1.1)

Definition

Beliefs/attitudes about and/or readiness to change food, nutrition, or nutrition-related behaviors

Monitoring

Changes in these Potential Indicators:

- Readiness to change
- Perceived consequence of change
- Perceived costs versus benefits of change
- Perceived risk
- Outcome expectancy
- Conflict with personal/family value system
- Self-efficacy
  - o Breastfeeding self-efficacy
  - o Eating self-efficacy
  - o Weight loss self-efficacy

Examples of the measurement methods or data sources for these outcome indicators

Patient/client self-report, client/patient assessment questionnaire or interview

Typically used to monitor and evaluate change in the following domains of nutrition interventions

Nutrition education, nutrition counseling

Typically used to monitor and evaluate change in the following nutrition diagnoses

Harmful beliefs/attitudes about food- or nutrition-related topics; not ready for diet/lifestyle change; inability to manage self-care; excess or inadequate oral food/beverage, energy, macronutrient, micronutrient or bioactive substance intake; imbalance of nutrients; inappropriate intake of amino acids; inappropriate fat foods; inappropriate intake of nutrients; underweight; overweight/obesity; disordered eating pattern; physical inactivity; excess exercise.

Clinical judgment must be used to select indicators and determine the appropriate measurement techniques and reference standards for a given patient population and setting. Once identified, these indicators, measurement techniques, and reference standards should be identified in policies and procedures or other documents for use in patient/client records, quality or performance improvement, or in formal research projects.

252

BELIEFS AND ATTITUDES (BE-1.1)

Evaluation

Criteria for evaluation
Comparison to Goal or Reference Standard:

1. Goal (tailored to individual's needs)

OR

2. Reference standard

Patient/Client Example(s)

Example(s) of one or two of the Nutrition Care Indicators for this outcome (*includes sample initial and re-assessment documentation for one of the indicators*)

Indicator(s) selected
Readiness to change

Criteria for evaluation
Comparison to Goal or Reference Standard:

1. Goal: Patient/client is currently in the precontemplation stage of change. Intervention goal is to move patient to the contemplation stage of change (recognition of the need to change) within 3 months.

OR

2. Reference standard: No validated standard exists.

Sample monitoring and evaluation documentation

Initial encounter with patient/client	Assessment results indicate patient/client is currently in the precontemplation stage of change related to need for DASH diet adherence. Will reassess in eight weeks.
Re-assessment after nutrition intervention	Reassessment indicates that patient/client has moved from the precontemplation stage to the contemplation stage related to need for DASH diet adherence. Will reassess in eight weeks.

Behavioral

253

Behavioral

BEHAVIORAL-ENVIRONMENTAL OUTCOMES DOMAIN · Knowledge/Beliefs

BELIEFS AND ATTITUDES (BE-1.1)

References

The following are some suggested references for indicators, measurement techniques, and reference standards for the outcome; other references may be appropriate.

1. Clark MM, Abrams DB, Niaura RS. Self-efficacy in weight management. *J Consult Clin Psychol.* 1991;59:739-744.
2. Irwin C, Guyton R. Eating self-efficacy among college students in a behavioral-based weight control program. *Am J Health Studies.* 1997;13:141-151.
3. Celio AA, Wilfley DE, Crow SJ, Mitchell J, Walsh BT. A comparison of the binge eating scale, questionnaire of eating and weight patterns-revised, and eating disorder examination with instructions with the eating disorder examination in the assessment of binge eating disorder and its symptoms. *Int J Eat Disord.* 2004;36:434-444.
4. Kitsantas, A. The role of self-regulation strategies and self-efficacy perceptions in successful weight loss maintenance. *Psychol Health.* 2000;15:811-820.
5. Sutton K, Logue E, Jarjoura D, Baughman K, Smucker W, Capers C. Assessing dietary and exercise stage of change to optimize weight loss interventions. *Obes Re.s* 2003;11:641-652.
6. Kristal AR, Glanz K, Curry SJ, Patterson RE. How can stages of change be best used in dietary interventions? *J Am Diet Assoc.* 1999; 99: 679-684.
7. Watson K;Baranowski T;Thompson D. Item response modeling: an evaluation of the children's fruit and vegetable self-efficacy questionnaire. *Health Educ Res.* 2006;21 Suppl 1:i47-i57
8. Perri MG, Corsica JA. Improving the maintenance of weight lost in behavioral treatment of obesity. In: Wadden TA, Stunkard AJ (eds). *Handbook of Obesity Treatment.* New York, NY: Guilford Press; 2002:357-379.
9. Miller WR, Rollnick S. *Motivational Interviewing* (2ⁿᵈ ed). New York, NY: Guilford Press; 2002.
10. Dennis C. The breastfeeding self-efficacy scale: psychometric assessment of the short form. *J Obstet Gynecol Neonatal Nurs.* 2003; 32:734-744.

FOOD AND NUTRITION KNOWLEDGE (BE-1.2)

Definition

Level of knowledge about food, nutrition and health, or nutrition-related information and guidelines relevant to patient/client needs

Monitoring

Changes in these Potential Indicators:

- Level of knowledge (e.g., none, limited, minimal, substantial, and extensive)
- Areas of knowledge
  - o Food/nutrient requirements
  - o Physiological functions
  - o Disease/condition
  - o Nutrition recommendations
  - o Food products
  - o Consequences of food behavior
  - o Food label understanding/knowledge
  - o Self-management parameters

NOTE: There are two dimensions of knowledge: level and area.

Examples of the measurement methods or data sources for this outcome

Pre- and/or post-tests administered orally, on paper or by computer, scenario discussions, patient/client restate key information, review of food records, practical demonstration/test

Typically used to monitor and evaluate change in the following domains of nutrition interventions

Nutrition education, nutrition counseling

Typically used to monitor and evaluate change in the following nutrition diagnoses

Food- and nutrition-related knowledge deficit, limited adherence to nutrition-related recommendations, intake domain

Clinical judgment must be used to select indicators and determine the appropriate measurement techniques and reference standards for a given patient population and setting. Once identified, these indicators, measurement techniques, and reference standards should be identified in policies and procedures or other documents for use in patient/client records, quality or performance improvement, or in formal research projects.

255

Behavioral

FOOD AND NUTRITION KNOWLEDGE (BE-1.2)

Evaluation

Criteria for evaluation
Comparison to Goal or Reference Standard:

1. Goal (tailored to individual's needs)

OR

2. Reference standard

Patient/Client Example(s)
Example(s) of one or two of the Nutrition Care Indicators for this outcome (*includes sample initial and re-assessment documentation for one of the indicators*)

Indicator(s) selected
Area of knowledge (carbohydrate counting)

Criteria for evaluation
Comparison to Goal or Reference Standard:

1. Goal: Patient/client will be able to accurately read a food label and identify the total number of grams of carbohydrate per serving.

OR

2. Reference standard: No validated standard exists.

Sample monitoring and evaluation documentation

Initial encounter with patient/client	Patient/client with newly diagnosed diabetes with limited knowledge regarding carbohydrate counting.
Re-assessment after nutrition intervention	Patient/client with moderate knowledge regarding carbohydrate counting. Able to apply knowledge to common scenarios, but not consistently able to apply knowledge to solve problems. Will continue to monitor at next encounter in one week.

256

FOOD AND NUTRITION KNOWLEDGE (BE-1.2)

References

The following are some suggested references for indicators, measurement techniques, and reference standards for the outcome; other references may be appropriate.

1. Snetselaar LG. *Nutrition Counseling Skills for Medical Nutrition Therapy.* Gaithersburg, MD: 1997:133,209.

2. ADA Evidence Analysis Library. Available at: www.adaevidencelibrary.com. Accessed 11/3/2006.

3. Kessler H, Wunderlich SM. Relationship between use of food labels and nutrition knowledge of people with diabetes. *Diabetes Educ.* 1999; 25.

4. Chapman-Novakofski K, Karduck J. Improvement in knowledge, social cognitive theory variables, and movement through stages of change after a community-based diabetes education program. *J Am Diet Assoc.* 2005; 105:1613-1616.

5. International Diabetes Center. *Type 2 Diabetes BASICS Pre/Post Knowledge Test. 2nd ed.* Minneapolis, MN: International Diabetes Center, 2004.

6. Powers MA, Carstensen K, Colon K, Rickheim P, Bergenstal RM. Diabetes BASICS: Education, innovation, revolution. *Diabetes Spectrum.* 2006;19:90-98.

7. Obayashi S, Bianchi LJ, Song WO. Reliability and validity of nutrition knowledge, social-psychological factors, and food label use scales from the 1995 Diet and Health Knowledge Survey. *J Nutr Educ Behav.* 2003;35:83-92.

8. Kunkel ME, Bell LB, Luccia BHD. Peer Nutrition Education Program To Improve Nutrition Knowledge Of Female Collegiate Athletes. *J Nutr Educ Behav.* 2001; 33:114-115.

Behavioral

Edition: 2008

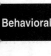

BEHAVIORAL-ENVIRONMENTAL OUTCOMES DOMAIN • Behavior

ABILITY TO PLAN MEALS/SNACKS (BE-2.1)

Definition
Patient/client ability level related to planning healthy meals and snacks, which are compatible with dietary goals

Monitoring
Changes in these Potential Indicators:

• Meal/snack planning ability (e.g., may include ability to use planning tools, plan a menu, create/tailor a meal plan, create/use a shopping list)

Examples of the measurement methods or data sources for these outcome indicators
Food intake records, self-report or caregiver report, 24-hour recall, menu review, targeted questionnaire

Typically used to measure the outcomes for the following domains of nutrition interventions
Nutrition education, nutrition counseling

Typically used to monitor and evaluate change in the following nutrition diagnosis
Excessive or inadequate oral food/beverage intake, underweight, overweight/obesity, limited adherence to nutrition related recommendations, inability or lack of desire to manage self-care

Clinical judgment must be used to select indicators and determine the appropriate measurement techniques and reference standards for a given patient population and setting. Once identified, these indicators, measurement techniques, and reference standards should be identified in policies and procedures or other documents for use in patient/client records, quality or performance improvement, or in formal research projects.

Evaluation

Criteria for evaluation
Comparison to Goal or Reference Standard:

1. Goal (tailored to individual's needs)

OR

2. Reference standard

Edition: 2008

ABILITY TO PLAN MEALS/SNACKS (BE-2.1)

Patient/Client Example(s)

Example(s) of one or two of the Nutrition Care Indicators for this outcome (*includes sample initial and re-assessment documentation for one of the indicators*)

Indicator(s) selected

Meal/snack planning ability (e.g., may include ability to use planning tools, plan a menu, create/tailor a meal plan, create/use a shopping list)

Criteria for evaluation

Comparison to Goal or Reference Standard:

1. Goal: Patient/client states that lack of planning impedes her progress. Patient/client currently never preplans meals/snacks and set a goal to develop or tailor a meal plan and follow it 6 days per week.

OR

2. Reference standard: No validated standard exists.

Sample monitoring and evaluation documentation

Initial encounter with patient/client	Patient/client states that lack of planning is a barrier to success. She rated herself a 2 on a scale of 1-10 on her ability to plan meals/snacks. Patient/client set goal to develop a meal plan prior to the beginning of each week. Will assess meal-planning skill at next encounter in two weeks.
Re-assessment after nutrition intervention	Significant progress made toward goal. Patient/client rated herself an 8 on a scale of 1-10 on her ability to plan meals at the beginning of each week. She tailored a meal plan she found in a magazine to her family's lifestyle. Patient/client would like to add more variety at the dinner meal. Will continue to monitor patient/client goal to preplan meals at next encounter in two weeks.

References

The following is a suggested reference for indicators, measurement techniques, and reference standards for the outcome; other references may be appropriate.

1. Snetselaar LG. *Nutrition Counseling Skills for Medical Nutrition Therapy.* 2nd ed. Gaithersburg, MD: Aspen Press; 2007.

Behavioral

259

BEHAVIORAL-ENVIRONMENTAL OUTCOMES DOMAIN • Behavior

ABILITY TO SELECT HEALTHFUL FOOD/MEALS (BE-2.2)

Definition

Patient/client ability level related to making selections at food stores and/or restaurants that are compatible with dietary goals

Monitoring

Changes in these Potential Indicators:

- Food/meal selection (e.g., may include ability to do the following: Interpret food labels, select healthful menu items, select healthful versions of food items, tailor/modify portion sizes)

Examples of the measurement methods or data sources for these outcome indicators

Food intake records, self-report or caregiver report, 24-hour recall, food frequency questionnaire, menu analysis, targeted questionnaires and monitoring devices

Typically used to measure the outcomes for the following domains of nutrition interventions

Nutrition education, nutrition counseling

Typically used to monitor and evaluate change in the following nutrition diagnosis

Excessive or inadequate oral food/beverage intake, overweight/obesity, disordered eating pattern, undesirable food choices, limited adherence to nutrition related recommendations, inability or lack of desire to manage self-care

Clinical judgment must be used to select indicators and determine the appropriate measurement techniques and reference standards for a given patient population and setting. Once identified, these indicators, measurement techniques, and reference standards should be identified in policies and procedures or other documents for use in patient/client records, quality or performance improvement, or in formal research projects

Evaluation

Criteria for evaluation:
Comparison to Goal or Reference Standard:

1. Goal (tailored to individual's needs)

OR

2. Reference standard

ABILITY TO SELECT HEALTHFUL FOOD/MEALS (BE-2.2)

Patient/Client Example(s)

Example(s) of one or two of the Nutrition Care Indicators for this outcome (*includes sample initial and re-assessment documentation for one of the indicators*)

Indicator(s) selected

Food/meal selection (e.g., may include ability to do the following: Interpret food labels, select healthful menu items, select healthful versions of food items, tailor/modify portion sizes)

Criteria for evaluation

Comparison to Goal or Reference Standard:

1. Goal: Patient/client currently selects high-fat entrees at lunch 5 days per week and has a goal of selecting low-fat entrees at lunch 5 day per week.

OR

2. Reference standard: No validated standard exists.

Sample monitoring and evaluation documentation

Initial encounter with patient/client	Based on patient/client food diary, patient/client consuming high-fat entrees at lunch 5 days/week. Will monitor quality of food selections at lunch at next encounter in one week.
Re-assessment at a later date	Some progress toward goal. Based upon lunch diary, patient/client selected low-fat entrees 3 of 5 days. Will continue to monitor quality of lunch menu selections.

References

The following is a suggested reference for indicators, measurement techniques, and reference standards for the outcome; other references may be appropriate.

1. Snetselaar LG. *Nutrition Counseling Skills for Medical Nutrition Therapy.* 2nd ed. Gaithersburg, MD: Aspen Press; 2007.

261

Behavioral

Edition: 2008

BEHAVIORAL-ENVIRONMENTAL OUTCOMES DOMAIN • Behavior

ABILITY TO PREPARE HEALTHFUL FOOD/MEALS (BE-2.3)

Definition
Patient/client ability level related to preparing food and meals that are compatible with dietary goals

Monitoring
Changes in these Potential Indicators:

• Food/meal preparation ability (e.g., may include meat, grain/starch, vegetable preparation, dinner preparation, recipe modification, recipe implementation)

Examples of the measurement methods or data sources for these outcome indicators
Food intake records, self-report or caregiver report, 24-hour recall, menu review, targeted questionnaire

Typically used to measure the outcomes for the following domains of nutrition interventions
Nutrition education, nutrition counseling

Typically used to monitor and evaluate change in the following nutrition diagnosis
Impaired ability to prepare foods/meals, excessive or inadequate oral food/beverage intake, underweight, overweight/obesity, limited adherence to nutrition related recommendations, inability or lack of desire to manage self-care

Clinical judgment must be used to select indicators and determine the appropriate measurement techniques and reference standards for a given patient population and setting. Once identified, these indicators, measurement techniques, and reference standards should be identified in policies and procedures or other documents for use in patient/client records, quality or performance improvement, or in formal research projects.

Evaluation

Criteria for evaluation:
Comparison to Goal or Reference Standard:

1. Goal (tailored to individual's needs)

   OR

2. Reference standard

Edition: 2008

ABILITY TO PREPARE HEALTHFUL FOOD/MEALS (BE-2.3)

Patient/Client Example(s)

Example(s) of one or two of the Nutrition Care Indicators for this outcome (*includes sample initial and re-assessment documentation for one of the indicators*)

Indicator(s) selected

Food/meal preparation ability (e.g., may include meat, grain/starch, vegetable preparation,; dinner preparation; recipe modification; recipe implementation)

Comparison to Goal or Reference Standard

1. Goal: Patient/client states that she does not know how to prepare vegetables so her family will eat them. Set goal to try three new ways to prepare vegetables, which may be acceptable to her family.

   OR

2. Reference standard: No validated standard exists.

Sample monitoring and evaluation documentation

Initial encounter with patient/client	Patient/client states that she is unable prepare vegetables in a healthy way (not fried) acceptable to herself and her family. She set goal to try three new techniques or recipes for vegetable preparation this week. Will monitor vegetable preparation skill at next encounter in two weeks.
Re-assessment after nutrition intervention	Some progress made. Patient/client tried one new recipe for preparing vegetables and it was highly acceptable to family. Will continue to monitor patient/client's goal to try new vegetable preparation techniques at next encounter in two weeks.

References

The following is ae suggested reference for indicators, measurement techniques, and reference standards for the outcome; other references may be appropriate.

1. Napier K, ed. American Dietetic Association *Cooking Healthy Across America.* Hoboken, NJ: John Wiley & Sons, Inc; 2005.

263

Behavioral

Edition: 2008

BEHAVIORAL-ENVIRONMENTAL OUTCOMES DOMAIN • Behavior

ADHERENCE (BE-2.4)

Definition
Level of compliance with nutrition-related recommendations or behavioral changes agreed upon by patient/client to achieve nutrition-related goals

Monitoring
Changes in these Potential Indicators:

- Self-reported adherence score
- Biochemical marker for adherence

NOTE: Use in conjunction with appropriate outcomes from Food and Nutrition Intake and Nutrition-Related Sign/Symptom outcome domains. May be useful in relapse prevention treatment (analyze and control factors that caused the lapse).

Examples of the measurement methods or data sources for these outcome indicators
Attendance, self-monitoring records, patient/client self-report, adherence tools or questionnaires, provider assessment

Typically used to measure the outcomes for the following domains of nutrition interventions
Food and/or nutrient delivery, nutrition education, nutrition counseling

Typically used to monitor and evaluate change in the following nutrition diagnosis
Limited adherence to nutrition-related recommendations

Clinical judgment must be used to select indicators and determine the appropriate measurement techniques and reference standards for a given patient population and setting. Once identified, these indicators, measurement techniques, and reference standards should be identified in policies and procedures or other documents for use in patient/client records, quality or performance improvement, or in formal research projects.

Evaluation

Criteria for evaluation
Comparison to Goal or Reference Standard:

1. Goal (tailored to individual's needs)

OR

2. Reference standard

Edition: 2008

ADHERENCE (BE-2.4)

Patient/Client Example(s)

Example(s) of one or two of the Nutrition Care Indicators for this outcome (*includes sample initial and re-assessment documentation for one of the indicators*)

Indicator(s) selected

Self-reported adherence score

Criteria for evaluation

Comparison to Goal or Reference Standard:

1. Goal: Patient/client rates herself a 4 on a scale of 1 to 10 (1 meaning never and 10 meaning always) on her level of compliance with nutrition-related goals. Patient/client desires to get self to a rating of 8.

OR

2. Reference standard: No validated standard exists.

Sample monitoring and evaluation documentation

Initial encounter with patient/client	Patient/client rates herself a 1 on a scale of 1-10 on her ability to adhere to her meal plan. Patient/client set a goal to adhere to her meal plan 5 days per week. Will evaluate adherence at the next encounter.
Re-assessment after nutrition intervention	Some progress toward goal. Patient/client rated herself a 6 on a scale of 1-10 on her ability to meet her adherence goal of following her meal plan 5 days per week. Is doing well on weekdays, but states she must improve on weekends. Will monitor at next encounter in two weeks.

References

The following are some suggested references for indicators, measurement techniques, and reference standards for the outcome; other references may be appropriate.

1. Haynes RB. Improving patient adherence: State of the art, with a special focus on medication taking for cardiovascular disorders. In: Burke LE, Ockene IS (eds). *Compliance in Healthcare and Research.* Armonk, NY: Futura Publishing Company, Inc.; 2001:3-21.

2. Milas N, Nowalk MP, Akpele L, Castoldo L, Coyne T, Doroshenko L, Kigawa L, Korzec-Ramirez D, Scherch LK, Snetselaar L. Factors Associated with Adherence to the Dietary Protein Intervention in the Modification of Diet in Renal Disease Study. *J Am Diet Assoc.* 1995; 95:1295-1300.

3. Snetselaar LG. *Nutrition Counseling Skills for Medical Nutrition Therapy. 2nd ed.* Gaithersburg, MD: Aspen Press; 2007.

4. Schlundt DG, Rea MR, Kline SS, Pichert JW. Situational obstacles to dietary adherence for adults with diabetes. *J Am Diet Assoc.* 1994;94:874-876.

5. DiMatteo MR, Giordani PJ, Lepper HS, Croghan TW. Patient adherence and medical treatment outcomes: a meta-analysis. *Med Care.* 2002;40:794-811.

6. Rushe H, McGee HM. Assessing adherence to dietary recommendations for hemodialysis patients: the Renal Adherence Attitudes Questionnaire (RAAQ) and the Renal Adherence Behaviour Questionnaire (RABQ). *J Psychosom Res.* 1998;45:149-157.

7. Sharma S, Murphy SP, Wilkens LR, Shen L, Hankin JH, Henderson B, Kolonel LN. Adherence to the Food Guide Pyramid recommendations among Japanese Americans, Native Hawaiians, and whites: Results from the Multiethnic Cohort Study. *J Am Diet Assoc.* 2003;103:1195-1198.

8. Tinker LF, Perri MG, Patterson RE, Bowen DJ, McIntosh M, Parker LM, Sevick MA, Wodarski LA. The effects of physical and emotional status on adherence to a low-fat dietary pattern in the Women's Health Initiative. *J Am Diet Assoc.* 2002;102:789-800.

Behavioral

BEHAVIORAL-ENVIRONMENTAL OUTCOMES DOMAIN • Behavior

GOAL SETTING (BE-2.5)

Definition

Patient/client ability level related to setting specific, realistic (in light of current skill level and beliefs), positive goals pertinent to food- and nutrition-related behaviors

Monitoring

Changes in these Potential Indicators:

- Goal setting ability (e.g., may include the ability to set specific, measurable, attainable, realistic, time-sensitive goals)

Examples of the measurement methods or data sources for these outcome indicators

Self-monitoring records, client/patient self-report, goal tracking tools

Typically used to monitor and evaluate change in the following domains of nutrition interventions

Nutrition education, nutrition counseling

Typically used to monitor and evaluate change in the following nutrition diagnosis

Excess oral food/beverage intake, excess or inadequate energy, macronutrient, micronutrient or bioactive substance intake, overweight/obesity, disordered eating pattern, inability or lack of desire to manage self-care, limited adherence to nutrition-related recommendations

Clinical judgment must be used to select indicators and determine the appropriate measurement techniques and reference standards for a given patient population and setting. Once identified, these indicators, measurement techniques, and reference standards should be identified in policies and procedures or other documents for use in patient/client records, quality or performance improvement, or in formal research projects.

Evaluation

Criteria for evaluation

Comparison to Goal or Reference Standard:

1. Goal (tailored to individual's needs)

OR

2. Reference standard

266

GOAL SETTING (BE-2.5)

Patient/Client Example(s)

Example(s) of one or two of the Nutrition Care Indicators for this outcome *(includes sample initial and re-assessment documentation for one of the indicators)*

Indicator(s) selected

Goal setting ability (e.g., may include the ability to set specific, measurable, attainable, realistic, time-sensitive goals)

Criteria for evaluation

Comparison to Goal or Reference Standard:

1. Goal: Patient/Client's current goal is to loss 30 pounds in 8 weeks. Following counseling, patient/client will be able to define a realistic weight loss goal and behavioral steps to achieve that long-term goal.

OR

2. Reference standard: No validated standard exists.

Sample monitoring and evaluation documentation

Initial encounter with patient/client	Patient/client frequently sets unrealistic goals and verbalizes frustration. Current goal is to loss 30 pounds in 8 weeks with no clear strategy.
Re-assessment after nutrition intervention	Some progress toward goal. Patient/client set goal to limit sweets to 1 serving/day and lose two pounds per week. Patient/client set goal to limit sweets to 1 serving/day and lose two pounds per week. Will continue to assess goal-setting skill at next encounter in two weeks.

References

The following are some suggested references for indicators, measurement techniques, and reference standards for the outcome; other references may be appropriate.

1. Laquatra I. Counseling skills for behavior change. In: Helm KK, Klawitter B. *Nutrition Therapy: Advanced Counseling Skills.* Lake Dallas, TX: Helm Seminars; 1995:129-132.
2. Snetselaar LG. *Nutrition Counseling Skills for Medical Nutrition Therapy.* 2nd ed. Gaithersburg, MD: Aspen Press; 2007.
3. Estabrooks P, Nelson C, Xu S, King D, Bayliss E, Gaglio B, Nutting P, Glasgow R. The frequency and behavioral outcomes of goal choices in the self-management of diabetes. *Diabetes Educ.* 2005:31:391-400.
4. Knäuper B, Cheema S, Rabiau M, Borten O. Self-set dieting rules: adherence and prediction of weight loss success. *Appetite.* 2005;44:283-288.
5. International Diabetes Center: *My Diabetes Success Plan (for Goal-Setting).* Minneapolis, MN: International Diabetes Center; 2004.

Behavioral

BEHAVIORAL-ENVIRONMENTAL OUTCOMES DOMAIN • Behavior

PORTION CONTROL (BE-2.6)

Definition
Patient/client ability level related to selecting and eating appropriate quantities of food (portion sizes) for a meal or snack, compatible with dietary goals

Monitoring
Changes in these Potential Indicators:

- Portion size eaten

Examples of the measurement methods or data sources for these outcome indicators
Food intake records, 24 hour recall, observation, response to questionnaire or interview questions

Typically used to monitor and evaluate change in the following domains of nutrition interventions
Food and/or nutrient delivery, nutrition education, nutrition counseling

Typically used to monitor and evaluate change in the following nutrition diagnoses
Excess or inadequate oral food/beverage intake, excess or inadequate energy, macronutrient, micronutrient or bioactive substance intake, imbalance of nutrients, inappropriate intake of types of carbohydrate, inconsistent carbohydrate intake, inappropriate fat foods, inappropriate intake of amino acids, underweight, overweight/obesity, disordered eating pattern, inability or lack of desire to manage self-care

Clinical judgment must be used to select indicators and determine the appropriate measurement techniques and reference standards for a given patient population and setting. Once identified, these indicators, measurement techniques, and reference standards should be identified in policies and procedures or other documents for use in patient/client records, quality or performance improvement, or in formal research projects.

Evaluation

Criteria for evaluation
Comparison to Goal or Reference Standard:

1. Goal (tailored to individual's needs): Compare progress to patient's baseline.

   OR

2. Reference standard

PORTION CONTROL (BE-2.6)

Patient/Client Example(s)

Example(s) of one or two of the Nutrition Care Indicators for this outcome (*includes sample initial and re-assessment documentation for one of the indicators*)

Indicator(s) selected

Portion size eaten

Criteria for evaluation

Comparison to Goal or Reference Standard:

1. Nutrition prescription or goal: Patient/client eats out for lunch 5 days per week and consumes all food served. Patient/client goal is to ask restaurant server to serve a half portion of the entrée and wrap the remainder to take home.

OR

2. Reference standard: No validated standard exists.

Sample monitoring and evaluation documentation

Initial encounter with patient/client	Patient/client identified portion control as a significant diet problem. Discussed portion control strategies and will monitor patient/client's success in implementing these at the next encounter.
Re-assessment after nutrition intervention	Significant progress toward goal. Patient/client rated herself a 6 on a scale of 1-10 on her ability to control portions. Is doing well at home, but states she must do better at restaurants. Discussed strategies that may be helpful at restaurants. Will monitor at next encounter in two weeks.

References

The following are some suggested references for indicators, measurement techniques, and reference standards for the outcome; other references may be appropriate.

1. ADA Evidence Analysis Library, Adult Weight Management Recommendation 8 Portion control., Available at: http://www.adaevidencelibrary.com/template.cfm?template=guide_summary&key=632, Accessed Feb 28, 2007.

2. National Heart Lung and Blood Institute, Department of Health and Human Services, National Institutes of Health. Portion Distortion and Serving Size. Available at: http://nhlbi.nih.gov/health/public/heart/obesity/wecan/learn-it/distortion.htm, Accessed February 28, 2007.

3. Rolls BJ, Roe LS, Meengs JS. Reductions in portion size and energy density of foods are additive and lead to sustained decreases in energy intake. *Am J Clin Nutr.* 2006;83:11-17.

4. Ledikwe JH, Ello-Martin JA, Rolls BJ. Portion sizes and the obesity epidemic. *J Nutr.* 2005;135:905-909.

5. Nothwehr F, Dennis L, Wu H. Measurement of behavioral objectives for weight management. *Health Education & Behavior* Online First, June 2006.

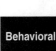

Behavioral

269

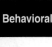

BEHAVIORAL-ENVIRONMENTAL OUTCOMES DOMAIN • Behavior

SELF-CARE MANAGEMENT (BE-2.7)

Definition

Alteration in ability to make judgments and implement action on a day-to-day basis to control a nutrition-related condition.

Monitoring

Changes in these Potential Indicators:

- Self-care management ability (e.g., may include interpreting results, problem solving, initiating appropriate action, symptom management and emergency prevention)

NOTE: Self-monitoring ability is covered on Self-Monitoring Reference Sheet.

Examples of the measurement methods or data sources for these outcome indicators

Client/patient self-report, caregiver report, self-care management tools, lab values, weight, ability to demonstrate using a scenario

Typically used to measure the outcomes for the following domains of nutrition interventions

Nutrition education, nutrition counseling

Typically used to monitor and evaluate change in the following nutrition diagnosis

Inability or lack of desire to manage self-care, excessive oral food/beverage intake, excess energy intake, excess macronutrient and micronutrient intake, involuntary weight loss, poor nutrition quality of life, self-feeding difficulty

Clinical judgment must be used to select indicators and determine the appropriate measurement techniques and reference standards for a given patient population and setting. Once identified, these indicators, measurement techniques, and reference standards should be identified in policies and procedures or other documents for use in patient/client records, quality or performance improvement, or in formal research projects.

Evaluation

Criteria for evaluation

Comparison to Goal or Reference Standard:

1. Goal (tailored to individual's needs)

   OR

2. Reference standard

Edition: 2008

SELF-CARE MANAGEMENT (BE-2.7)

Patient/Client Example(s)

Example(s) of one or two of the Nutrition Care Indicators for this outcome *(includes sample initial and re-assessment documentation for one of the indicators)*

Indicator(s) selected

Self-care management ability (e.g., may include interpreting results, problem solving, initiating appropriate action, symptom management and emergency prevention)

Criteria for evaluation

Comparison to Goal or Reference Standard:

1. Goal: Patient/Client with diabetes reaching stage to accept greater responsibility in self-management of type 1 diabetes. Patient to monitor blood glucose and adjust carbohydrate intake at lunch and meals away from home.

OR

2. Reference standard: No validated standard exists.

Sample monitoring and evaluation documentation

Initial encounter with patient/client	Patient/client states that he has not participated in diabetes self-care management in the past and rates himself a 1 on a scale of 1-10 on his ability to do self-care management. Patient/client set goal to monitoring blood glucose and adjust carbohydrate intake in the afternoons, 5 days per week. Will evaluate self-care management skill at the next encounter.
Re-assessment after nutrition intervention	Some progress toward goal. Patient/client rated himself a 5, on a scale of 1-10, on his ability to meet his self-care management goal of monitoring blood glucose and adjusting carbohydrate intake in the afternoon, 5 days per week. Is doing well on weekdays, but states he must do better on weekends. Will monitor at next encounter in two weeks.

References

The following are some suggested references for indicators, measurement techniques, and reference standards for the outcome; other references may be appropriate.

1. Balamurugan A, Ohsfeldt R, Hughes T, Phillips M. Diabetes self-management education program for Medicaid recipients: a continuous quality improvement process. *Diabetes Educ.* 2006;32:893-900.
2. Nelson RG, Tuttle KR. The New KDOQI Clinical Practice Guidelines and Clinical Practice Recommendations for Diabetes and CKD. *Blood Purif.* 2007;25:112-114. Epub 2006 Dec 14.
3. Williams PD, Piamjariyakul U, Ducey K, Badura J, Boltz KD, Olberding K, Wingate A, Williams AR. Cancer treatment, symptom monitoring, and self-care in adults: pilot study. *Cancer Nurs.* 2006;29:347-355.
4. Mensing C (ed). *Art and Science of Diabetes Self-management Education.* Chicago, IL: American Association of Diabetes Educators; 2006.
5. Willey T. *The Power of Choice: A Guide to Personal and Professional Self-Management.* Denver, CO: Training Company, Inc/Berwick House; 1988.

Edition: 2008

Behavioral

BEHAVIORAL-ENVIRONMENTAL OUTCOMES DOMAIN • Behavior

SELF-MONITORING (BE-2.8)

Definition

Ability level related to using techniques to observe and document feelings, behaviors, weight or blood/urine values to achieve a goal

Monitoring

Changes in these Potential Indicators:

- Self-monitoring ability (e.g., may include completeness of monitoring and frequency of monitoring)

NOTE: Application of self-monitoring information is covered on Self-Care Management Reference Sheet.

Examples of the measurement methods or data sources for these outcome indicators

Food diaries/records, weight records, blood glucose monitoring, physical activity record, behavior checklists

Typically used to measure the outcomes for the following domains of nutrition interventions

Nutrition education, nutrition counseling

Typically used to monitor and evaluate change in the following nutrition diagnoses

Underweight, overweight/obesity, disordered eating pattern, undesirable food choices, physical inactivity, inability or lack of desire to manage self-care, self-monitoring deficit, not ready for lifestyle change, limited adherence, excessive exercise

Clinical judgment must be used to select indicators and determine the appropriate measurement techniques and reference standards for a given patient population and setting. Once identified, these indicators, measurement techniques, and reference standards should be identified in policies and procedures or other documents for use in patient/client records, quality or performance improvement, or in formal research projects.

Evaluation

Criteria for evaluation

Comparison to Goal or Reference Standard:

1. Goal (tailored to individual's needs)

   OR

2. Reference standard

Edition: 2008

SELF-MONITORING (BE-2.8)

Patient/Client Example(s)

Example(s) of one or two of the Nutrition Care Indicators for this outcome (*includes sample initial and re-assessment documentation for one of the indicators*)

Indicator(s) selected

Self-monitoring ability (e.g., may include completeness of monitoring and frequency of monitoring)

Criteria for evaluation

Comparison to Goal or Reference Standard:

1. Goal: Patient/client enrolled in lifestyle change program and has never kept a food diary. Patient/client goal is to maintain a food intake record 5 days per week recording time, food, portion size, calorie and fat content.

OR

2. Reference standard: No validated standard exists.

Sample monitoring and evaluation documentation

Initial encounter with patient/client	Based upon patient/client records, patient/client monitoring blood glucose 1 day/wk and is not monitoring carbohydrate intake. Will evaluate blood glucose and carbohydrate counting records at the next encounter.
Re-assessment after nutrition intervention	Some progress toward self-monitoring goal. Patient/client recording blood glucose levels 2 day/wk and carbohydrate intake 2 times/week. Will continue to monitor self-monitoring at next encounter in 2 weeks.

References

The following are some suggested references for indicators, measurement techniques, and reference standards for the outcome; other references may be appropriate.

1. Tinker LF, Paterson RE, Kristal AR, Bowen DJ, Kuniyuki A, Henry H, Shattuck A. Measurement characteristics of 2 different self-monitoring tools used in a dietary intervention study. *J Am Diet Assoc.* 2001;101:1031-1040.
2. Tate DF, Jackvony EH, Wing RR. Effects of internet behavioral counseling on weight loss in adults at risk for type 2 diabetes: a randomized trial. *JAMA.* 2003;289:1833-1836.
3. Milas NC, Nowalk MP, Akpee L, Castaldo L, Coyne T, Doroshenko L, Kigawa L, Korzec-Ramirez D, Scherch LK, Snetselaar L. Factors associated with adherence to the dietary protein intervention in the modification of diet in renal disease study. *J Am Diet Assoc.* 1995;95:1295-1300.
4. Boutelle KN, Kirschenbaum DS. Further support for consistent self-monitoring as a vital component of successful weight control. *Obes Res.* 1998; 52: 219-224.

Behavioral

273

Edition: 2008

BEHAVIORAL-ENVIRONMENTAL OUTCOMES DOMAIN • Behavior

SOCIAL SUPPORT (BE-2.9)

Definition

Ability level related to building and utilizing a network of family, friends, colleagues, health professionals, and community resources for encouragement, emotional support and enhancing environment to support behavior change

Monitoring

Changes in these Potential Indicators:

- Ability to build and utilize social support (e.g., may include perceived social support, social integration, and assertiveness)

Examples of the measurement methods used or data sources for these outcome indicators
Self-monitoring records, client/patient self-report, goal tracking tools

Typically used to monitor and evaluate change in the following domains of nutrition interventions
Nutrition counseling

Typically used to monitor and evaluate change in the following nutrition diagnosis
Intake domain, underweight, overweight/obesity, disordered eating pattern, undesirable food choices, inability or lack of desire to manage self-care, breastfeeding difficulty, not ready for diet/lifestyle change, limited adherence to nutrition-related recommendations

Clinical judgment must be used to select indicators and determine the appropriate measurement techniques and reference standards for a given patient population and setting. Once identified, these indicators, measurement techniques, and reference standards should be identified in policies and procedures or other documents for use in patient/client records, quality or performance improvement, or in formal research projects.

Evaluation

Criteria for evaluation
Comparison to Goal or Reference Standard:

1. Goal (tailored to individual's needs)

OR

2. Reference standard

SOCIAL SUPPORT (BE-2.9)

Patient/Client Example(s)

Example(s) of one or two of the Nutrition Care Indicators for this outcome (*includes sample initial and re-assessment documentation for one of the indicators*)

Indicator(s) selected

Ability to build and utilize social support (e.g., may include perceived social support, social integration, and assertiveness)

Criteria for evaluation

Comparison to Goal or Reference Standard:

1. Goal: Overweight patient/client's wife adds fat to all foods prepared at home. Goal is reduce the amount of fat in meals prepared at home by asking wife to not dress the salad or add fat seasoning to vegetables before serving.

OR

2. Reference standard: No validated standard exists.

Sample monitoring and evaluation documentation

Initial encounter with patient/client	Patient/client states that he rarely verbalizes his nutrition-related desires/needs in family or social situations and rates his ability to elicit social support a 3 on a scale of 1 to 10. Will evaluate at the next encounter.
Re-assessment at a later date	Some progress toward goal. Patient/client rated himself a 5, on a scale of 1-10, on his ability to elicit social support. Has begun to verbalize his needs and plans to research restaurants that meet his needs that others will enjoy. Will monitor at next encounter in two weeks.

References

The following are some suggested references for indicators, measurement techniques, and reference standards for the outcome; other references may be appropriate.

1. Barrera M, Toobert D, Angell K, Glasgow R, Mackinnon D. Social support and social-ecological resources as mediators of lifestyle intervention effects for type 2 diabetes. *J Health Psychol.* 2006;11:483-495.
2. Sherbourne CD, Stewart AI. The MOS Social Support Survey. *Social Sci Med.* 1991;32:706-714.
3. Barrera M Jr, Glasgow RE, McKay HG, Boles SM, Feil E. Do internet-based support interventions change perceptions of social support?: an experimental trial of approaches for supporting diabetes self-management. *Am J Comm Psychol.* 2002; 30:637-654.
4. LaGreca AM, Bearman KJ. The diabetes social support questionnaire-family version: evaluating adolescents' diabetes-specific support from family members. *J Pediatr Psychol.* 2002;27:665-676.
5. Glasgow RE, Strycker LA, Toobert DJ, Eakin E. A social-ecologic approach to assessing support for disease self-management: the Chronic Illness Resources Survey. *J Behav Med.* 2000;23:559-583.

Behavioral

275

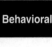

BEHAVIORAL-ENVIRONMENTAL OUTCOMES DOMAIN • Behavior

STIMULUS CONTROL (BE-2.10)

Definition
Ability level related to developing/implementing strategies to manage eating behavior and physical activity in response to stimuli

Monitoring
Changes in these Potential Indicators:

- Ability to manage behavior in response to stimuli (e.g., may include ability to identify triggers/cues, develop a plan, modify environment or behavior)

Examples of the measurement methods or data sources for these outcome indicators
Self-monitoring records, client/patient self-report

Typically used to monitor and evaluate change in the following domains of nutrition interventions
Nutrition education, nutrition counseling

Typically used to monitor and evaluate change in the following nutrition diagnosis
Excess oral food/beverage, energy, macronutrient or bioactive substance intake; imbalance of nutrients; inappropriate intake of types of carbohydrate; inconsistent carbohydrate intake; inappropriate fat foods; underweight; overweight/obesity; disordered eating pattern; undesirable food choices; inability or lack of desire to manage self-care; physical inactivity; excess exercise

Clinical judgment must be used to select indicators and determine the appropriate measurement techniques and reference standards for a given patient population and setting. Once identified, these indicators, measurement techniques, and reference standards should be identified in policies and procedures or other documents for use in patient/client records, quality or performance improvement, or in formal research projects.

Evaluation

Criteria for evaluation
Comparison to Goal or Reference Standard:

1. Goal (tailored to individual's needs)

OR

2. Reference standard

STIMULUS CONTROL (BE-2.10)

Patient/Client Example(s)

Example(s) of one or two of the Nutrition Care Indicators for this outcome (*includes sample initial and re-assessment documentation for one of the indicators*)

Indicator(s) selected

Ability to build and utilize social support (e.g., may include perceived social support, social integration, and assertiveness)

Criteria for evaluation

Comparison to Goal or Reference Standard:

1. Goal: After monitoring behavior using a self-monitoring record, patient becomes aware that she is over eating while watching the 10 PM news and realizes every time the TV is on she feels hungry. She sets a goal to no longer eat while watching TV.

OR

2. Reference standard: No validated standard exists.

Sample monitoring and evaluation documentation

Initial encounter with patient/client	Based upon self-monitoring, patient/client identified that she eats while watching TV, 7 days per week and desires to eliminate the TV as a trigger for inappropriate eating. Patient/client currently rates herself a 2, on a scale of 1–10 on ability to manage eating while watching TV (trigger). Will monitor patient/client's achievement of goal at next encounter in one week.
Re-assessment after nutrition intervention	Met stimulus control goal. Patient/client rated herself a 9 on a scale of 1-10 on ability to eat appropriately while watching TV. She has started using the treadmill and knitting in front of the TV rather than eating. Will continue to monitor progress over the next few weeks to ensure sustainment of behavior change.

References

The following is a suggested reference for indicators, measurement techniques, and reference standards for the outcome; other references may be appropriate.

1. Fabricatore AN. Behavior therapy and cognitive-behavioral therapy of obesity: Is there a difference? *J Am Diet Assoc.* 2007;107:92-99.

277

Behavioral

BEHAVIORAL-ENVIRONMENTAL AND FUNCTIONAL OUTCOMES DOMAIN • Access

ACCESS TO A SUFFICIENT, RELIABLE SUPPLY OF SAFE, HEALTHFUL FOOD (BE-3.1.1)

Definition

Degree to which enough healthful, safe food is available

Monitoring

Changes in these Potential Indicators:

- Access to a sufficient supply of healthful food

  (e.g., access to federal programs, such as, WIC and the Food Stamp Program and/or community programs, such as food pantries and meal sites; access to financial resources, school/community food programs with healthful food choices, and/or to transportation; assistance in securing food; caregiver support and access to food; participation in federal and/or community food programs)

- Access to safe food

  (e.g., procurement, identification of safe food, preparation and/or storage techniques)

Examples of the measurement methods or data sources for these outcome indicators

Patient/client report overall food availability/food consumed during the week, referral information, home evaluation

Typically used to measure the outcomes for the following domains of nutrition interventions

Nutrition education, nutrition counseling, coordination of nutrition care

Typically used to monitor and evaluate change in the following nutrition diagnoses

Access to food, access to safe food, inadequate or excessive energy intake

Clinical judgment must be used to select indicators and determine the appropriate measurement techniques and reference standards for a given patient population and setting. Once identified, these indicators, measurement techniques, and reference standards should be identified in policies and procedures or other documents for use in patient/client records, quality or performance improvement, or in formal research projects.

Evaluation

Criteria for evaluation

Comparison to Goal or Reference Standard:

1. Goal (tailored to patient/client needs)

   OR

2. Reference standard

Edition: 2008

ACCESS TO A SUFFICIENT, RELIABLE SUPPLY OF SAFE, HEALTHFUL FOOD (BE-3.1.1)

Patient/Client Example(s)

Example(s) of one or two of the Nutrition Care Indicators for this outcome (*includes sample initial and re-assessment documentation for one of the indicators*)

Indicator(s) selected

Access to a sufficient supply of healthful food

Criteria for evaluation

Comparison to Goal or Reference Standard:

1. Goal: Patient/client has limited access to a sufficient quantity of food when substantial or extensive access to a sufficient, reliable supply of food is the goal.

   OR

2. Reference standard: No validated standard exists.

Sample monitoring and evaluation documentation

Initial encounter with patient/client	The patient/client has limited access to a sufficient, reliable supply of food. Will monitor change in access to food at next appointment.
Re-assessment after nutrition intervention	Some progress toward goal as patient/client has moderate access to a sufficient, reliable supply of food.

References

The following are some suggested references for indicators, measurement techniques, and reference standard for the outcome; other references may be appropriate.

1. Department of Health and Human Services (HHS) Poverty Guidelines, 2006. Available at: http://aspe.hhs.gov/poverty/06poverty.shtml. Accessed November 14, 2006.
2. Dietary Guidelines for Americans, 2005. Available at: http://www.health.gov/dietaryguidelines/dga2005/document/html/executivesummary.htm. Accessed October 25, 2006.
3. Granger LE, Holben DH. Self-identified food security knowledge and practices of family physicians in Ohio. *Top Clin Nutr.* 2004;19:280-285.
4. Holben DH. Incorporation of food security learning activities into dietetics curricula. *Top Clin Nutr.* 2005;20:339-350.
5. Holben DH, Myles W. Food Insecurity in the United States: How It Affects Our Patients. *Am Fam Physician.* 2004;69;1058-1063.
6. Partnership for Food Safety Education. Available at: http://www.fightbac.org. Accessed October 19, 2006.
7. Position of the American Dietetic Association on Food Insecurity and Hunger in the United States. *J Am Diet Assoc.* 2006;106:446-458.
8. Position of the American Dietetic Association: Addressing world hunger, malnutrition, and food insecurity. *J Am Diet Assoc.* 2003;103:1046-1057.
9. Position of the American Dietetic Association: Food and water safety. *J Am Diet Assoc.* 2003;103:1203-1218.
10. Tscholl E, Holben DH. Knowledge and Practices of Ohio Nurse Practitioners and Its Relationship to Food Access of Patients. *J Am Acad Nusr Pract.* 2006;18:335-342.
11. U.S. Department of Agriculture, Economic Research Service. Food security in the United States. Available at: http://www.ers.usda.gov/Briefing/FoodSecurity/. Accessed February 28, 2007.
12. U.S. Environmental Protection Agency, Ground Water and Drinking Water Frequently Asked Questions. Available at: http://www.epa.gov/safewater/faq/faq.html#safe. Accessed November 14, 2006.

279

Behavioral

BEHAVIORAL-ENVIRONMENTAL OUTCOMES DOMAIN • Physical Activity and Function

BREASTFEEDING SUCCESS (BE-4.1)

Definition

Degree to which breastfeeding plans and experience meet nutritional and other needs of the infant and mother

Monitoring

Changes in these Potential Indicators:

- Initiation of breastfeeding
- Duration of breastfeeding
- Exclusive breastfeeding
- Breastfeeding problems

NOTE: Infant/child growth can be found on the Body Composition/Growth Reference Sheet.
Breastfeeding self-efficacy and intention to breastfeed can be found on the Beliefs and Attitudes Reference Sheet.

Examples of the measurement methods or data sources for these outcome indicators

Patient/client report, practitioner observation of breastfeeding dyad, self-monitoring records, infant weight trends

Typically used to measure the outcomes for the following domains of nutrition interventions

Nutrition education, nutrition counseling, coordination of nutrition care

Typically used to monitor and evaluate change in the following nutrition diagnoses

Maternal breastfeeding difficulty, food- and nutrition-related knowledge deficit, harmful beliefs/attitudes about food- or nutrition-related topics; and infant underweight, involuntary weight loss, inadequate fluid intake

Clinical judgment must be used to select indicators and determine the appropriate measurement techniques and reference standards for a given patient population and setting. Once identified, these indicators, measurement techniques, and reference standards should be identified in policies and procedures or other documents for use in patient/client records, quality or performance improvement, or in formal research projects.

Edition: 2008

BREASTFEEDING SUCCESS (BE-4.1)

Evaluation

Criteria for evaluation
Comparison to Goal or Reference Standard:

1. Goal (tailored to patient/client's needs)

OR

2. Reference standard

Patient/Client Example(s)
Example(s) of one or two of the Nutrition Care Indicators for this outcome (*includes sample initial and re-assessment documentation for one of the indicators*)

Indicator(s) selected
Initiation of breastfeeding

Criteria for evaluation
Comparison to Goal or Reference Standard:

1. Goal: Patient/client currently fears her breast milk supply is not adequate and worries about how she will manage when she returns to work in four weeks. Goal is for mother to breastfeed for six months.

OR

2. Reference standard: No validated standard exists.

Sample monitoring and evaluation documentation

Initial encounter with patient/client	Postpartum patient/client states she is planning to use a combination of formula and breastfeed and start solids at 3 months. Will educate and refer to lactation support group.
Re-assessment after nutrition intervention	Patient/client reports she has exclusively breast fed for three months and plans to delay introduction of solids. Will reinforce and educate. Continue to monitor.

References
The following are some suggested references for indicators, measurement techniques, and reference standards for the outcome; other references may be appropriate.
1. Riordan, J. *Breastfeeding and Human Lactation.* 3rd ed. Sudbury, MA: Jones and Bartlett Publishers; 2005:219.
2. Leff EW, Gagne MP, Jefferis SC. Maternal perceptions of successful breastfeeding. *J Hum Lact.* 2004;10:99-104.
3. Avery M, Duckett L, Dodgson J, Savik K, Henly SJ. Factors associated with very early weaning among primiparas intending to breastfeed. *Maternal Child Health J.* 1998;2:167-179.
4. American Academy of Pediatrics. Policy statement: Breastfeeding and the use of human milk, section on breastfeeding. *Pediatrics.* 2005;115:496-506.
5. CAPPA Position Paper. The lactation educator's role in providing breastfeeding information and support. 2002. Available at: http://www.cappa.net. Accessed March13, 2007.

Edition: 2008

Behavioral

NUTRITION-RELATED ACTIVITIES OF DAILY LIVING AND INSTRUMENTAL ACTIVITIES OF DAILY LIVING (BE-4.2)

Definition

Level of cognitive and physical ability to perform nutrition-related activities of daily living and instrumental activities of daily living by older and/or disabled persons

Monitoring

Changes in these Potential Indicators:

- Acceptance of assistance with eating
- Ability to use adaptive eating devices
- Time taken to eat and consume meals
- Ability to shop for food
- Nutrition-related activities of daily living (ADL) score
- Nutrition-related instrumental activities of daily living (IADL) score

NOTE: Sufficient intake of food can be found on the Food Intake Reference Sheet.

Sufficient intake of fluid can be found on the Fluid/Beverage Intake Reference Sheet.

Food security and ability to maintain sanitation can be found on the Access to Food Reference Sheet.

Ability to prepare/cook food can be found on the Ability to Prepare Healthy Food/Meals Reference Sheet.

Examples of the measurement methods or data sources for these outcome indicators

Self-report, caregiver report, home visit, targeted questionnaires and monitoring devices, ADL and/or IADL measurement tool, congregate meal site attendance records

Typically used to monitor and evaluate change in the following domains of nutrition interventions

Coordination of nutrition care

Typically used to monitor and evaluate change in the following nutrition diagnoses

Inability to manage self-care, impaired ability to prepare foods/meals

Clinical judgment must be used to select indicators and determine the appropriate measurement techniques and reference standards for a given patient population and setting. Once identified, these indicators, measurement techniques, and reference standards should be identified in policies and procedures or other documents for use in patient/client records, quality or performance improvement, or in formal research projects.

282

Edition: 2008

NUTRITION-RELATED ACTIVITIES OF DAILY LIVING AND INSTRUMENTAL ACTIVITIES OF DAILY LIVING (BE-4.2)

Evaluation

Criteria for evaluation

Comparison to Goal or Reference Standard:

1. Goal (tailored to patient/client's needs)

OR

2. Reference standard

Patient/Client Example(s)

Example(s) of one or two of the Nutrition Care Indicators for this outcome (*includes sample initial and re-assessment documentation for one of the indicators*)

Indicator(s) selected

Nutrition-related instrumental activities of daily living (IADL) score

Criteria for evaluation

Comparison to Goal or Reference Standard:

1. Goal: Patient/client with decreased food intake because of impaired ability to use eating utensils sets goal to utilize adaptive eating devices at meals to decrease eating difficulty.

OR

2. Reference standard: No validated standard exists.

Sample monitoring and evaluation documentation

Initial encounter with patient/client	Patient/client with inadequate food intake due to inability to drive, no close relative living in vicinity, subsequent weight loss and difficulties in performing ADLs and IADLs due to weakness. Client is to use new strategies and community resources to facilitate attendance at senior center congregate meals 5 times per week, use of community provided transportation offered to grocery store 1 x per week and attendance in strength training at senior center.
Re-assessment after nutrition intervention	Significant progress in nutrition-related activities of daily living. Patient/client able to attend senior center for meals and strength training 3 times this week. Goal is 5 times. Will continue to assess at next encounter. Client going to grocery store 1 x per week.

References

The following are some suggested references for indicators, measurement techniques, and reference standards for the outcome; other references may be appropriate.

1. ADL/IADL evaluation tools used for Administration on Aging (AoA) nutrition programs available from AoA. Performance Outcomes Management Project, Physical Functioning and Health Survey. Available at: https://www.gpra.net/PFmain.asp . Accessed March 18, 2007

2. Kretser A, Voss T, Kerr W, Cavadini C, Friedmann J. Effects of two models of nutritional intervention on homebound older adults at nutritional risk. *J Am Diet Assoc.* 2003;103:329-336.

Edition: 2008

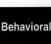

Behavioral

BEHAVIORAL-ENVIRONMENTAL OUTCOMES DOMAIN • Physical Activity and Function

PHYSICAL ACTIVITY (BE-4.3)

Definition
Level of physical activity and/or amount of exercise performed

Monitoring
Change in these Potential Indicators :

- Consistency/frequency
- Duration
- Intensity
- Strength

Examples of the measurement methods or data sources for these outcome indicators
Exercise log, watch, pedometer with a time function, and other electronic monitoring devices that detect time and intensity; attendance at strength training, balance training (for older adults), and/or aerobic classes

Typically used to measure the outcomes for the following domains of nutrition interventions
Nutrition education, nutrition counseling

Typically used to monitor and evaluate change in the following nutrition diagnoses
Physical inactivity, excessive exercise, underweight, overweight/obesity, involuntary weight loss or weight gain

Clinical judgment must be used to select indicators and determine the appropriate measurement techniques and reference standards for a given patient population and setting. Once identified, these indicators, measurement techniques, and reference standards should be identified in policies and procedures or other documents for use in patient/client records, quality or performance improvement, or in formal research projects.

Evaluation

Criteria for evaluation
Comparison to Goal or Reference Standard:

1. Goal (tailored to patient/client's needs)

OR

2. Reference standard

PHYSICAL ACTIVITY (BE-4.3)

Patient/Client Example(s)

Example(s) of one or two of the Nutrition Care Indicators for this outcome (*includes sample initial and re-assessment documentation for one of the indicators*)

Indicator(s) selected
Consistency and duration

Criteria for evaluation
Comparison to Goal or Reference Standard:

1. Goal: Patient/client is currently completely sedentary, but established a goal to walk 10 minutes per day, 6 days per week.

OR

2. Reference standard: Patient/client's typical 10-minute walk, twice a week is well below the recommended 30 minutes of moderate-intensity physical activity, but above usual activity, at work or home most days/wk (Dietary Guidelines for Americans 2005).

Sample monitoring and evaluation documentation

Initial encounter with patient/client	Based upon exercise log, patient/client doing moderate-intensity physical activities 30 minutes/day, 2 days/week. Goal is to exercise 30 minutes/day, moderate-intensity activities, 5 or more days/wk. Will monitor physical activity level at next appointment.
Re-assessment after nutrition intervention	Significant progress toward goal of exercising 30 minutes/day, moderate-intensity activities, 5 or more days/wk. Patient/client reports doing moderate-intensity activities 30 minutes per day, 4 days/week

References
The following are some suggested references for indicators, measurement techniques, and reference standards for the outcome; other references may be appropriate.

1. United States Department of Health and Human Services, United States Department of Agriculture. Dietary Guidelines for Americans 2005. Available at: www.healthierus.gov/dietaryguidelines. Accessed December 9, 2006.
2. National Heart, Lung, and Blood Institute. Clinical guidelines on the identification, evaluation, and treatment of overweight and obesity in adults: The evidence report. *Obes Res.* 1998;6(suppl 2):51S-210S.
3. American College of Sports Medicine Position Stands. Available at: http://www.acsm-msse.org. Accessed March 14, 2007.
4. Department of Health and Human Services, Centers for Disease Control and Prevention, Growing Stronger–Strength Training for Older Adults. Available at: http://www.cdc.gov/nccdphp/dnpa/physical/growing_stronger/index.htm. Accessed March 18, 2007.
5. American College of Sports Medicine, National Blueprint: Increasing physical activity among adults aged 50 and older. Available at: http://www.agingblueprint.org/overview.cfm. Accessed March 18, 2007.
6. Exercise Guidelines During Pregnancy. American Pregnancy Association. Available at: http://www.americanpregnancy.org/pregnancyhealth/exerciseguidelines.html. Accessed March 14, 2007.
7. Perri MG, Martin AD, Leermakers EA, Sears SF, Notelovitz M. Effects of group- versus home-based exercise in treatment of obesity. *J Consult Clin Psychol.* 1997;65:278-285.
8. Jakicic JM, Wing RR, Butler BA, Robertson RJ. Prescribing exercise in multiple short bouts versus one continuous bout: Effects on adherence, cardiorespiratory fitness, and weight loss in overweight women. *Int J Obes Relat Metab Disord.* 1995;19:893-901.
9. Fabricatore AN. Behavior therapy and cognitive-behavioral therapy of obesity: Is there a difference? *J Am Diet Assoc.* 2007;107:92-99.

Edition: 2008

285

Behavioral

FOOD AND NUTRIENT INTAKE OUTCOMES DOMAIN • Energy Intake

ENERGY INTAKE (FI-1.1)

Definition

Amount of energy intake from all sources (e.g., food, beverages, supplements, and via enteral and parenteral routes)

Monitoring

Changes in these Potential Indicators:

• Total energy intake

Examples of the measurement methods or data sources for these outcome indicators

Food intake records, 24-hour recall, 3-5 day food diary, food frequency questionnaire, caretaker intake records, menu analysis, intake and output records

Typically used to measure the outcomes for the following domains of nutrition interventions

Food and/or nutrient delivery, nutrition education, nutrition counseling, coordination of nutrition care

Typically used to monitor and evaluate change in the following nutrition diagnosis

Inadequate energy intake, excessive energy intake, evident protein-calorie malnutrition, inadequate protein-energy intake, underweight, involuntary weight loss, overweight/obesity, involuntary weight gain, swallowing difficulty, breastfeeding difficulty, altered GI function, limited adherence to nutrition-related recommendations

Clinical judgment must be used to select indicators and determine the appropriate measurement techniques and reference standards for a given patient population and setting. Once identified, these indicators, measurement techniques, and reference standards should be identified in policies and procedures or other documents for use in patient/client records, quality or performance improvement, or in formal research projects.

Evaluation

Criteria for evaluation

Comparison to Goal or Reference Standard:

1. Goal (tailored to individual's needs)

   OR

2. Reference standard

ENERGY INTAKE (FI-1.1)

Patient/Client Example(s)

Example(s) of one or two of the Nutrition Care Indicators for this outcome (*includes sample initial and re-assessment documentation for one of the indicators*)

Indicator(s) selected

Total energy intake

Criteria for evaluation

Comparison to Goal or Reference Standard:

1. Goal: Food diary indicates patient/client consumes 2600 kcal/day. Patient/client to target an intake of 1800 kcal/day.

   OR

2. Reference standard: Patient/client's I & O indicates patient/client's intake at 2000 kcal, 75% of goal based on an estimated energy requirement of 2665 kcal/day.

Sample monitoring and evaluation documentation

Initial encounter with patient/client	Based on patient/client food diary, patient/client consuming approximately 2600 kcal/day, 144% of recommended level of 1800 kcals. Will evaluate calorie intake at next encounter in two weeks.
Re-assessment after nutrition intervention	Significant progress toward recommended kcal intake. Based upon food diary, patient/client decreased calorie consumption to 2100 kcal, 117% recommended level. Will assess kcal intake in four weeks.

References

The following are some suggested references for indicators, measurement techniques, and reference standards for the outcome; other references may be appropriate.

1. Institute of Medicine, Food and Nutrition Board. Dietary Reference Intakes for Energy, Carbohydrate, Fiber, Fat, Fatty Acids, Cholesterol, Protein and Amino Acids. Washington, DC: National Academy Press; 2002. Available at: www.iom.edu/Object.File/Master/21/372/DRI%20Tables%20after%20electrolytes%20plus%20micro-macroEAR_2.pdf.

2. Frankenfield D, Roth-Yousey L, Compher C. Comparison of predictive equations for resting metabolic rate in healthy nonobese adults: A systematic review. *J Am Diet Assoc*. 2005;105:775-789.

3. Charney P, Malone A, eds. *ADA Pocket Guide to Nutrition Assessment*. Chicago, IL: American Dietetic Association; 2004.

4. Compher C, Frankenfield D, Keim N, Roth-Yousey L. Best practice methods to apply to measurement of resting metabolic rate in adults: A systematic review. *J Am Diet Assoc*. 2006;106:881-903.

5. ADA Evidence Analysis Library. Accessed on: 10/28/2006 from http://ada.portalxm.com/eal/template.cfm? key=1309&cms_preview=1

6. American Society for Parenteral and Enteral Nutrition Board of Directors and The Clinical Guidelines Task Force. Guidelines for the use of parenteral and enteral nutrition in adult and pediatric patients: Life cycle and metabolic conditions. *J Parenter Enteral Nutr*. 2002;26(Suppl):S45-S60.

7. American Society for Parenteral and Enteral Nutrition Board of Directors and The Clinical Guidelines Task Force. Guidelines for the use of parenteral and enteral nutrition in adult and pediatric patients: Specific guidelines for disease—adults. *J Parenter Enteral Nutr*. 2002;26(Suppl):S61-S96.

8. American Society for Parenteral and Enteral Nutrition Board of Directors and The Clinical Guidelines Task Force. Guidelines for the use of parenteral and enteral nutrition in adult and pediatric patients: Specific guidelines for disease—pediatrics. *J Parenter Enteral Nutr*. 2002;26(Suppl):S111-S138.

9. American Dietetic Association. *ADA Nutritional Care Manual*. Available at: http://nutritioncaremanual.org.

Edition: 2008

Food & Nutrient

FLUID/BEVERAGE INTAKE (FI-2.1)

Definition

Amount and type of fluid/beverage intake from all sources (e.g., beverages, supplements, and via enteral and parenteral routes)

Monitoring

Changes in these Potential Indicators:

- Oral fluid amounts
  - o Water
  - o Coffee and tea
  - o Juice
  - o Milk
  - o Soda (regular or artificial sweetened)
- Food-derived fluids
- IV fluids
- Liquid meal replacement

Examples of the measurement methods or data sources for these outcome indicators

Food intake records, 24-hour recall, food frequency questionnaire, menu analysis, intake and output data, number of urinations per day

Typically used to measure the outcomes for the following domains of nutrition interventions

Food and/or nutrient delivery, nutrition education, nutrition counseling, coordination of nutrition care

Typically used to monitor and evaluate change in the following nutrition diagnosis

Excessive or inadequate oral food/beverage intake, food-medication interaction, underweight, overweight/obesity, disordered eating pattern, undesirable food choices, limited adherence to nutrition related recommendations, inability or lack of desire to manage self-care, swallowing difficulty, breastfeeding difficulty, altered GI function

Clinical judgment must be used to select indicators and determine the appropriate measurement techniques and reference standards for a given patient population and setting. Once identified, these indicators, measurement techniques, and reference standards should be identified in policies and procedures or other documents for use in patient/client records, quality or performance improvement, or in formal research projects.

Food & Nutrient

Edition: 2008

FLUID/BEVERAGE INTAKE (FI-2.1)

Evaluation

Criteria for evaluation
Comparison to Goal or Reference Standard:

1. Goal (tailored to patient/client's needs)

OR

2. Reference standard

Patient/Client Example(s)

Example(s) of one or two of the Nutrition Care Indicators for this outcome (*includes sample initial and re-assessment documentation for one of the indicators*)

Indicator(s) selected
Oral fluid amounts

Criteria for evaluation
Comparison to Goal or Reference Standard:

1. Goal: Patient /client currently drinks 12 oz of water per day and has a goal of consuming 64 oz of water per day.

OR

2. Reference standard: Patient/client's intake of 1000 mL of free water (0.8 mL/kcal) is below the 1mL/kcal guideline.

Sample monitoring and evaluation documentation

Initial encounter with patient/client	Based on patient/client food diary, patient/client consuming approximately 1000 mL water per day. Will monitor water intake at next encounter.
Re-assessment after nutrition intervention	Significant progress toward recommended water intake. Based upon fluid intake records, patient/client increased consumption of water from 1000 mL to 2600 mL per day.

References
The following are some suggested references for indicators, measurement techniques, and reference standards for the outcome; other references may be appropriate.

1. Institute of Medicine, Food and Nutrition Board. Dietary Reference Intakes for Energy, Carbohydrate, Fiber, Fat, Fatty Acids, Cholesterol, Protein and Amino Acids. Washington, DC: National Academy Press; 2002. Available at: www.iom.edu/report.asp?id=4340.

2. American Society for Parenteral and Enteral Nutrition Board of Directors and The Clinical Guidelines Task Force. Guidelines for the use of parenteral and enteral nutrition in adult and pediatric patients: Specific guidelines for disease—adults. *J Parenter Enteral Nutr.* 2002;26(Suppl):S61-S96.

3. Queen PM, Lang CE. *Handbook of Pediatric Nutrition.* Gaitherburg, MD: Aspen Press; 1993.

4. American Society for Parenteral and Enteral Nutrition Board of Directors and The Clinical Guidelines Task Force. Guidelines for the use of parenteral and enteral nutrition in adult and pediatric patients: Specific guidelines for disease—pediatrics. *J Parenter Enteral Nutr.* 2002:26(Suppl):S111-S138.

5. Fluid needs in nephrolithiasis. *ADA Nutritional Care Manual.* 2006. Available at: http://nutritioncaremanual.org.

6. American College of Sports Medicine Web site. Available at: http://www.acsm.org.

Edition: 2008

Food & Nutrient

FOOD INTAKE (FI-2.2)

Definition

Amount, type and quality of food consumed orally

Monitoring

Changes in these Potential Indicators

- Food variety
- Number of food group servings
  - o Grains
  - o Fruits
  - o Vegetables
  - o Milk/Dairy Foods
  - o Meat/Protein Substitutes (beans, eggs. peanut butter, tofu)
- Healthy Eating Index (HEI)
- Children's Diet Quality Index (C-DQI)
- Revised Children's Diet Quality Index (RC-DQI)

Examples of the measurement methods or data sources for these outcome indicators

Food intake records, 24-hour recall, food frequency questionnaire, menu analysis, MyPyramid Tracker, Healthy Eating Index, C-DQI, RC-DQI

Typically used to measure the outcomes for the following domains of nutrition interventions

Food and/or nutrient delivery, nutrition education, nutrition counseling, coordination of nutrition care

Typically used to monitor and evaluate change in the following nutrition diagnosis

Excessive or inadequate oral food/beverage intake, food-medication interaction, underweight, overweight/obesity, disordered eating pattern, undesirable food choices, limited adherence to nutrition related recommendations, inability or lack of desire to manage self-care.

Clinical judgment must be used to select indicators and determine the appropriate measurement techniques and reference standards for a given patient population and setting. Once identified, these indicators, measurement techniques, and reference standards should be identified in policies and procedures or other documents for use in patient/client records, quality or performance improvement, or in formal research projects.

Edition: 2008

FOOD INTAKE (FI-2.2)

Evaluation

Criteria for evaluation
Comparison to Goal or Reference Standard:

1. Goal (tailored to patient/client needs)

OR

2. Reference standard

Patient/Client Example(s)

Example(s) of one or two of the Nutrition Care Indicators for this outcome (*includes sample initial and re-assessment documentation for one of the indicators*)

Indicator(s) selected
Number of food group servings

Criteria for evaluation
Comparison to Goal or Reference Standard:

1. Goal: Patient/client currently eats approximately 1-2 fruit and vegetable servings per day. Goal is to increase fruit and vegetable intake to 5 servings per day.

OR

2. Reference standard: Patient/client's current intake of 1-2 servings of fruit and vegetable servings per day is below the 2005 *Dietary Guidelines for Americans* recommendation of 2 cups of fruit and 2 ½ cups of vegetables per day.

Sample monitoring and evaluation documentation

Initial encounter with patient/client	Based on patient/client recall, patient/client consuming approximately 1-2 servings of fruits and vegetables per day. Will monitor fruit and vegetable intake at next encounter.
Re-assessment after nutrition intervention	Significant progress toward goal of 5 servings of fruit and vegetables per day. Based upon food records, patient/client increased consumption of fruits and vegetables from approximately 1 to 4 servings per day.

Food & Nutrient

FOOD AND NUTRIENT INTAKE OUTCOMES DOMAIN • Food and Beverage Intake

Food &
Nutrient

FOOD INTAKE (FI-2.2)

References
The following are some suggested references for indicators, measurement techniques, and reference standards for the outcome; other references may be appropriate.

1. US Departments of Agriculture and Health and Human Services. *Dietary Guidelines for Americans 2005.* Available at: www.healthierus.gov/dietaryguidelines.

2. US Department of Agriculture Center for Nutrition Policy and Promotion. *The Food Guide Pyramid for Young Children 2 to 6 Years Old.* Bethesda, MD: US Department of Agriculture; Center for Nutrition Policy and Promotion; 1998.

3. United States Department of Agriculture Human Nutrition Information Service. My Pyramid. 2005. Available at: http://www.mypyramid.gov. Accessed January 9, 2007.

4. *ADA Nutrition Care Manual.* 2006. Available at: www.nutritioncaremanual.org. Accessed December 11, 2006.

5. Ledikwe JH, Blanck HM, Khan LK, Serdula MK, Seymour JD, Tohill BC, Rolls BJ. Low-energy-density diets are associated with high diet quality in adults in the United States. *J Am Diet Assoc.* 2006;106:1172-1180.

6. Rolls B. *The Volumetrics Eating Plan.* New York, NY: HarperCollins Publishers, Inc; 2005.

7. American Academy of Pediatrics Committee on Nutrition. *Pediatric Nutrition Handbook. 5th ed.* Elk Grove Village, IL: American Academy of Pediatrics; 2004.

8. Kranz S, Hartman T, Siega-Riz AM, Herring AH. A diet quality index for American preschoolers based on current dietary intake recommendations and an indicator of energy balance. *J Am Diet Assoc.* 2006;106:1594-1604.

Edition: 2008

ENTERAL AND PARENTERAL NUTRITION INTAKE (FI-3.1)

Definition

Amount or type of enteral and/or parenteral nutrition

Monitoring

Changes in these Potential Indicators:

- Access
- Formula/solution
- Discontinuation
- Initiation
- Rate/schedule

Examples of the measurement methods or data sources for these outcome indicators

Patient/client report/recall, patient/client record, home evaluation, pharmacy report

Typically used to measure the outcomes for the following domains of nutrition interventions

Food and/or nutrient delivery, coordination of nutrition care

Typically used to monitor and evaluate change in the following nutrition diagnoses

Inadequate or excess intake of enteral or parenteral nutrition

Clinical judgment must be used to select indicators and determine the appropriate measurement techniques and reference standards for a given patient population and setting. Once identified, these indicators, measurement techniques, and reference standards should be identified in policies and procedures or other documents for use in patient/client records, quality or performance improvement, or in formal research projects.

Evaluation

Criteria for evaluation

Comparison to Goal or Reference Standard:

1. Goal (tailored to patient/client needs)

   OR

2. Reference standard

Edition: 2008

Food &
Nutrient

FOOD AND NUTRIENT INTAKE OUTCOMES DOMAIN • Enteral/Parenteral Nutrition

ENTERAL AND PARENTERAL NUTRITION INTAKE (FI-3.1)

Patient/Client Example(s)

Example(s) of one or two of the Nutrition Care Indicators for this outcome (*includes sample initial and re-assessment documentation for one of the indicators*)

Indicator (s) selected

Rate/schedule

Criteria for evaluation

Comparison to Goal or Reference Standard:

1. Goal: Patient/client's enteral nutrition is at a rate of 50 mL per hour of 1 calorie per mL formula compared to the nutrition prescription of 80 mL/hour to meet estimated nutrition needs.

OR

2. Reference standard: There is no reference standard for this outcome because the provision of EN/PN is individualized.

Sample monitoring and evaluation documentation

Initial encounter with patient/client	Monitor enteral nutrition initiation and rate advancement.
Re-assessment after nutrition intervention	Enteral nutrition at 70 mL per hour. Significant progress toward nutrition prescription of 1 calorie per mL formula at 80 mL per hour.

References

The following are some suggested references for indicators, measurement techniques, and reference standards for the outcome; other references may be appropriate.

1. Charney P, Malone A, eds. *ADA Pocket Guide to Enteral Nutrition.* Chicago, IL: American Dietetic Association; 2006.
2. Charney P, Malone A, eds. *ADA Pocket Guide to Nutrition Assessment.* Chicago, IL: American Dietetic Association; 2004.
3. *ADA Nutrition Care Manual.* 2006. Available at: www.nutritioncaremanual.org. Accessed November 29, 2006.
4. Cavicchi M, Philippe Beau P, Crenn P, Degott C, Messing B. Prevalence of liver disease and contributing factors in patients receiving home parenteral nutrition for permanent intestinal failure. *Intern Med.* 2000;132:525-532.
5. Centers for Medicare and Medicaid Services. National coverage determination (NCD) for enteral and parenteral nutrition therapy. Available at: http://www.cms.hhs.gov/mcd/viewncd.asp?ncd_id=180.2&ncd_version=1&basket=ncd%3A180%2E2%E2%3A1%3AEnteral+and+Parenteral+Nutritional+Therapy. Accessed December 22, 2006.
6. Compher C, Frankenfield D, Keim N, Roth-Yousey L. Best practice methods to apply to measurement of resting metabolic rate in adults: A systematic review. *J Am Diet Assoc.* 2006;106:881-903.
7. Guidelines for the use of parenteral and enteral nutrition in adult and pediatric patients: Administration of specialized nutrition support—issues unique to pediatrics. *J Parenter Enteral Nutr.* 2002;26(Suppl):S97-S110.
8. Guidelines for the use of parenteral and enteral nutrition in adult and pediatric patients: Specific guidelines for disease—adults. *J Parenter Enteral Nutr.* 2002;26(Suppl):S61-S96.
9. Guidelines for the use of parenteral and enteral nutrition in adult and pediatric patients: Access for administration of nutrition support. *J Parenter Enteral Nutr.* 2002;26(1 Suppl):33SA-41SA.
10. Guidelines for the use of parenteral and enteral nutrition in adult and pediatric patients: Specific guidelines for disease—pediatrics. *J Parenter Enteral Nutr.* 2002;26(Suppl):S111-S138.
11. Guidelines for the use of parenteral and enteral nutrition in adult and pediatric patients: Life cycle and metabolic conditions. *J Parenter Enteral Nutr.* 2002;26(Suppl):S45-S60.
12. Steiger E; HPEN Working Group. Consensus statements regarding optimal management of home parenteral nutrition (HPN) access. *J Parenter Enteral Nutr.* 2006;30(1 Suppl):S94-S95.
13. Kovacevich DS, Frederick A, Kelly D, Nishikawa R, Young L; American Society for Parenteral and Enteral Nutrition Board of Directors; Standards for Specialized Nutrition Support Task Force. Standards for specialized nutrition support: home care patients. *Nutr Clin Pract.* 2005;20:579-590.

Edition: 2008

CHANGE IN ALCOHOL INTAKE (FI-4.1)

Definition

Alteration in alcohol consumption and pattern

Monitoring

Changes in these Potential Indicators:

- Drink size/volume
- Frequency

Examples of the measurement methods or data sources for these outcome indicators

Patient/client report/recall, three item questionnaire, self-monitoring log, 24 hour recall

Typically used to measure the outcomes for the following domains of nutrition interventions

Nutrition education, nutrition counseling

Typically used to monitor and evaluate change in the following nutrition diagnoses

Excess intake of alcohol; excess or inadequate intake of energy; altered nutrition-related laboratory values; impaired nutrient utilization; overweight/obesity

Clinical judgment must be used to select indicators and determine the appropriate measurement techniques and reference standards for a given patient population and setting. Once identified, these indicators, measurement techniques, and reference standards should be identified in policies and procedures or other documents for use in patient/client records, quality or performance improvement, or in formal research projects.

Evaluation

Criteria for evaluation

Comparison to Goal or Reference Standard:

1. Goal (tailored to patient/client needs)

OR

2. Reference standard

Food & Nutrient

Edition: 2008

FOOD AND NUTRIENT INTAKE OUTCOMES DOMAIN • Bioactive Substances

CHANGE IN ALCOHOL INTAKE (FI-4.1)

Patient/Client Example(s)

Example(s) of one or two of the Nutrition Care Indicators for this outcome (*includes sample initial and re-assessment documentation for one of the indicators*)

Indicator(s) selected

- Drink size/volume
- Frequency

Criteria for evaluation

Comparison to Goal or Reference Standard:

1. Goal: Patient/client's intake of one 5-ounce glass of wine 2-3 times per week is significantly above and noncompliant with the goal to abstain from alcohol during pregnancy.

   OR.

2. Reference standard: Patient/client's intake of three to four 5-ounce glasses of wine per day is significantly above* the reference standard of one 5-ounce glass of wine per day for women.

Sample monitoring and evaluation documentation

Initial encounter with patient/client	Based upon recall, patient/client consuming three to four 5-ounce glasses of wine per day. Will monitor change in alcohol intake at next encounter.
Re-assessment after nutrition intervention	Significant progress toward reference standard one 5-ounce glass of wine per day. Based upon 3-day record, patient/client consuming 8 ounces of wine total over the 3-day period.

References

The following are some suggested references for indicators, measurement techniques, and reference standards for the outcome; other references may be appropriate.

1. *Dietary Guidelines for Americans*, 2005. Available at: http://www.health.gov/dietaryguidelines/dga2005/document/html/executivesummary.htm. Accessed October 27, 2006.
2. National Institutes of Health, National Institute on Alcoholism and Alcohol Abuse. Task Force on Recommended Alcohol Questions, National Council on Alcohol Abuse and Alcoholism Recommended Sets of Alcohol Consumption Questions. Available at: http://www.niaaa.nih.gov/Resources/ResearchResources/TaskForce.htm. Accessed October 27, 2006.

*Could be specified as "above," "below," or a "percent of" the reference value.

Food & Nutrient

BIOACTIVE SUBSTANCE INTAKE (FI-4.2)

Definition

Amount and type of bioactive substances consumed

NOTE: Working definition of bioactive substances—physiologically active components of foods that may offer health benefits beyond traditional macro- or micronutrient requirements. Note: There is no scientific consensus about a definition for bioactive substances/components.

Monitoring

Changes in these Potential Indicators :

- Plant sterol and stanol esters
- Soy protein
- Psyllium and β-glucan

Examples of the measurement methods or data sources for these outcome indicators

Patient/client report/recall, self-monitoring log

Typically used to measure the outcomes for the following domains of nutrition interventions

Nutrition education, nutrition counseling

Typically used to monitor and evaluate change in the following nutrition diagnoses

Inadequate or excess intake of bioactive substances, food-medication interaction

Clinical judgment must be used to select indicators and determine the appropriate measurement techniques and reference standards for a given patient population and setting. Once identified, these indicators, measurement techniques, and reference standards should be identified in policies and procedures or other documents for use in patient/client records, quality or performance improvement, or in formal research projects.

Evaluation

Criteria for evaluation

Comparison to Goal or Reference Standard:

1. Goal (tailored to patient/client needs)

    OR

2. Reference standard

Edition: 2008

FOOD AND NUTRIENT INTAKE OUTCOMES DOMAIN • Bioactive Substances

BIOACTIVE SUBSTANCE INTAKE (FI-4.2)

Patient/Client Example(s)

Example(s) of one or two of the Nutrition Care Indicators for this outcome (*includes sample initial and re-assessment documentation for one of the indicators*)

Indicator(s) selected
Plant sterol and stanol esters

Criteria for evaluation
Comparison to Goal or Reference Standard:

1. Goal: The patient/client does not consume plant sterol or stanol esters compared to the goal intake of 2-3 grams per day.

OR

2. Reference standard: No validated standard exists.

Sample monitoring and evaluation documentation

Initial encounter with patient/client	Based upon recall, patient/client consuming approximately 0 grams of stanol/sterol ester per day. Will monitor change in stanol/sterol ester intake at next encounter.
Re-assessment after nutrition intervention	No progress toward the goal of 2-3 g/day of stanol/sterol ester. Based upon 3-day diet record, patient/client still consuming 0 grams stanol/sterol ester per day.

References
The following are some suggested references for indicators, measurement techniques, and reference standards for the outcome; other references may be appropriate.

1. ADA Disorders of Lipid Metabolism Evidence-Based Nutrition Practice Guideline, 2006. Available at: http://www.adaevidencelibrary.com/topic.cfm?cat=301. Accessed November 5, 2005.
2. Position of the American Dietetic Association: Functional foods. *J Am Diet Assoc.* 2004;104:814-826.

FOOD AND NUTRIENT INTAKE OUTCOMES DOMAIN • Bioactive Substance Intake

CAFFEINE INTAKE (FI-4.3)

Definition

Amount of caffeine intake from all sources (e.g., food, beverages, supplements, and via enteral and parenteral routes)

Monitoring

Changes in these Potential Indicators:

- Total caffeine intake
  (e.g., naturally occurring caffeine in leaves, seeds, fruits of plants and sources with added caffeine such as, water/beverages, medications)

Examples of the measurement methods or data sources for these outcome indicators

Patient/client report/recall, self-monitoring log

Typically used to measure the outcomes for the following domains of nutrition interventions

Nutrition education, nutrition counseling

Typically used to monitor and evaluate change in the following nutrition diagnoses

Food- and nutrition-related knowledge deficit

Clinical judgment must be used to select indicators and determine the appropriate measurement techniques and reference standards for a given patient population and setting. Once identified, these indicators, measurement techniques, and reference standards should be identified in policies and procedures or other documents for use in patient/client records, quality or performance improvement, or in formal research projects.

Evaluation

Criteria for evaluation

Comparison to Goal or Reference Standard:

1. Goal (tailored to patient/client needs)

OR

2. Reference standard

Food & Nutrient

Edition: 2008

FOOD AND NUTRIENT INTAKE OUTCOMES DOMAIN • Bioactive Substance Intake

CAFFEINE INTAKE (FI-4.3)

Patient/Client Example(s)

Example(s) of one or two of the Nutrition Care Indicators for this outcome *(includes sample initial and re-assessment documentation for one of the indicators)*

Indicator(s) selected
Total caffeine intake

Criteria for evaluation
Comparison to Goal or Reference Standard:

1. Goal: The patient/client's intake is 600 mg of caffeine per day, which is above the goal of < 300 mg caffeine per day.

OR

2. Reference standard: The patient/client's intake is approximately 600 mg of caffeine per day which is 150%* of the reference standard of 400 mg caffeine per day.

Sample monitoring and evaluation documentation

Initial encounter with patient/client	Based upon recall, patient/client consuming approximately 600 mg caffeine per day. Will monitor change in caffeine intake at next encounter.
Re-assessment after nutrition intervention	No progress toward the reference standard of 400 mg for caffeine. Based upon 3-day diet record, patient/ client still consuming 600 mg caffeine per day.

References
The following are some suggested references for indicators, measurement techniques, and reference standards for the outcome; other references may be appropriate.

1. Department of Health and Human Services, National Institute of Environmental Health Sciences, National Toxicology Program. Center for the Evaluation of Risks to Human Reproduction (CERHR). Available at: http://cerhr.niehs.nih.gov/common/caffeine.html. Accessed October 31, 2006.
2. Frary CD, Johnson RK, Wang MQ. Food sources and intakes of caffeine in the diets of persons in the United States. *J Am Diet Assoc.* 2005;105:110-113.
3. Kaiser LL, Allen L. Position of the American Dietetic Association: Nutrition and lifestyle for a healthy pregnancy outcome. *J Am Diet Assoc.* 2002;102:1479-1490.
4. Nawrot P, Jordan S, Eastwood J, Rotstein J, Hugenholtz A, Feeley M. Effects of caffeine on human health. *Food Addit Contam.* 2003;20:1–30.
5. Nutrient Data Laboratory. USDA National Nutrient Database for Standard Reference. Available at: http://www.nal.usda.gov/fnic/foodcomp/search/. Accessed on October 30, 2006.
6. Organization of Teratology Information Services (OTIS). Caffeine and Pregnancy. Available at: http://www.otispregnancy.org/pdf/caffeine.pdf. Accessed November 11, 2006.
7. Winkelmayer WC, Stampfer MJ, Willett WC, Curhan GC. Habitual caffeine intake and the risk of hypertension in women *JAMA.* 2005;294:2330-2335.

*Could be specified as "above," "below," or a "percent of" the reference value.

Food & Nutrient

Edition: 2008

FAT AND CHOLESTEROL INTAKE (FI-5.1)

Definition

Fat and cholesterol consumption from all sources, e.g., food, beverages, supplements, and via enteral and parenteral routes

Monitoring

Changes in these Potential Indicators:

- Total fat (grams or % of calories)
- Saturated fat (grams or % of calories)
- *Trans* fatty acids (grams or % of calories)
- Polyunsaturated fat (grams or % of calories)
- Monounsaturated fat (grams or % of calories)
- Omega-3 fatty acids
  - o Marine-derived
  - o Plant-derived
    - Alpha-linolenic acid (amount or % of calories)
- Dietary cholesterol

NOTE: Plant sterol and stanol esters can be found on the Bioactive Substance Intake Reference Sheet.

Examples of the measurement methods or data sources for these outcome indicators

Food intake records, 24-hour recall, food frequency questionnaires, menu analysis, fat and cholesterol targeted questionnaires and monitoring devices

Typically used to measure the outcomes for the following domains of nutrition interventions

Food and/or nutrient delivery, nutrition education, nutrition counseling

Typically used to monitor and evaluate change in the following nutrition diagnosis

Inadequate and excessive fat intake, inappropriate intake of food fats, overweight/obesity, altered nutrition-related lab values, altered food and nutrition-related knowledge deficit

Clinical judgment must be used to select indicators and determine the appropriate measurement techniques and reference standards for a given patient population and setting. Once identified, these indicators, measurement techniques, and reference standards should be identified in policies and procedures or other documents for use in patient/client records, quality or performance improvement, or in formal research projects.

301

Food &
Nutrient

FAT AND CHOLESTEROL INTAKE (FI-5.1)

Evaluation

Criteria for evaluation
Comparison to Goal or Reference Standard:

1. Goal (tailored to patient/client's needs)

OR

2. Reference standard

Patient/Client Example(s)
Example(s) of one or two of the Nutrition Care Indicators for this outcome (*includes sample initial and re-assessment documentation for one of the indicators*)

Indicator(s) selected
- Total fat (grams or % of calories)
- Dietary cholesterol

Criteria for evaluation
Comparison to Goal or Reference Standard:

1. Goal: Patient/client currently consumes 50% of calories from fat. Goal is to decrease fat intake to 40% of calories.

OR

2. Reference standard: Patient/client's intake of 350 mg of cholesterol per day is 175% of the Adult Treatment Panel III guidelines of less than 200 mg of dietary cholesterol per day.

Sample monitoring and evaluation documentation

Initial encounter with patient/client	Based upon a three-day food diary, patient/client is consuming approximately 50% of calories from fat. Patient/client goal is to reduce total fat intake to 40% of calories. Will monitor fat and calorie intake at next appointment.
Re-assessment after nutrition intervention	Significant progress toward the goal intake of 40% calories from fat. Based on a three-day food diary patient/client's total fat intake decreased from approximately 50% to 44% calories from fat/day. Will continue to monitor progress at next encounter in 6 weeks.

Food &
Nutrient

302

FAT AND CHOLESTEROL INTAKE (FI-5.1)

References

The following are some suggested references for indicators, measurement techniques, and reference standards for the outcome; other references may be appropriate.

1. American Heart Association Nutrition Committee: Lichtenstein, A, Appel, L, Brands M, Carnethon M, Daniels S, Franch HA, Franklin B, Kris-Etherton P, Harris WS, Howard B, Karanja N, Lefevre M, Rudel L, Sacks F, Van Horn L, Winston M, Wylie-Rosett J. Diet and lifestyle recommendations revision 2006: a scientific statement from the American Heart Association Nutrition Committee. *Circulation.* 2006;114:82-96.

2. Bantle JP, Wylie-Rosett J, Albright AL, Apovian CM, Clark NG, Franz MJ, Hoogwerf BJ, Lichtenstein AH, Mayer-Davis E, Mooradian AD, Wheeler ML. Nutrition recommendations and interventions for diabetes-2006: a position statement of the American Diabetes Association. *Diabetes Care.* 2006;29:2140-2157.

3. Committee on Nutrient Relationships in Seafood—National Academies. *Seafood choices: Balancing Benefits and Risks.* National Academies Press; 2006.

4. US Departments of Agriculture and Health and Human Services. Dietary Guidelines for Americans 2005. Available at: www.healthierus.gov/dietaryguidelines/.

5. US Department of Health and Human Services. National Institutes of Health. *Third Report of the Expert Panel on Detection, Evaluation, and Treatment of High Blood Cholesterol in Adults (Adult Treatment Panel III).* Bethesda, MD: National Institutes of Health; 2001

6. Institute of Medicine, Food and Nutrition Board. Dietary Reference Intakes for Energy, Carbohydrate, Fiber, Fat, Fatty Acids, Cholesterol, Protein and Amino Acids. Washington, DC: National Academy Press; 2002. Available at: www.iom.edu/report.asp?id=4340.

7. American Society for Parenteral and Enteral Nutrition Board of Directors and The Clinical Guidelines Task Force. Guidelines for the use of parenteral and enteral nutrition in adult and pediatric patients: Specific guidelines for disease—adults. *J Parenter Enteral Nutr.* 2002;26(Suppl):S61-S96.

8. *ADA Nutrition Care Manual.* 2006. Available at: www.nutritioncaremanual.org. Accessed December 11, 2006.

303

Food & Nutrient

FOOD AND NUTRIENT INTAKE OUTCOMES DOMAIN • Macronutrients

PROTEIN INTAKE (FI-5.2)

Definition

Protein intake from all sources (e.g., food, beverages, supplements, and via enteral and parenteral routes)

Monitoring

Changes in these Potential Indicators:

- Total protein
- High biological value protein
- Casein
- Whey
- Soy protein*
- Amino acids
- Essential amino acids

*Soy protein can be found on the Bioactive Substance Intake Reference Sheet.

Examples of the measurement methods or data sources for these outcome indicators

Food intake records, 24-hour recall, food frequency questionnaires, menu analysis, protein intake collection tools

Typically used to measure the outcomes for the following domains of nutrition interventions

Food and/or nutrient delivery, nutrition education, nutrition counseling, coordination of nutrition care

Typically used to monitor and evaluate change in the following nutrition diagnosis

Inadequate and excessive protein intake, inappropriate intake of amino acids, evident protein-energy malnutrition, inadequate protein-energy intake, swallowing difficulty, breastfeeding difficulty, altered GI function, limited adherence to nutrition-related recommendations

Clinical judgment must be used to select indicators and determine the appropriate measurement techniques and reference standards for a given patient population and setting. Once identified, these indicators, measurement techniques, and reference standards should be identified in policies and procedures or other documents for use in patient/client records, quality or performance improvement, or in formal research projects.

Evaluation

Criteria for evaluation

Comparison to Goal or Reference Standard:

1. Goal (tailored to patient/client's needs)
   OR
2. Reference standard

Edition: 2008

FOOD AND NUTRIENT INTAKE OUTCOMES DOMAIN • Macronutrients

PROTEIN INTAKE (FI-5.2)

Patient/Client Example(s)

Example(s) of one or two of the Nutrition Care Indicators for this outcome *(includes sample initial and re-assessment documentation for one of the indicators)*

Indicator(s) selected

Total protein

Criteria for evaluation

Comparison to Goal or Reference Standard:

1. Goal: Patient/client's current intake of 25 g protein per day is below the recommended level of 55–65 g per day.

OR

2. Reference standard: (Used when patient goal is based on the population standard) Patient/client's intake of 12 g protein/day is less then the DRI of 53 g/day (0.8 g/kg BW). Patient/client's goal is to increase protein intake to approximately 55 g/day.

Sample monitoring and evaluation documentation

Initial encounter with patient/client	Enteral feeding currently providing 25 g protein/day, well below the recommended level of 55–65 g/day (1-1.2 g/kg BW). Will continue to monitor protein intake daily.
Re-assessment after nutrition intervention	Some progress toward goal intake of 55–65 g protein/day. Current intake approximately 30 g protein/day, 25 g protein below desired level. Will continue to monitor protein intake daily.

References

The following are some suggested references for indicators, measurement techniques, and reference standards for the outcome; other references may be appropriate.

1. Institute of Medicine, Food and Nutrition Board. *Dietary Reference Intakes for Energy, Carbohydrate, Fiber, Fat, Fatty Acids, Cholesterol, Protein and Amino Acids.* Washington, DC: National Academy Press; 2002. Available at: www.iom.edu/report.asp?id=4340.
2. Young VR, Borgouha S. Adult human amino acid requirements. *Curr Opin Clin Metab Care.* 1999;2:39-45.
3. Charney P, Malone A, eds. *ADA Pocket Guide to Nutrition Assessment.* Chicago, IL.: American Dietetic Association; 2004.
4. American Society for Parenteral and Enteral Nutrition Board of Directors and The Clinical Guidelines Task Force. Guidelines for the use of parenteral and enteral nutrition in adult and pediatric patients: Specific guidelines for disease—adults. *J Parenter Enteral Nutr.* 2002:26(Suppl):S61-S96
5. American Society for Parenteral and Enteral Nutrition Board of Directors and The Clinical Guidelines Task Force. Guidelines for the use of parenteral and enteral nutrition in adult and pediatric patients: Life cycle and metabolic conditions. *J Parenter Enteral Nutr.* 2002:26(Suppl):S45-S60.
6. American Society for Parenteral and Enteral Nutrition Board of Directors and The Clinical Guidelines Task Force. Guidelines for the use of parenteral and enteral nutrition in adult and pediatric patients: Specific guidelines for disease—pediatrics. *J Parenter Enteral Nutr.* 2002:26(Suppl):S111-S138
7. *ADA Nutrition Care Manual.* 2006. Available at: www.nutritioncaremanual.org. Accessed December 14, 2006.

Edition: 2008

305

Food & Nutrient

FOOD AND NUTRIENT INTAKE OUTCOMES DOMAIN • Macronutrients

CARBOHYDRATE INTAKE (FI-5.3)

Definition

Carbohydrate consumption from all sources, (e.g., food, beverages, supplements, and via enteral and parenteral routes)

Monitoring

Changes in these Potential Indicators:

- Total carbohydrate
- Sugar
- Starch
- Glycemic index
- Glycemic load

NOTE: Fiber intake is listed on the Fiber Intake Reference Sheet.

Examples of the measurement methods or data sources for these outcome indicators

Food intake records, 24-hour recall, food frequency questionnaires, menu analysis, carbohydrate counting tools

Typically used to measure the outcomes for the following domains of nutrition interventions

Food and/or nutrient delivery, nutrition education, nutrition counseling, coordination of nutrition care

Typically used to monitor and evaluate change in the following nutrition diagnosis

Inadequate and excessive carbohydrate intake, inappropriate intake of types of carbohydrate, inconsistent carbohydrate intake

Clinical judgment must be used to select indicators and determine the appropriate measurement techniques and reference standards for a given patient population and setting. Once identified, these indicators, measurement techniques, and reference standards should be identified in policies and procedures or other documents for use in patient/client records, quality or performance improvement, or in formal research projects.

Evaluation

Criteria for evaluation

Comparison to Goal or Reference Standard:

1. Goal (tailored to patient/client's needs)

   OR

2. Reference standard

Edition: 2008

306

CARBOHYDRATE INTAKE (FI-5.3)

Patient/Client Example(s)

Example(s) of one or two of the Nutrition Care Indicators for this outcome (*includes sample initial and re-assessment documentation for one of the indicators*)

Indicator(s) selected

Total carbohydrate (distribution by meal)

Criteria for evaluation

Comparison to Goal or Reference Standard:

1. Goal: Patient/client's current carbohydrate intake in the morning is inconsistent. Patient/client will consume approximately 30 g carbohydrate at breakfast.

OR

2. Reference standard: No validated standard exists.

Sample monitoring and evaluation documentation

Initial encounter with patient/client	Based upon carbohydrate counting tools, patient/client consumes 30 g carbohydrate at breakfast 2 days/ week. Goal is to consume 30 g carbohydrate 6 days per week.
Re-assessment after nutrition intervention	Based upon carbohydrate counting tools, patient/client consumed 30 g carbohydrate at breakfast 2 days/week. No progress made in this indicator. Will monitor carbohydrate intake at breakfast at next encounter.

References

The following are some suggested references for indicators, measurement techniques, and reference standards for the outcome; other references may be appropriate.

1. Institute of Medicine, Food and Nutrition Board. *Dietary Reference Intakes for Energy, Carbohydrate, Fiber, Fat, Fatty Acids, Cholesterol, Protein and Amino Acids.* Washington, DC: National Academy Press; 2002. Available at: www.iom.edu/report.asp?id=4340.

2. American Society for Parenteral and Enteral Nutrition Board of Directors and The Clinical Guidelines Task Force. Guidelines for the use of parenteral and enteral nutrition in adult and pediatric patients: Specific guidelines for disease—adults. *J Parenter Enteral Nutr.* 2002;26(Suppl):S61-S96.

3. *ADA Nutrition Care Manual.* 2006. Available at: www.nutritioncaremanual.org. Accessed December 14, 2006.

4. The American Diabetes Association. Standards of Medical Care in Diabetes—2006. *Diabetes Care.* 2006;29:S4-S42.

5. US Departments of Agriculture and Health and Human Services. Dietary Guidelines for Americans 2005. Available at: www.healthierus.gov/dietaryguidelines.

Food &
Nutrient

307

FIBER INTAKE (FI-5.4)

Definition

Amount and/or type of indigested carbohydrate from all sources (e.g., food, beverages, supplements, and via enteral routes)

Monitoring

Changes in these Potential Indicators:

- Total Fiber
- Soluble Fiber
- Insoluble Fiber
  - o Fructooligosaccharides

NOTE: Psyllium and β-glucan can be found on the Bioactive Substance Intake Reference Sheet

Examples of the measurement methods or data sources for these outcome indicators

Food intake records, 24-hour recall, food frequency questionnaires, menu analysis, fiber counting tools

Typically used to measure the outcomes for the following domains of nutrition interventions

Food and/or nutrient delivery, nutrition education, nutrition counseling, coordination of nutrition care

Typically used to monitor and evaluate change in the following nutrition diagnosis

Inadequate and excessive fiber intake, altered GI function

Clinical judgment must be used to select indicators and determine the appropriate measurement techniques and reference standards for a given patient population and setting. Once identified, these indicators, measurement techniques, and reference standards should be identified in policies and procedures or other documents for use in patient/client records, quality or performance improvement, or in formal research projects.

Evaluation

Criteria for evaluation

Comparison to Goal or Reference Standard:

1. Goal (tailored to patient/client's needs)

   OR

2. Reference standard

Food &
Nutrient

FIBER INTAKE (FI-5.4)

Patient/Client Example(s)

Example(s) of one or two of the Nutrition Care Indicators for this outcome *(includes sample initial and re-assessment documentation for one of the indicators)*

Indicator(s) selected
Total fiber

Criteria for evaluation
Comparison to Goal or Reference Standard:

1. Goal: Patient/client with current fiber intake of 15 g per day. Goal is to increase fiber intake to approximately 25 g per day.

OR

2. Reference standard: Patient/client's current intake of 15 g of dietary fiber per day is below the DRI of 25 g/day for a 40-year-old woman.

Sample monitoring and evaluation documentation

Initial encounter with patient/client	Based upon patient/client's food diary, patient/client is consuming approximately 15 g of fiber/day. Will monitor fiber intake at next encounter in three weeks.
Re-assessment after nutrition intervention	Goal achieved. Patient/client's intake of 27 g fiber exceeded goal intake of 25 g/day. Will continue to monitor to ensure success is sustained.

References
The following are some suggested references for indicators, measurement techniques, and reference standards for the outcome; other references may be appropriate.

1. Institute of Medicine, Food and Nutrition Board. *Dietary Reference Intakes for Energy, Carbohydrate, Fiber, Fat, Fatty Acids, Cholesterol, Protein and Amino Acids.* Washington, DC: National Academy Press; 2002. Available at: www.iom.edu/report.asp?id=4340.

2. US Department of Health and Human Services. National Institutes of Health. National Heart, Lung and Blood Institute. *Third Report of the Expert Panel on Detection, Evaluation, and Treatment of High Blood Cholesterol in Adults (Adult Treatment Panel III).* Bethesda, MD: National Institutes of Health; 2001

3. *ADA Nutrition Care Manual.* 2006. Available at: www.nutritioncarema. Accessed December 14, 2006.

309

Food & Nutrient

VITAMIN INTAKE (FI-6.1)

Definition

Vitamin intake from all sources (e.g., food, beverages, supplements, and via enteral and parenteral routes)

Monitoring

Changes in these Potential Indicators:

- Vitamin A
- Vitamin C
- Vitamin D
- Vitamin E
- Vitamin K
- Thiamin
- Riboflavin

- Niacin
- Vitamin B6
- Folate
- Vitamin B12
- Pantothenic acid
- Biotin
- Choline

Examples of the measurement methods or data sources for these outcome indicators

Patient/client report or recall, food frequency, home evaluation, supplement use questionnaire

Typically used to measure the outcomes for the following domains of nutrition interventions

Food and/or nutrient delivery, nutrition education, nutrition counseling, coordination of nutrition care

Typically used to monitor and evaluate change in the following nutrition diagnoses

Excess or inadequate intake of vitamins, parenteral, or enteral nutrition

Clinical judgment must be used to select indicators and determine the appropriate measurement techniques and reference standards for a given patient population and setting. Once identified, these indicators, measurement techniques, and reference standards should be identified in policies and procedures or other documents for use in patient/client records, quality or performance improvement, or in formal research projects.

Evaluation

Criteria for evaluation

Comparison to Goal or Reference Standard:

1. Nutrition prescription or goal (tailored to patient/client needs)
   OR
2. Reference standard

310

VITAMIN INTAKE (FI-6.1)

Patient/Client Example(s)

Example(s) of one or two of the Nutrition Care Indicators for this outcome (*includes sample initial and re-assessment documentation for one of the indicators*)

Indicator(s) selected
Vitamin D

Criteria for evaluation
Comparison to Goal or Reference Standard:

1. Nutrition prescription or goal: Use if patient/client's nutrition prescription/goal is different from the reference standard.

OR

2. Reference standard: The patient/client's intake of 2 µg of vitamin D is 20%* of the adequate intake (AI) for men age 51 and older.

Sample monitoring and evaluation documentation

Initial encounter with patient/client	Based upon recall, patient/client consuming approximately 20% of the adequate intake (AI) for vitamin D per day. Will monitor vitamin D intake at next encounter.
Re-assessment after nutrition intervention	Significant progress toward the adequate intake of 10 µg for vitamin D. Based upon 3-day diet record, patient/client has increased consumption of vitamin D from 50% to 75% of the adequate intake per day.

References

The following are some suggested references for indicators, measurement techniques, and reference standards for the outcome; other references may be appropriate.

1. ADA Nutrition Care Manual. 2006. Available at: www.nutritioncaremanual.org. Accessed December 11, 2006.
2. Gartner LM, Greer FR, American Academy of Pediatrics Committee on Nutrition. Prevention of rickets and vitamin D deficiency: new guidelines for vitamin D Intake. *Pediatrics.* 2003:111:908-910.
3. Guidelines for the use of parenteral and enteral nutrition in adult and pediatric patients: Normal requirements—adults. *J Parenter Enteral Nutr.* 2002:26(Suppl):S22-S24.
4. Guidelines for the use of parenteral and enteral nutrition in adult and pediatric patients: Normal requirements—pediatrics. *J Parenter Enteral Nutr.* 2002:26(Suppl):S25-S32.
5. Institute of Medicine. *Dietary Reference Intakes for Calcium, Phosphorus, Magnesium, Vitamin D, and Fluoride.* Washington, DC: National Academy Press; 1997.
6. Institute of Medicine. *Dietary Reference Intakes: Thiamin, Riboflavin, Niacin, Vitamin B6, Folate, Vitamin B12, Pantothenic Acid, Biotin, and Choline.* Washington, DC: National Academy Press; 1998.
7. Institute of Medicine. *Dietary Reference Intakes for Vitamin A, Vitamin K, Arsenic, Boron, Chromium, Copper, Iodine, Iron, Manganese, Molybdenum, Nickel, Silicon, Vanadium, and Zinc.* Washington, DC: National Academy Press; 2001.
8. Institute of Medicine. *Dietary Reference Intakes: Vitamin C, Vitamin E, Selenium, and Carotenoids.* Washington, DC: National Academy Press; 2000.

*Could be specified as "above," "below," or a "percent of" the reference value.

Food & Nutrient

FOOD AND NUTRIENT INTAKE OUTCOMES DOMAIN • Micronutrients

MINERAL/ELEMENT INTAKE (FI-6.2)

Definition
Mineral/element intake from all sources (e.g., food, beverages, supplements, and via enteral and parenteral routes)

Monitoring
Changes in these Potential Indicators:

- Calcium
- Copper
- Fluoride
- Iodine
- Iron
- Magnesium
- Phosphorus

- Selenium
- Zinc
- Potassium
- Sodium
- Chloride
- Chromium

Examples of the measurement methods or data sources for these outcome indicators
Patient/client report or recall, food frequency, home evaluation, home care or pharmacy report, supplement use questionnaire

Typically used to measure the outcomes for the following domains of nutrition interventions
Food and/or nutrient delivery, nutrition education, nutrition counseling, coordination of nutrition care

Typically used to monitor and evaluate change in the following nutrition diagnoses
Excess or inadequate intake of minerals

Clinical judgment must be used to select indicators and determine the appropriate measurement techniques and reference standards for a given patient population and setting. Once identified, these indicators, measurement techniques, and reference standards should be identified in policies and procedures or other documents for use in patient/client records, quality or performance improvement, or in formal research projects.

Evaluation

Criteria for evaluation
Comparison to Goal or Reference Standard:

1. Nutrition prescription or goal (tailored to individual's needs)

OR

2. Reference standard

Edition: 2008

MINERAL/ELEMENT INTAKE (FI-6.2)

Patient/Client Example(s)

Example(s) of one or two of the Nutrition Care Indicators for this outcome (*includes sample initial and re-assessment documentation for one of the indicators*)

Indicator(s) selected

- Sodium
- Calcium

Criteria for evaluation

Comparison to Goal or Reference Standard:

1. Nutrition prescription or goal: The patient/client's intake of sodium is approximately 6000 mg per day compared to the nutrition prescription of 4000 mg per day.

OR

2. Reference standard: The patient/client's intake of calcium is 500 mg per day which is 50%* of the Adequate Intake (AI) for women 31-50 years of age.

Sample monitoring and evaluation documentation

Initial encounter with patient/client	Based upon recall, patient/client consuming approximately 50% of the adequate intake for calcium per day. Will monitor calcium intake at next encounter.
Re-assessment after nutrition intervention	Significant progress toward the adequate intake of 1000 mg of calcium per day. Based upon 3-day diet record, patient/client has increased consumption from 50% to 75% of the adequate daily intake for calcium.

References

The following are some suggested references for indicators, measurement techniques, and reference standards for the outcome; other references may be appropriate.

1. ADA Adult Weight Management Evidence-Based Guideline, 2006. Available at: http://www.adaevidencelibrary.com/topic.cfm?cat=2798. Accessed October 30, 2006.
2. ADA Nutrition Care Manual. 2006. Available at: www.nutritioncaremanual.org. Accessed December 12, 2006.
3. Appel LJ, Moore TJ, Obarzanek E, Vollmer WM, Svetkey LP, Sacks FM, Bray GA, Vogt TM, Cutler JA, Windhauser MM, Lin P, Karanja N, Simons-Morton D, McCullough M, Swain J, Steele P, Evans MA, Miller ER, Harsha DW. A clinical trial of the effects of dietary patterns on blood pressure. *New Engl J Med.* 1997;336:1117-1124.
4. Dietary Guidelines for Americans, 2005. Available at: http://www.health.gov/dietaryguidelines/dga2005/document/html/executivesummary.htm. Accessed October 27, 2006.
5. Guidelines for the use of parenteral and enteral nutrition in adult and pediatric patients: Normal requirements—adults. *J Parenter Enteral Nutr.* 2002;26(Suppl):S22-S24.
6. Guidelines for the use of parenteral and enteral nutrition in adult and pediatric patients: Normal requirements—pediatrics. *J Parenter Enteral Nutr:* 2002;26(Suppl):S25-S32.
7. Institute of Medicine. *Dietary Reference Intakes for Calcium, Phosphorus, Magnesium, Vitamin D, and Fluoride.* Washington, DC: National Academy Press; 1997.
8. Institute of Medicine. *Dietary Reference Intakes for Vitamin A, Vitamin K, Arsenic, Boron, Chromium, Copper, Iodine, Iron, Manganese, Molybdenum, Nickel, Silicon, Vanadium, Zinc.* Washington, DC: National Academy Press; 2001.
9. Institute of Medicine. *Dietary Reference Intakes for Vitamin C, Vitamin E, Selenium, and Carotenoids.* Washington, DC: National Academy Press; 2000.
10. Institute of Medicine. *Dietary Reference Intakes for Water, Potassium, Sodium, Chloride, and Sulfate,* Washington DC: National Academy Press; 2004.
11. Your Guide to Lowering Your Blood Pressure. Available at: http://www.nhlbi.nih.gov/hbp/prevent/h_eating/h_eating.htm. Accessed November 16, 2006.

*Could be specified as "above," "below," or a "percent of" the reference value.

Edition: 2008

Food & Nutrient

313

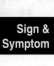

Sign &
Symptom

BODY COMPOSITION/GROWTH (S-1.1)

Definition
The body's fat, muscle, and bone tissue, including growth

Monitoring
Changes in these Potential Indicators:

- Body mass index
- Ideal body weight (IBW) or usual body weight (UBW) percentage
- Growth pattern (head circumference, length/height, weight for length/stature, BMI percentile/age (*Also see Weight change below*)
- Weight, weight change (e.g., % change for adults, weight gain [e.g., g/day for neonates])
- Lean body mass, fat free mass
- Mid-arm muscle circumference
- Body fat percentage
- Triceps skin fold
- Waist circumference
- Waist hip ratio
- Bone age
- Bone mineral density

Examples of the measurement methods or data sources for these outcome indicators
Direct measurement, patient/client report, medical record

Typically used to measure the outcomes for the following domains of nutrition interventions
Food and nutrient delivery, nutrition education, nutrition counseling

Typically used to monitor and evaluate change in the following nutrition diagnoses
Excess or inadequate intake of energy, fat, protein, carbohydrate, alcohol, and/or mineral intake; underweight, overweight, physical inactivity, excessive exercise

Clinical judgment must be used to select indicators and determine the appropriate measurement techniques and reference standards for a given patient population and setting. Once identified, these indicators, measurement techniques, and reference standards should be identified in policies and procedures or other documents for use in patient/client records, quality or performance improvement, or in formal research projects.

BODY COMPOSITION/GROWTH (S-1.1)

Evaluation

Criteria for evaluation
Comparison to Goal or Reference Standard:

1. Goal (tailored to patient/client's needs)

OR

2. Reference standard

Patient/Client Example(s)
Example(s) of one or two of the Nutrition Care Indicators for this outcome (*includes sample initial and re-assessment documentation for one of the indicators*)

Indicator(s) selected
- Weight gain/day
- BMI percentile/age

Criteria for evaluation
Comparison to Goal or Reference Standard:

1. Goal: The infant is only gaining, on average, 10 grams per day compared with a goal weight gain of 20–30 grams per day.

OR

2. Reference standard: Child's (> age 3 years) BMI percentile/age per growth curves has crossed 2 percentiles from 50% to 10% in last 6 months.

Sample monitoring and evaluation documentation

Initial encounter with patient/client	Child's BMI percentile/age per growth curves has crossed 2 percentiles from 50% to 10% in last 6 months. Will monitor BMI percentile/age at next encounter.
Re-assessment after nutrition intervention	Child's BMI percentile/age per growth curves is unchanged from baseline measure.

Sign & Symptom

315

BODY COMPOSITION/GROWTH (S-1.1)

References

The following are some suggested references for indicators, measurement techniques, and reference standards for the outcome; other references may be appropriate.

1. ACSM's *Guidelines for Exercise Testing and Prescription*. 6th ed. Indianapolis, IN: American College of Sports Medicine; 2000.
2. Charney P, Malone A, eds. *ADA Pocket Guide to Nutrition Assessment*. Chicago, IL: American Dietetic Association; 2004.
3. American Dietetic Association. Adult Weight Management Evidence-Based Nutrition Practice Guideline, 2006. Available at: http://www.adaevidencelibrary.com/topic.cfm?cat=2798. Accessed December 28, 2006.
4. Barlow SE, Dietz WH. Obesity evaluation and treatment: expert committee recommendations. *Pediatrics*. 1998;102:7. [Note. Barlow SE, et.al., will publish Expert Committee Recommendations of Childhood Obesity Prevention, Assessment and Treatment: Summary Paper in *Pediatrics* in 2007.
5. Bone Health and Osteoporosis: A Report of the Surgeon General. Available at: http://www.surgeongeneral.gov/library/bonehealth/. Accessed December 10, 2006.
6. Callaway CW et al. Circumferences. In: Lohman TG et al. *Anthropometric Standardization Reference Manual*. Champaign, IL: Human Kinetics, 1988: 39-54.
7. Centers for Disease Control, Bone Health Campaign. Powerful Bones. Powerful Girls. Available at: http://www.cdc.gov/nccdphp/dnpa/bonehealth/. Accessed December 10, 2006.
8. Frankel HM. Body mass index graphic for children. *Pediatrics*. 2004;113:425-426.
9. Going S. Optimizing techniques for determining body composition. Available at: http://www.gssiweb.com/Article_Detail.aspx?articleid=720. Accessed on December 29, 2006.
10. Guidelines for the use of parenteral and enteral nutrition in adult and pediatric patients: Normal requirements—adults. *J Parenter Enteral Nutr*. 2002;26(Suppl):S22-S24.
11. Guidelines for the use of parenteral and enteral nutrition in adult and pediatric patients: Normal requirements—pediatrics. *J Parenter Enteral Nutr*. 2002;26(Suppl):S25-S32.
12. Heyward V, Wagner D, eds. *Applied Body Composition and Assessment*. 2nd ed. Champaign, IL: Human Kinetics; 2004.
13. The Johns H Johns Hopkins Hospital. *The Harriet Lane Handbook: A Manual for Pediatric House Officers*. 17th ed. St. Louis, MO: Mosby; 2005.
14. Kleinman RE, ed. *Pediatric Nutrition Handbook*. 5th ed. Chicago, IL: American Academy of Pediatrics; 2004.
15. Leonberg BL. *ADA Pocket Guide to Pediatric Nutrition Assessment*. Chicago, IL: American Dietetic Association; 2008.
16. Modlesky CM. Assessment of body size and composition. In: Dunford M *Sports Nutrition: A Practice Manual for Professionals*. 4th ed. Chicago, IL: American Dietetic Association; 2006.
17. Institute of Medicine. *Dietary Reference Intakes for Calcium, Phosphorus, Magnesium, Vitamin D, and Fluoride*. Washington, DC: National Academy Press; 1997.
18. NIDDK Weight control information network. Available at: http://win.niddk.nih.gov/publications/tools.htm. Accessed October 24, 2006.
19. NHLBI Guidelines on Overweight and Obesity, Online Textbook, 1998. Available at: http://www.nhlbi.nih.gov/guidelines/obesity/e_txtbk/index.htm. Accessed October 24, 2006.
20. NIH, National Center for Health Statistics (NCHS). Clinical Growth Charts, 2000. Available at: www.cdc.gov/nchs/about/major/nhanes/growthcharts/clinical_charts.htm. Accessed October 25, 2006.
21. Nevin-Folino N. *Pediatric Manual of Clinical Dietetics*. 2nd ed. Chicago, IL: American Dietetic Association; 2003.
22. World Health Organization Child Growth Standards. Available at: http://www.who.int/childgrowth/en/. Accessed March 28, 2007.

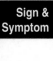

ACID-BASE BALANCE (S-2.1)

Definition

Degree of acidity and alkalinity in the blood as measured by the systemic arterial pH

Monitoring

Changes in these Potential Indicators:

- pH, serum
- Bicarbonate (HCO_3)
- Partial pressure of carbon dioxide in arterial blood ($PaCO_2$)

NOTE: Sodium and Chloride can be found on the Electrolyte and Renal Profile reference sheet.

Examples of the measurement methods or data sources for these outcome indicators

Biochemical measurement, laboratory report

Typically used to measure the outcomes for the following domains of nutrition interventions

Food and/or nutrient delivery, coordination of nutrition care

Typically used to monitor and evaluate change in the following nutrition diagnoses

Excess intake of parenteral or enteral nutrition

Clinical judgment must be used to select indicators and determine the appropriate measurement techniques and reference standards for a given patient population and setting. Once identified, these indicators, measurement techniques, and reference standards should be identified in policies and procedures or other documents for use in patient/client records, quality or performance improvement, or in formal research projects.

Evaluation

Criteria for evaluation

Comparison to Goal or Reference Standard:

1. Goal (tailored to patient/client's needs)

OR

2. Reference standard

Sign & Symptom

Edition: 2008

ACID-BASE BALANCE (S-2.1)

Patient/Client Example(s)

Example(s) of one or two of the Nutrition Care Indicators for this outcome (*includes sample initial and re-assessment documentation for one of the indicators*)

Indicator(s) selected

pH

Criteria for evaluation

Comparison to Goal or Reference Standard:

1. Goal: Not generally used for this outcome.

OR

2. Reference standard: The patient/client pH is 7.48 which is above* the reference standard (7.35-7.45).

Sample monitoring and evaluation documentation

Initial encounter with patient/client	Patient/client's pH is 7.48. Will monitor change in pH at next blood gas.
Re-assessment after nutrition intervention	Significant progress toward reference standard. Patient/client's pH is 7.45.

References

The following are some suggested references for indicators, measurement techniques, and reference standards for the outcome; other references may be appropriate.

1. Charney P, Malone A, eds. *ADA Pocket Guide to Nutrition Assessment*. Chicago, IL: American Dietetic Association; 2004.
2. The Johns H Johns Hopkins Hopkital. *The Harriet Lane Handbook: A Manual for Pediatric House Officers*. 17th ed. St. Louis MO: Mosby; 2005.
3. Kasper DL, Braunwald E, Fauci AS, Hauser SL, Longo DL, Jameson JL, Isselbacher KJ, eds. *Harrison's Principle of Internal Medicine*, 16th ed. Columbus, OH: The McGraw-Hill Co.; 2005.

*Could be specified as "above," "below," or a "percent of" the reference value.

Sign & Symptom

Edition: 2008

ELECTROLYTE AND RENAL PROFILE (S-2.2)

Definition

Laboratory measures associated with electrolyte balance and kidney function

Monitoring

Changes in these Potential Indicators:

- BUN
- Creatinine
- BUN:creatinine ratio
- Glomerular filtration rate
- Sodium
- Chloride
- Potassium
- Magnesium
- Calcium
- Calcium, ionized
- Phosphorus
- Serum osmolality
- Parathyroid hormone

NOTE: Bicarbonate can be found on the Acid Base Balance reference sheet.

Examples of the measurement methods or data sources for these outcome indicators

Biochemical measurement, laboratory report

Typically used to measure the outcomes for the following domains of nutrition interventions

Food and/or nutrient delivery, coordination of nutrition care

Typically used to monitor and evaluate change in the following nutrition diagnoses

Excess or inadequate intake of protein or minerals

Clinical judgment must be used to select indicators and determine the appropriate measurement techniques and reference standards for a given patient population and setting. Once identified, these indicators, measurement techniques, and reference standards should be identified in policies and procedures or other documents for use in patient/client records, quality or performance improvement, or in formal research projects.

319

Edition: 2008

ELECTROLYTE AND RENAL PROFILE (S-2.2)

Evaluation

Criteria for evaluation
Comparison to Goal or Reference Standard:

1. Goal (tailored to patient/client's needs)

OR

2. Reference standard

Patient/Client Example(s)

Example(s) of one or two of the Nutrition Care Indicators for this outcome (*includes sample initial and re-assessment documentation for one of the indicators*)

Indicator(s) selected
Potassium

Criteria for evaluation
Comparison to Goal or Reference Standard:

1. Goal: Not generally used for this outcome.

OR

2. Reference standard: The patient/client's potassium is 2.9 mEq/L which is below* the reference standard (3.5-5.0 mEq/L).

Sample monitoring and evaluation documentation

Initial encounter with patient/client	Patient/client's serum potassium is 2.9 mEq/L. Will monitor change in potassium at next encounter.
Re-assessment after nutrition intervention	Regression from reference standard. Patient/client's potassium is 2.7 mEq/L.

References

The following are some suggested references for indicators, measurement techniques, and reference standards for the outcome; other references may be appropriate.

1. Charney P, Malone A, eds. *ADA Pocket Guide to Nutrition Assessment.* Chicago, IL: American Dietetic Association; 2004.
2. American Dietetic Association. *Chronic Kidney Disease (Non-dialysis) Medical Nutrition Therapy Protocol.* Chicago, IL: American Dietetic Association; 2002.
3. ADA Nutrition Care Manual. 2006. Available at: www.nutritioncaremanual.org. Accessed December 11, 2006.
4. The Johns H Johns Hopkins Hospital. *The Harriet Lane Handbook: A Manual for Pediatric House Officers.* 17th ed. St. Louis, MO: Mosby; 2005.
5. National Institutes of Health, Clinical Center Test Guide. Available at: http://cclnprod.cc.nih.gov/dlm/testguide.nsf/TestIndex?OpenForm&Count=5000. Accessed October 19, 2006.
6. National Kidney Foundation K/DOQI. Clinical practice guidelines for nutrition in chronic renal failure. *Am J Kid Dis.* 2000;35:S1-S104.
7. National Kidney Foundation K/DOQI Workgroup. National Kidney Foundation K/DOQI Guidelines on bone metabolism and disease in chronic kidney disease. *Am J Kid Dis.* 2003;42(4 Suppl 3): S1-S201.
8. Wiggins KL. *Guidelines for Nutrition Care of Renal Patients.* Chicago, IL: American Dietetic Association; 2001.

*Could be specified as "above," "below," or a "percent of" the reference value.

Edition: 2008

Sign & Symptom

320

ESSENTIAL FATTY ACID PROFILE (S-2.3)

Definition
Laboratory measures of essential fatty acids

Monitoring
Changes in these Potential Indicators:

- Triene:Tetraene ratio

Examples of the measurement methods or data sources for these outcome indicators
Biochemical measurement, laboratory report/record

Typically used to measure the outcomes for the following domains of nutrition interventions
Food and/or nutrient delivery, coordination of nutrition care

Typically used to monitor and evaluate change in the following nutrition diagnoses
Inadequate intake of fat, parenteral nutrition; inappropriate intake of parenteral nutrition; altered nutrition-related laboratory values; impaired nutrient utilization

Clinical judgment must be used to select indicators and determine the appropriate measurement techniques and reference standards for a given patient population and setting. Once identified, these indicators, measurement techniques, and reference standards should be identified in policies and procedures or other documents for use in patient/client records, quality or performance improvement, or in formal research projects.

Evaluation

Criteria for evaluation
Comparison to Goal or Reference Standard:

1. Goal (tailored to patient/client's needs)

   OR

2. Reference standard

Sign &
Symptom

Edition: 2008

ESSENTIAL FATTY ACID PROFILE (S-2.3)

Sign & Symptom

Patient/Client Example(s)

Example(s) of one or two of the Nutrition Care Indicators for this outcome (*includes sample initial and re-assessment documentation for one of the indicators*)

Indicator(s) selected

Triene:Tetraene ratio

Criteria for evaluation

Comparison to Goal or Reference Standard:

1. Goal: Not generally used for this outcome.

   OR

2. Reference standard: The patient/client's Triene:Tetraene ratio is 0.45, which is above* the reference standard (> 0.2-0.4) indicating essential fatty acid deficiency.

Sample monitoring and evaluation documentation

Initial encounter with patient/client	Patient/client's Triene:Tetraene ratio is 0.45. Will monitor change in Triene:Tetraene ratio at next encounter.
Re-assessment after nutrition intervention	Significant progress toward reference standard. Patient/client's Triene:Tetraene ratio is 0.1.

References

The following is a suggested reference for indicators, measurement techniques, and reference standards for the outcome; other references may be appropriate.

1. Charney P, Malone A, eds. *ADA Pocket Guide to Nutrition Assessment.* Chicago, IL: American Dietetic Association; 2004.

*Could be specified as "above," "below," or a "percent of" the reference value.

Edition: 2008

322

GASTROINTESTINAL PROFILE (S-2.4)

Definition
Laboratory measures associated with function of the gastrointestinal tract and related organs

Monitoring
Changes in these Potential Indicators:

- Amylase
- Alkaline phophatase
- Alanine aminotransferase (ALT)
- Aspartate aminotransferase (AST)
- Gamma Glutamyl Transferase (GGT)
- Bilirubin, total
- Ammonia, serum
- Prothrombin time (PT)
- Partial thromboplastin time (PTT)
- INR (ratio)
- Fecal fat

Examples of the measurement methods or data sources for these outcome indicators
Biochemical measurement, laboratory report

Typically used to measure the outcomes for the following domains of nutrition interventions
Food and/or nutrient delivery, nutrition education, nutrition counseling

Typically used to monitor and evaluate change in the following nutrition diagnoses
Altered nutrition-related laboratory values, excess intake of protein or fat

Clinical judgment must be used to select indicators and determine the appropriate measurement techniques and reference standards for a given patient population and setting. Once identified, these indicators, measurement techniques, and reference standards should be identified in policies and procedures or other documents for use in patient/client records, quality or performance improvement, or in formal research projects.

Sign & Symptom

Edition: 2008

GASTROINTESTINAL PROFILE (S-2.4)

Sign & Symptom

Evaluation

Criteria for evaluation
Comparison to Goal or Reference Standard:

1. Goal (tailored to patient/client's needs)

    OR

2. Reference standard

Patient/Client Example(s)

Example(s) of one or two of the Nutrition Care Indicators for this outcome (*includes sample initial and re-assessment documentation for one of the indicators*)

Indicator(s) selected
Ammonia, serum

Criteria for evaluation
Comparison to Goal or Reference Standard:

1. Goal: The patient/client's serum ammonia is 105 µg/dL, which is above the goal (< 75 µg/dL) for this patient/client with end-stage liver disease.

    OR

2. Reference standard: The patient/client serum ammonia is 85 µg/dL which is above* the reference standard (11-35 µg/dL).

Sample monitoring and evaluation documentation

Initial encounter with patient/client	Patient/client's serum ammonia is 85 µg/dL. Will monitor change in serum ammonia at next encounter.
Re-assessment after nutrition intervention	Significant progress toward reference standard. Patient/client's serum ammonia 45 µg/dL.

References
The following are some suggested references for indicators, measurement techniques, and reference standards for the outcome; other references may be appropriate.
1. National Institutes of Health, Clinical Center Test Guide. Available at: http://cclnprod.cc.nih.gov/dlm/testguide.nsf/TestIndex?OpenForm&Count=5000. Accessed October 19, 2006.
2. The Johns H Johns Hopkins Hospital. The Harriet Lane Handbook: *A Manual for Pediatric House Officers.* 17th ed. St. Louis, MO: Mosby; 2005.

*Could be specified as "above," "below," or a "percent of" the reference value.

GLUCOSE PROFILE (S-2.5)

Definition

Laboratory measures associated with glycemic control

Monitoring

Changes in these Potential Indicators:

- Glucose, fasting
- Glucose, casual
- HgbA1c
- Preprandial capillary plasma glucose
- Peak postprandial capillary plasma glucose

Examples of the measurement methods or data sources for these outcome indicators

Biochemical measurement, laboratory report

Typically used to measure the outcomes for the following domains of nutrition interventions

Food and/or nutrient delivery, nutrition education, nutrition counseling

Typically used to monitor and evaluate change in the following nutrition diagnoses

Excess or inadequate intake of carbohydrate, energy; inappropriate intake of types of carbohydrates; or inconsistent carbohydrate intake

Clinical judgment must be used to select indicators and determine the appropriate measurement techniques and reference standards for a given patient population and setting. Once identified, these indicators, measurement techniques, and reference standards should be identified in policies and procedures or other documents for use in patient/client records, quality or performance improvement, or in formal research projects.

Evaluation

Criteria for evaluation

Comparison to Goal or Reference Standard:

1. Goal (tailored to patient/client's needs)

   OR

2. Reference standard

325

Edition: 2008

GLUCOSE PROFILE (S-2.5)

Sign &
Symptom

Patient/Client Example(s)

Example(s) of one or two of the Nutrition Care Indicators for this outcome (*includes sample initial and re-assessment documentation for one of the indicators*)

Indicator(s) selected
HgbA1c

Criteria for evaluation
Comparison to Goal or Reference Standard:

1. Goal: The patient/client's HgbA1c is 7.8%, which is above the reference standard; however, acceptable in this pediatric patient.
OR
2. Reference standard: The patient/client's HgbA1c is 11%, which is above* the reference standard (<6%).

Sample monitoring and evaluation documentation

Initial encounter with patient/client	Patient/client's HgbA1c is 9%. Will monitor change in HgbA1c at next encounter.
Re-assessment after nutrition intervention	Regression from reference standard. Patient/client's HgbA1c is 9.5%.

References
The following are some suggested references for indicators, measurement techniques, and reference standards for the outcome; other references may be appropriate.

1. American Diabetes Association. Diagnosis and classification of diabetes mellitus. *Diabetes Care.* 2006: 29;S43-S48. Available at: http://care.diabetesjournals.org/cgi/content/full/29/suppl_1/s43. Accessed October 20, 2006.
2. American Diabetes Association. Standards of medical care in diabetes. *Diabetes Care.* 2006: 29;S4-S42. Available at: http://care.diabetesjournals.org/cgi/content/full/29/suppl_1/s4. Accessed October 20, 2006.
3. American Dietetic Association. Critical illness evidence-based nutrition guideline, 2006. Available at: http://www.adaevidencelibrary.com/topic.cfm?cat=2809. Accessed November 1, 2006.
4. International Diabetes Center. Type 2 diabetes practice guidelines, 2003. Available at: http://www.guideline.gov/summary/summary.aspx?doc_id=4159&nbr=3187. Accessed November 1, 2006.
5. Joslin Diabetes Center. Clinical Guidelines for Adults. Available at: http://www.joslin.org/managing_your_diabetes_joslin_clinical_guidelines.asp. Accessed January 10, 2007.

*Could be specified as "above," "below," or a "percent of" the reference value.

LIPID PROFILE (S-2.6)

Definition
Laboratory measures associated with lipid disorders

Monitoring
Changes in these Potential Indicators:

- Cholesterol, serum
- Cholesterol, HDL
- Cholesterol, LDL
- Triglycerides, serum

Examples of the measurement methods or data sources for these outcome indicators
Biochemical measurement, laboratory report, patient/client report

Typically used to measure the outcomes for the following domains of nutrition interventions
Nutrition education, nutrition counseling

Typically used to monitor and evaluate change in the following nutrition diagnoses
Excess or inadequate intake of fat, energy

Clinical judgment must be used to select indicators and determine the appropriate measurement techniques and reference standards for a given patient population and setting. Once identified, these indicators, measurement techniques, and reference standards should be identified in policies and procedures or other documents for use in patient/client records, quality or performance improvement, or in formal research projects.

Evaluation

Criteria for evaluation
Comparison to Goal or Reference Standard:

1. Goal (tailored to patient/client's needs)

   OR

2. Reference standard

Edition: 2008

Sign & Symptom

NUTRITION SIGN AND SYMPTOM OUTCOMES DOMAIN • Biochemical and Medical Tests

LIPID PROFILE (S-2.6)

Patient/Client Example(s)

Example(s) of one or two of the Nutrition Care Indicators for this outcome (*includes sample initial and re-assessment documentation for one of the indicators*)

Indicator(s) selected

LDL–cholesterol

Criteria for evaluation

Comparison to Goal or Reference Standard:

1. Goal: The patient/client's LDL–cholesterol is 200 mg/dL, compared to a goal of < 100 mg/dL. (Note: Although reference standards are generally used for laboratory measures, a goal might be used in a special situation such as this example. The patient/client has a familial hypercholesterolemia where a normal reference standard may not be realistic.)

OR

2. Reference standard: The patient/client's LDL–cholesterol is 159 mg/dL, which is above* the NHLBI recommended level of < 100 mg/dL.

Sample monitoring and evaluation documentation

Initial encounter with patient/client	The patient/client LDL–cholesterol is 159 mg/dL, compared to the NHLBI recommended level of < 100 mg/dL. Will monitor LDL–cholesterol at next encounter.
Re-assessment after nutrition intervention	Some progress toward goal/reference standard as patient/client's LDL–cholesterol is 145 mg/dL.

References

The following are some suggested references for indicators, measurement techniques, and reference standards for the outcome; other references may be appropriate.

1. National Institutes of Health, National Heart, Lung, and Blood Institute (NHLBI). Third Report of the Expert Panel on Detection, Evaluation, and Treatment of High Cholesterol in Adults, May 2001. Available at: http://www.nhlbi.nih.gov/guidelines/cholesterol/index.htm. Accessed October 18, 2006.
2. National Kidney Foundation, K/DOQI Guidelines, 2000. Maintenance Dialysis, Evaluation of Protein-Energy Nutrition Status. Available at: http://www.kidney.org/professionals/kdoqi/guidelines/nut_a06.html. Accessed October 28, 2006.
3. Onder G, Landi F, Volpato S, Fellin R, Carbonin P, Gambassi G, Bernabei R. Serum cholesterol levels and in-hospital mortality in the elderly. *Am J Med.* 2003;115:265-271.
4. Position of the American Dietetic Association and Dietitians of Canada: Nutrition intervention in the care of persons with human immunodeficiency virus infection. *J Am Diet Assoc.* 2004;104:1425-1441.

*Could be specified as "above," "below," or a "percent of" the reference value.

MINERAL PROFILE (S-2.7)

Definition

Laboratory measures associated with body mineral status

Monitoring

Changes in these Potential Indicators :

- Copper, serum
- Iodine, urinary excretion
- Thyroid stimulating hormone (TSH) (↑ TSH as an indicator of excess iodine supplementation)
- Zinc, plasma

NOTE: Calcium, magnesium, phosphorus, and potassium can be found on the Electrolyte and Renal Profile reference sheet

Serum iron, serum ferritin, and transferrin saturation can be found on the Nutritional Anemia Profile reference sheet

Examples of the measurement methods or data sources for these outcome indicators

Biochemical measurement, laboratory record

Typically used to measure the outcomes for the following domains of nutrition interventions

Food and/or nutrient delivery, nutrition education, nutrition counseling

Typically used to monitor and evaluate change in the following nutrition diagnoses

Excess or inadequate intake of minerals, parenteral nutrition

Clinical judgment must be used to select indicators and determine the appropriate measurement techniques and reference standards for a given patient population and setting. Once identified, these indicators, measurement techniques, and reference standards should be identified in policies and procedures or other documents for use in patient/client records, quality or performance improvement, or in formal research projects.

Evaluation

Criteria for evaluation

Comparison to Goal or Reference Standard:

1. Goal (tailored to patient/client's needs)

OR

2. Reference standard

Edition: 2008

329

NUTRITION SIGN AND SYMPTOM OUTCOMES DOMAIN • Biochemical and Medical Tests

MINERAL PROFILE (S-2.7)

Patient/Client Example(s)

Example(s) of one or two of the Nutrition Care Indicators for this outcome (*includes sample initial and re-assessment documentation for one of the indicators*)

Indicator(s) selected
Zinc, plasma

Criteria for evaluation
Comparison to Goal or Reference Standard:

1. Goal: There is no goal generally associated with mineral status.

   OR

2. Reference standard: The patient/client's plasma zinc is 40 µg/dL which is below* the reference standard (66–110 µg/dL) for adults.

Sample monitoring and evaluation documentation

Initial encounter with patient/client	Patient/client's plasma zinc is 40 µg/dL, which is below the reference standard for adults. Will monitor change in plasma zinc at next encounter.
Re-assessment after nutrition intervention	Goal/reference standard achieved as patient/client's plasma zinc is 90 µg/dL.

References

The following are some suggested references for indicators, measurement techniques, and reference standards for the outcome; other references may be appropriate.

1. Institute of Medicine. *Dietary Reference Intakes for Calcium, Phosphorus, Magnesium, Vitamin D, and Fluoride*. Washington, DC: National Academy Press; 1997.
2. Institute of Medicine. *Dietary Reference Intakes for Vitamin A, Vitamin K, Arsenic, Boron, Chromium, Copper, Iodine, Iron, Manganese, Molybdenum, Nickel, Silicon, Vanadium, Zinc*. Washington, DC: National Academy Press; 2001.
3. Institute of Medicine. *Dietary Reference Intakes for Vitamin C, Vitamin E, Selenium, and Carotenoids*. Washington, DC: National Academy Press; 2000.
4. Institute of Medicine. *Dietary Reference Intakes for Water, Potassium, Sodium, Chloride, and Sulfate*. Washington DC: National Academy Press; 2004.

*Could be specified as "above," "below," or a "percent of" the reference value.

330

NUTRITIONAL ANEMIA PROFILE (S-2.8)

Definition

Laboratory measures associated with nutritional anemias

Monitoring

Changes in these Potential Indicators:

- Hemoglobin
- Hematocrit
- Mean corpuscular volume (MCV)
- RBC folate
- Red cell distribution width (RDW)
- Serum B12
- Serum methylmalonic acid (MMA)
- Serum folate
- Serum homocysteine
- Serum ferritin
- Serum iron
- Total iron-binding capacity
- Transferrin saturation

Examples of the measurement methods or data sources for these outcome indicators

Biochemical measurement, patient/client laboratory record; national/state/local nutrition monitoring and surveillance data

Typically used to measure the outcomes for the following domains of nutrition interventions

Food and/or nutrient delivery, nutrition education, nutrition counseling

Typically used to monitor and evaluate change in the following nutrition diagnoses

Excess or inadequate intake of vitamins or minerals (e.g., iron, B12, folate); altered nutrition-related laboratory values; impaired nutrient utilization

Clinical judgment must be used to select indicators and determine the appropriate measurement techniques and reference standards for a given patient population and setting. Once identified, these indicators, measurement techniques, and reference standards should be identified in policies and procedures or other documents for use in patient/client records, quality or performance improvement, or in formal research projects.

Sign & Symptom

NUTRITIONAL ANEMIA PROFILE (S-2.8)

Evaluation

Criteria for evaluation

Comparison to Goal or Reference Standard:

1. Goal (tailored to patient/client's needs)

OR

2. Reference standard

Patient/Client Example(s)

Example(s) of one or two of the Nutrition Care Indicators for this outcome (*includes sample initial and re-assessment documentation for one of the indicators*)

Indicator(s) selected

- Hemoglobin
- Serum ferritin

Criteria for evaluation

Comparison to Goal or Reference Standard:

1. Goal: The patient/client's hemoglobin and hematocrit are below the reference standard for adult males, but are within the goal range for a patient/client receiving hemodialysis.

OR

2. Reference standard: The patient/client's serum ferritin is 8 ng/mL which is below* the reference standard for women.

Sample monitoring and evaluation documentation

Initial encounter with patient/client	Patient/client's serum ferritin is 8 ng/mL which is below the reference standard for adult females. Will monitor change in serum ferritin at next encounter.
Re-assessment after nutrition intervention	Goal/reference standard achieved as patient/client's serum ferritin is 10.9 ng/mL.

References

The following are some suggested references for indicators, measurement techniques, and reference standards for the outcome; other references may be appropriate.

1. Charney P, Malone A, eds. *ADA Pocket Guide to Nutrition Assessment.* Chicago, IL: American Dietetic Association; 2004.
2. Centers for Disease Control and Prevention. Recommendations to prevent and control iron deficiency anemia in the United States. *Morb Mortal Wkly Rep.* 2002;51:897-899.
3. The Johns H Johns Hopkins Hospital. *The Harriet Lane Handbook: A Manual for Pediatric House Officers.* 17th ed. St. Louis, MO: Mosby; 2005.
4. National Kidney Foundation, Dialysis Outcomes Quality Initiative. Available at: http://kidney.niddk.nih.gov/kudiseases/pubs/anemia/index.htm#diagnosis. Accessed October 23, 2006.
5. National Library of Medicine and NIH, Medline Plus Medical Encyclopedia. Available at: http://www.nlm.nih.gov/medlineplus/encyclopedia.html. Accessed October 25, 2006.
6. *Healthy People 2010* (Conference Edition, in Two Volumes). Washington, DC: US Department of Health and Human Services; 2000.

*Could be specified as "above," "below," or a "percent of" the reference value.

Edition: 2008

PROTEIN PROFILE (S-2.9)

Definition

Laboratory measures associated with hepatic and circulating proteins

Monitoring

Changes in these Potential Indicators:

- Albumin
- Prealbumin
- Transferrin
- Phenylalanine, plasma
- Tyrosine, plasma

Note: Hepatic proteins may be useful when monitoring nutritional status over time in conjunction with other markers/information about nutritional status (e.g., body weight, weight change, nutrient intake).

Examples of the measurement methods or data sources for these outcome indicators

Biochemical measurement, laboratory report

Typically used to measure the outcomes for the following domains of nutrition interventions

Food and/or nutrient delivery, nutrition education, nutrition counseling, coordination of nutrition care

Typically used to monitor and evaluate change in the following nutrition diagnoses

Increased nutrient needs, evident protein-energy malnutrition, inadequate intake of enteral/parenteral nutrition

Clinical judgment must be used to select indicators and determine the appropriate measurement techniques and reference standards for a given patient population and setting. Once identified, these indicators, measurement techniques, and reference standards should be identified in policies and procedures or other documents for use in patient/client records, quality or performance improvement, or in formal research projects.

Evaluation

Criteria for evaluation

Comparison to Goal or Reference Standard:

1. Goal (tailored to patient/client's needs)

OR

2. Reference standard

Edition: 2008

Sign & Symptom

NUTRITION SIGN AND SYMPTOM OUTCOMES DOMAIN • Biochemical and Medical Tests

Sign & Symptom

PROTEIN PROFILE (S-2.9)

Patient/Client Example(s)

Example(s) of one or two of the Nutrition Care Indicators for this outcome (*includes sample initial and re-assessment documentation for one of the indicators*)

Indicator(s) selected

Prealbumin

Criteria for evaluation

Comparison to Goal or Reference Standard:

1. Goal: Not generally used for this outcome.

OR

2. Reference standard: The patient/client's prealbumin is 7 mg/dL, which is below* the reference standard (16-40 mg/dL) for adults.

Sample monitoring and evaluation documentation

Initial encounter with patient/client	Patient/client's prealbumin is 7.0 mg/dL. Will monitor change in pre-albumin at next encounter.
Re-assessment after nutrition intervention	Significant progress toward goal/reference standard as patient/client's serum prealbumin is 13.0 mg/dL.

References

The following are some suggested references for indicators, measurement techniques, and reference standards for the outcome; other references may be appropriate.

1. Charney P, Malone A, eds. *ADA Pocket Guide to Nutrition Assessment.* Chicago, IL: American Dietetic Association; 2004.
2. ADA Nutrition Care Manual. 2006. Available at: www.nutritioncaremanual.org. Accessed December 10, 2006.
3. Fuhrman MP, Charney P, Mueller CM. Hepatic proteins and nutrition assessment. *J Am Diet Assoc.* 2004;104:1258-1264.
4. The Johns H Johns Hopkins Hospital. *The Harriet Lane Handbook: A Manual for Pediatric House Officers.* 17th ed. St. Louis, MO: Mosby; 2005.
5. National Kidney Foundation, Clinical Practice Guidelines for Nutrition in Chronic Renal Failure, 2000. Available at: http://www.kidney.org/professionals/kdoqi/guidelines/doqi_nut.html. Accessed October 19, 2006.

*Could be specified as "above," "below," or a "percent of" the reference value.

Edition: 2008

RESPIRATORY QUOTIENT (RQ) (S-2.10)

Definition
Ratio of the volume of carbon dioxide produced to the volume of oxygen consumed, which, under controlled conditions, is a reflection of net substrate utilization in the body

Monitoring
Changes in these Potential Indicators:

- Respiratory quotient ($RQ = CO_2$ produced/O_2 consumed)

Examples of the measurement methods or data sources for these outcome indicators
Direct measurement, medical record

Typically used to measure the outcomes for the following domains of nutrition interventions
Food and/or nutrient delivery

Typically used to monitor and evaluate change in the following nutrition diagnoses
Excessive or inadequate intake of parenteral/enteral nutrition; inappropriate infusion of enteral/parenteral nutrition

Clinical judgment must be used to select indicators and determine the appropriate measurement techniques and reference standards for a given patient population and setting. Once identified, these indicators, measurement techniques, and reference standards should be identified in policies and procedures or other documents for use in patient/client records, quality or performance improvement, or in formal research projects.

Evaluation

Criteria for evaluation
Comparison to Goal or Reference Standard:

1. Goal (tailored to patient/client's needs)

OR

2. Reference standard

Sign & Symptom

RESPIRATORY QUOTIENT (RQ) (S-2.10)

Patient/Client Example(s)

Example(s) of one or two of the Nutrition Care Indicators for this outcome (*includes sample initial and re-assessment documentation for one of the indicators*)

Indicator(s) selected

RQ

Criteria for evaluation

Comparison to Goal or Reference Standard:

1. Goal: There is no goal for RQ, only a reference standard.

OR

2. Reference standard: A patient/client on parenteral nutrition support with an RQ of 1.04 compared to the reference standard (0.7-1.0) with no apparent errors in the measurement.

Sample monitoring and evaluation documentation

Initial encounter with patient/client	Patient/client's RQ is 1.04. Will re-measure RQ and rule out measurement error.
Re-assessment after nutrition intervention	No progress toward reference standard as patient/client's RQ is 1.05 with no apparent measurement errors. Will monitor change in RQ after feeding adjustment.

References

The following are some suggested references for indicators, measurement techniques, and reference standards for the outcome; other references may be appropriate.

1. American Dietetic Association. *Critical Illness Adult Weight Management Evidence-Based Nutrition Practice Guideline.* Available at: http://www.adaevidencelibrary.com/topic.cfm?cat=2799. Accessed December 19, 2006.
2. Compher C, Frankenfield D, Keim N, Roth-Yousey L. Best practice methods to apply to measurement of resting metabolic rate in adults: A systematic review. *J Am Diet Assoc.* 2006;106:881-903.
3. Guidelines for the use of parenteral and enteral nutrition in adult and pediatric patients: Specific guidelines for disease—adults. *J Parenter Enteral Nutr.* 2002;26(Suppl):S61-S96.
4. Guidelines for the use of parenteral and enteral nutrition in adult and pediatric patients: Specific guidelines for disease—pediatrics. *J Parenter Enteral Nutr.* 2002;26(Suppl):S111-S138.
5. McClave SA, Lowen CC, Kleber MJ, McConnell JW, Jung LY, Goldsmith LJ. Clinical use of the respiratory quotient obtained from indirect calorimetry. *J Parenter Enteral Nutr.* 2003;27:21-26.

Sign & Symptom

URINE PROFILE (S-2.11)

Definition
Physical and/or chemical properties of urine

Monitoring
Changes in these Potential Indicators:

- Urine color
- Urine osmolality
- Urine specific gravity
- Urine tests (e.g., ketones, sugar, protein)
- Urine volume

Examples of the measurement methods or data sources for these outcome indicators
Observation, biochemical measurement, laboratory report, patient/client report

Typically used to measure the outcomes for the following domains of nutrition interventions
Food and/or nutrient delivery, coordination of nutrition care

Typically used to monitor and evaluate change in the following nutrition diagnoses
Inadequate or excessive fluid intake; inadequate or excessive enteral/parenteral nutrition

Clinical judgment must be used to select indicators and determine the appropriate measurement techniques and reference standards for a given patient population and setting. Once identified, these indicators, measurement techniques, and reference standards should be identified in policies and procedures or other documents for use in patient/client records, quality or performance improvement, or in formal research projects.

Evaluation

Criteria for evaluation
Comparison to Goal or Reference Standard:

1. Goal (tailored to patient/client's needs)

    OR

2. Reference standard

Edition: 2008

Sign & Symptom

URINE PROFILE (S-2.11)

Patient/Client Example Patient/Client Example(s)

Example(s) of one or two of the Nutrition Care Indicators for this outcome (*includes sample initial and re-assessment documentation for one of the indicators*)

Indicator(s) selected
Urine specific gravity

Criteria for evaluation
Comparison to Goal or Reference Standard

   1. Goal: Not generally used for this indicator.

   OR

   2. Reference standard: The patient/client's urine specific gravity is 1.050, which is above* the normal range (using the reference standard of 1.003-1.030).

Sample monitoring and evaluation documentation

Initial encounter with patient/client	Patient/client's urine specific gravity is 1.050, which is above the normal range compared to the reference standard of 1.003-1.030. Will monitor change in urine specific gravity at next encounter.
Re-assessment after nutrition intervention	Significant progress toward goal; patient/client's urine specific gravity is 1.035.

References

The following are some suggested references for indicators, measurement techniques, and reference standards for the outcome; other references may be appropriate.

1. Charney P, Malone A, eds. *ADA Pocket Guide to Nutrition Assessment.* Chicago, IL: American Dietetic Association; 2004.
2. Armstrong, LE. Hydration assessment techniques. *Nutr Rev.* 2005;63(6 pt 2):S40-54.
3. National Institutes of Health, Clinical Center Test Guide. Available at: http://cclnprod.cc.nih.gov/dlm/testguide.nsf/TestIndex?OpenForm&Count=5000. Accessed October 27, 2006.

*Could be specified as "above," "below," or a "percent of" the reference value.

Sign &
Symptom

VITAMIN PROFILE (S-2.12)

Definition

Laboratory measures associated with body vitamin status

Monitoring

Changes in these Potential Indicators:

- Vitamin A, serum or plasma retinol
- Vitamin C, plasma or serum
- Vitamin D (25-Hydroxy)
- Vitamin E (plasma alpha-tocopherol)
- Thiamin (activity coefficient for erythrocyte transketolase activity)
- Riboflavin (activity coefficient for erythrocyte glutathione reductase activity)
- Niacin (urinary N′methyl-nicotinamide concentration)
- Vitamin B6 (plasma or serum pyridoxal 5′phosphate) concentration

NOTE: Measures for folate and Vitamin B12 can be found on the Nutritional Anemia Profile reference sheet.

Measures related to Vitamin K (PT, PTT, INR) can be found on the GI Profile reference sheet.

Examples of the measurement methods or data sources for these outcome indicators

Biochemical measurement, patient/client record

Typically used to measure the outcomes for the following domains of nutrition interventions

Food and/or nutrient delivery, coordination of nutrition care

Typically used to monitor and evaluate change in the following nutrition diagnoses

Excess or inadequate intake of vitamins

Clinical judgment must be used to select indicators and determine the appropriate measurement techniques and reference standards for a given patient population and setting. Once identified, these indicators, measurement techniques, and reference standards should be identified in policies and procedures or other documents for use in patient/client records, quality or performance improvement, or in formal research projects.

Sign & Symptom

339

NUTRITION SIGN AND SYMPTOM OUTCOMES DOMAIN • Biochemical and Medical Tests

VITAMIN PROFILE (S-2.12)

Sign & Symptom

Evaluation

Criteria for evaluation
Comparison to Goal or Reference Standard:

1. Goal (tailored to patient/client's needs)

OR

2. Reference standard

Patient/Client Example(s)

Example(s) of one or two of the Nutrition Care Indicators for this outcome *(includes sample initial and re-assessment documentation for one of the indicators)*

Indicator(s) selected
Serum retinol

Criteria for evaluation
Comparison to Goal or Reference Standard:

1. Goal: Not generally used for this indicator.

OR

2. Reference standard: The patient/client's serum retinol is 95 µg/dL which is above* the reference standard (10-60 µg/dL).

Sample monitoring and evaluation documentation

Initial encounter with patient/client	Patient/client's serum retinol is 95 µg/dL. Will monitor change in serum retinol at next encounter.
Re-assessment at a later date	Significant progress toward reference standard. Patient/client's retinol is 70 µg/dL.

References
The following are some suggested references for indicators, measurement techniques, and reference standards for the outcome; other references may be appropriate.

1. ADA Nutrition Care Manual. 2006. Available at: www.nutritioncaremanual.org. Accessed December 11, 2006.
2. The Johns H Johns Hopkins Hospital. *The Harriet Lane Handbook: A Manual for Pediatric House Officers.* 17th ed. St. Louis, MO: Mosby; 2005.
3. Guidelines for the use of parenteral and enteral nutrition in adult and pediatric patients: Normal requirements—adults. *J Parenter Enteral Nutr.* 2002:26(Suppl):S22-S24.
4. Guidelines for the use of parenteral and enteral nutrition in adult and pediatric patients: Normal requirements—pediatrics. *J Parenter Enteral Nutr.* 2002:26(Suppl):S25-S32.
5. Institute of Medicine. *Dietary Reference Intakes for Calcium, Phosphorus, Magnesium, Vitamin D, and Fluoride.* Washington, DC: National Academy Press; 1997.
6. Institute of Medicine. *Dietary Reference Intakes: Thiamin, Riboflavin, Niacin, Vitamin B6, Folate, Vitamin B12, Pantothenic Acid, Biotin, and Choline.* Washington, DC: National Academy Press; 1998.
7. Institute of Medicine. *Dietary Reference Intakes for Vitamin A, Vitamin K, Arsenic, Boron, Chromium, Copper, Iodine, Iron, Manganese, Molybdenum, Nickel, Silicon, Vanadium, and Zinc.* Washington, DC: National Academy Press; 2001.
8. Institute of Medicine. *Dietary Reference Intakes: Vitamin C, Vitamin E, Selenium, and Carotenoids.* Washington, DC: National Academy Press; 2000.

*Could be specified as "above," "below," or a "percent of" the reference value.

Edition: 2008

NUTRITION PHYSICAL EXAM FINDINGS (S-3.1)

Definition

Nutrition-related physical characteristics associated with pathophysiological states derived from observation or the medical record

Monitoring

Changes in these Potential Indicators:

- Cardiovascular-pulmonary system
  - o edema, pulmonary (crackles or rales)
- Extremities and musculo-skeletal system
  - o bones, obvious prominence
  - o hands/feet, tingling and numbness
  - o muscle soreness
  - o nail beds, blue, clubbing, pale
  - o muscle wasting, subcutaneous fat loss
  - o excessive subcutaneous fat
  - o Russell's sign
- Gastrointestinal system
  - o ascites
  - o appetite, satiety
  - o bowel function
  - o bowel sounds
  - o distension, abdominal
  - o gastric residual volume (GRV)
  - o nausea
  - o taste alterations
  - o vomiting

- Head and neck
  - Eyes:
    - o bitot's spots
    - o night blindness
    - o xerophthalmia
  - Tongue:
    - o bright red or magenta
    - o dry or cracked
    - o glossitis
  - Mouth and throat:
    - o cheilosis
    - o dry mucus membranes
    - o gums, inflamed or bleeding
    - o ketone smell on breath
    - o lesions, oral
    - o lips, dry or cracked
    - o mucosa, edema
    - o stomatitis
  - Head:
    - o hair, brittle, lifeless, coiled, or loss
    - o headache
    - o lanugo hair formation
    - o mucosa, dry nasal
    - o temporal wasting

- Neurological system
  - o confusion, concentration
  - o cranial nerve evaluation
  - o motor, fine disturbance
  - o motor, gross and/or gait disturbance
  - o vibratory and position sense
- Skin
  - o acanthanosis nigricans
  - o edema, peripheral
  - o erythema, scaling and peeling
  - o ecchymosis
  - o follicular hyperkeratosis
  - o integrity, turgor
  - o seborrheic dermatitis
  - o perifolicular hemorrhages
  - o petechiae
  - o pressure ulcers (stage II-IV)
  - o wound healing
  - o xanthomas
- Vital signs
  - o blood pressure
  - o respiratory rate

341

Sign & Symptom

NUTRITION SIGN AND SYMPTOM OUTCOMES DOMAIN • Physical Examination

NUTRITION PHYSICAL EXAM FINDINGS (S-3.1)

Examples of the measurement methods or data sources for these outcome indicators
Direct observation, patient/client report, medical record

Typically used to measure the outcomes for the following domains of nutrition interventions
Nutrition education, nutrition counseling

Typically used to monitor and evaluate change in the following nutrition diagnoses
Excess or inadequate intake of sodium, vitamins/minerals, fluid, parenteral/enteral nutrition; overweight/obesity

Clinical judgment must be used to select indicators and determine the appropriate measurement techniques and reference standards for a given patient population and setting. Once identified, these indicators, measurement techniques, and reference standards should be identified in policies and procedures or other documents for use in patient/client records, quality or performance improvement, or in formal research projects.

Evaluation

Criteria for evaluation
Comparison to Goal or Reference Standard:

  1. Goal (tailored to patient/client's needs)

  OR

  2. Reference standard

Patient/Client Example(s)
Example(s) of one or two of the Nutrition Care Indicators for this outcome *(includes sample initial and re-assessment documentation for one of the indicators)*

Indicator(s) selected
Blood pressure

Criteria for evaluation
Comparison to Goal or Reference Standard:

  1. Goal: The patient/client has reduced blood pressure to goal of 135/85 mmHg with weight loss.

  OR

  2. Reference standard: The patient/client's blood pressure is 150/90 mmHg which is above* the reference standard (<120/80 mmHg), indicating stage I hypertension.

*Could be specified as "above," "below," or a "percent of" the reference value.

Edition: 2008

NUTRITION PHYSICAL EXAM FINDINGS (S-3.1)

Sample monitoring and evaluation documentation

Initial encounter with patient/client	Patient/client's blood pressure is 150/90 mmHg, stage I hypertension. Will monitor change in blood pressure at next encounter.
Re-assessment after nutrition intervention	Significant progress toward reference standard. Patient/client's blood pressure is 135/82 mmHg.

References

The following are some suggested references for indicators, measurement techniques, and reference standards for the outcome; other references may be appropriate.

1. American Dietetic Association. Critical illness evidence-based nutrition guideline, 2006. Available at: http://www.adaevidencelibrary.com/topic.cfm?cat=2809. Accessed November 5, 2006.
2. Charney P, Malone A, eds. *ADA Pocket Guide to Nutrition Assessment.* Chicago, IL: American Dietetic Association; 2004.
3. Centers for Medicare and Medicaid Services. Minimum Data Set (MDS)—Version 2.0 for Nursing Home Resident Assessment and Care Screening Basic Assessment Tracking Form. Available at: http://www.cms.hhs.gov/MDS20SWSpecs/Downloads/MDS%20Tracking%20Form.pdf. Accessed November 14, 2006.
4. Mackle TJ, Touger-Decker R, Maillet JO, Holland BK. Registered dietitians' use of physical assessment parameters in professional practice. *J Am Diet Assoc.* 2003;103:1632-1638.
5. National Institutes of Health, National Heart, Lung, and Blood Institute. The Seventh Report of the Joint National Committee on Prevention, Detection, Evaluation, and Treatment of High Blood Pressure. Available at: http://www.nhlbi.nih.gov/guidelines/hypertension/express.pdf. Accessed October 24, 2006.
6. Position of the American Dietetic Association: Oral health and nutrition. *J Am Diet Assoc.* 2007;107(in press).
7. U.S. Preventive Services Task Force (USPSTF). Screening for high blood pressure: recommendations and rationale. Rockville, MD: Agency for Healthcare Research and Quality (AHRQ), 2003. Available at: http://www.guideline.gov/summary/summary.aspx?doc_id=3853&nbr=003068&string=AHRQ+AND+guideline. Accessed on November 14, 2006.

Sign & Symptom

NUTRITION QUALITY OF LIFE (PC-1.1)

Definition

Extent to which the nutrition care process impacts a patient/client's physical, mental and social well-being related to food and nutrition

Monitoring

Changes in these Potential Indicators:

- Food impact (e.g., choice, available, enjoyable)
- Physical state (e.g., food-related condition impacted activity, sleep, breathing)
- Psychological factors (e.g., positive/negative feelings related to food)
- Self-image
- Self-efficacy (e.g., know what, how much to eat)
- Social/interpersonal factors
- Nutrition quality of life score

NOTE: A nutrition quality of life instrument has been developed and is being validated (Barr JT, et al 2003). Focused questioning around the six indicators using the 50 NQOL statements is recommended.

Self-efficacy can be found on the Beliefs and Attitudes Reference Sheet.

Social/interpersonal factors can be found Social Support Reference Sheet.

Food impact may entail monitoring certain aspects on the Access to Food Reference Sheet.

Physical state may entail monitoring physical activity using the Physical Activity Reference Sheet.

Examples of the measurement methods or data sources for these outcome indicators

Nutrition Quality of Life measurement tool, other quality of life tools

Typically used to monitor and evaluate change in the following domains of nutrition interventions

Food and/or nutrient delivery, supplements, nutrition education, nutrition counseling, coordination of nutrition care

Typically used to monitor and evaluate change in the following nutrition diagnoses

Poor nutrition quality of life, inadequate or excessive energy or macronutrient intake, underweight, involuntary weight loss, overweight/obesity, involuntary weight gain, disordered eating pattern, inability or lack of desire to manage self-care, swallowing difficulty, chewing difficulty, self-feeding difficulty, altered GI function, limited access to food

Clinical judgment must be used to select indicators and determine the appropriate measurement techniques and reference standards for a given patient population and setting. Once identified, these indicators, measurement techniques, and reference standards should be identified in policies and procedures or other documents for use in patient/client records, quality or performance improvement, or in formal research projects.

Patient/ Client- Centered

NUTRITION QUALITY OF LIFE (PC-1.1)

Evaluation

Criteria for evaluation
Comparison to Goal or Reference Standard:

1. Goal (tailored to patient/client's needs)

OR

2. Reference standard

Patient/Client Example(s)

Example(s) of one or two of the Nutrition Care Indicators for this outcome (*includes sample initial and re-assessment documentation for one of the indicators*)

Indicator(s) selected
Nutrition quality of life score

Criteria for evaluation
Comparison to Goal or Reference Standard:

1. Goal: Patient/client with chronic renal disease currently reports poor nutrition quality of life, especially decreased walking ability (physical) and limited food choices on renal diet (food impact). The goal of medical nutrition therapy is to educate and coach patient and his family on options and strategies to significantly enhance his nutrition quality of life.

OR

2. Reference standard: No validated standard exists.

Sample monitoring and evaluation documentation

Initial encounter with patient/client	Patient/client with chronic renal disease reports poor nutrition quality of life, particularly in physical and food impact aspects. Patient/client to receive intensive medical nutrition therapy with a goal to improve client's overall nutrition quality of life over a 6-month period. Will monitor nutrition quality of life in 6 months.
Re-assessment after nutrition intervention	Some progress toward goal. Patient/client's nutrition quality of life is increased, but further improvement is desired in the physical dimension. Will continue medical nutrition therapy and reassess in 3 months.

345

Patient/
Client-
Centered

NUTRITION QUALITY OF LIFE (PC-1.1)

References

The following are some suggested references for indicators, measurement techniques, and reference standards for the outcome; other references may be appropriate.

1. Barr JT, Schumacher GE. The need for a nutrition-related quality-of-life measure. *J Am Diet Assoc.* 2003;103:177–180.

2. Barr JT, Schumacher GE. Using focus groups to determine what constitutes quality of life in clients receiving medical nutrition therapy: First steps in the development of a nutrition quality-of-life survey. *J Am Diet Assoc.* 2003;103:844-851.

3. Ware JE, Sherbourne CD. The MOS 36-item short-form health survey (SF-36), I: Conceptual framework and item selection. *Med Care.* 1992;30:473-483.

4. Moorehead M,Ardelt-Gattinger E, Lechner H, Oria H. The validation of the Moorehead-Ardelt Quality of Life Questionnaire II. *Obes Surg.* 2003;13:684-692.

5. Groll D, Vanner S, Depew W, DaCosta L, Simon J, Groll A, Roblin N, Paterson W. The IBS-36: a new quality of life measure for irritable bowel syndrome. *Am J Gastroenterol.* 2002;97:962-971.

6. Diabetes Control and Complications Trial Research Group. Reliability and validity of a diabetes quality of life measure for the Diabetes Control and Complications Trial (DCCT). *Diabetes Care.* 1988;11:725–732.

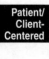

Patient/
Client-
Centered

346

INTERNATIONAL DIETETICS AND NUTRITION TERMINOLOGY (IDNT)
Standardized Language for the Nutrition Care Process

Bibliography and Resources

Publications

International Dietetics and Nutrition Terminology (IDNT) Reference Manual: Standardized Language for the Nutrition Care Process, First Edition. Chicago, IL: American Dietetic Association; 2008.

Pocket Guide for the International Dietetics and Nutrition Terminology Reference Manual, First Edition. Chicago, IL: American Dietetic Association; 2008.

American Dietetic Association. *Nutrition Diagnosis and Intervention: Standardized Language for the Nutrition Care Process.* Chicago, IL: American Dietetic Association; 2007.

American Dietetic Association. *Nutrition Diagnosis: A Critical Step in the Nutrition Care Process.* Chicago, IL: American Dietetic Association; 2006.

Journal articles

Mathieu J, Foust M, Ouellette P. Implementing nutrition diagnosis, step two in the nutrition care process and model: Challenges and lesions learned in two health care facilities. J Am Diet Assoc. 2005;105:1636-1640.

Lacey K, Pritchett E. Nutrition care process and model: ADA adopts road map to quality care and outcomes management. J Am Diet Assoc. 2003;103:1061-1072.

Web resources

Nutrition Care Process and Model Resources http://www.eatright.org/cps/rde/xchg/ada/hs.xsl/career_9706_ENU_HTML.htm.

NCP Frequently Asked Questions
http://www.eatright.org/cps/rde/xchg/ada/hs.xsl/career_9706_ENU_HTML.htm.

NCP Patient/Client Case Studies and Process Improvement Case Example
http://www.eatright.org/cps/rde/xchg/ada/hs.xsl/career_9706_ENU_HTML.htm.

Evidence-Based Nutrition Practice Guidelines, available using the "store" tab http://www.adaevidencelibrary.com/default.cfm?auth=1

Scope of Dietetic Practice Framework, Standards of Practice in Nutrition Care and Updated Standards of Professional Performance, and the Standards of Practice in Nutrition Care Appendix http://www.eatright.org/cps/rde/xchg/ada/hs.xsl/home_7232_ENU_HTML.htm

Edition: 2008

Nutrition Care Process and Model: ADA adopts road map to quality care and outcomes management

KAREN LACEY, MS, RD; ELLEN PRITCHETT, RD

The establishment and implementation of a standardized Nutrition Care Process (NCP) and Model were identified as priority actions for the profession for meeting goals of the ADA Strategic Plan to "Increase demand and utilization of services provided by members" and "Empower members to compete successfully in a rapidly changing environment" (1). Providing high-quality nutrition care means doing the right thing at the right time, in the right way, for the right person, and achieving the best possible results. Quality improvement literature shows that, when a standardized process is implemented, less variation and more predictability in terms of outcomes occur (2). When providers of care, no matter their location, use a process consistently, comparable outcomes data can be generated to demonstrate value. A standardized Nutrition Care Process effectively promotes the dietetics professional as the unique provider of nutrition care when it is consistently used as a systematic method to think critically and make decisions to provide safe and effective nutrition care (3).

This article describes the four steps of ADA's Nutrition Care Process and the overarching framework of the Nutrition Care Model that illustrates the context within which the Nutrition Care Process occurs. In addition, this article provides the rationale for a standardized process by which nutrition care is provided, distinguishes between the Nutrition Care Process and Medical Nutrition Therapy (MNT), and discusses future implications for the profession.

BACKGROUND

Prior to the adoption of this standardized Nutrition Care Process, a variety of nutrition care processes were utilized by practitioners and taught by dietetics educators. Other allied health professionals, including nursing, physical therapy, and occupational therapy, utilize defined care processes specific to their profession (4-6). When asked whether ADA should develop a standardized Nutrition Care Process, dietetics professionals were overwhelmingly in favor and strongly supportive of having a standardized Nutrition Care Process for use by registered dietitians (RD) and dietetics technicians, registered (DTR).

The Quality Management Committee of the House of Delegates (HOD) appointed a Nutrition Care Model Workgroup in May 2002 to develop a nutrition care process and model. The first draft was presented to the HOD for member input and review in September 2002. Further discussion occurred during the October 2002 HOD meeting, in Philadelphia. Revisions were made accordingly, and the HOD unanimously adopted the final version of the Nutrition Care Process and Model on March 31, 2003 "for implementation and dissemination to the dietetics profession and the Association for the enhancement of the practice of dietetics."

SETTING THE STAGE

Definition of Quality/Rationale for a Standardized Process

The National Academy of Science's (NAS) Institute of Medicine (IOM) has defined quality as "The degree to which health services for individuals and populations increase the likelihood of desired health outcomes and are consistent with current professional knowledge" (7,8). The quality performance of providers can be assessed by measuring the following: (a) their patients' outcomes (end-results) or (b) the degree to which providers adhere to an accepted care process (7,8). The Committee on Quality of Health Care in America further states that it is not acceptable to have a wide quality chasm, or a gap, between *actual* and *best possible* performance (9). In an effort to ensure that dietetics professionals can meet both requirements for quality performance noted above, the American Dietetic Association (ADA) supports a standardized Nutrition Care Process for the profession.

Standardized Process versus Standardized Care

ADA's Nutrition Care Process is a standardized process for dietetics professionals and not a means to provide standardized care. A standardized process refers to a consistent structure and framework used to provide nutrition care, whereas stan-

K. Lacey is lecturer and Director of Dietetic Programs at the University of Wisconsin–Green Bay, Green Bay. She is also the Chair of the Quality Management Committee. E. Pritchett is Director, Quality and Outcomes at ADA headquarters in Chicago, IL.

If you have questions regarding the Nutrition Care Process and Model, please contact Ellen Pritchett, RD, CPHQ, Director of Quality and Outcomes at ADA, epritchett@eatright.org

Resources

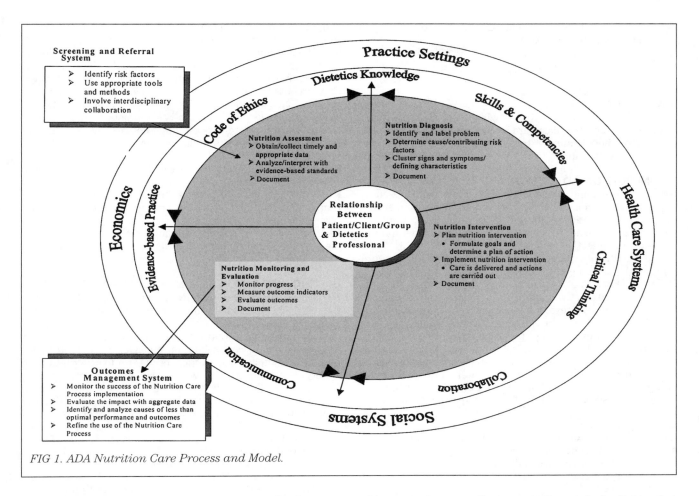

FIG 1. ADA Nutrition Care Process and Model.

dardized care infers that all patients/clients receive the same care. This process supports and promotes individualized care, not standardized care. As represented in the model (Figure 1), the relationship between the patient/client/group and dietetics professional is at the core of the nutrition care process. Therefore, nutrition care provided by qualified dietetics professionals should always reflect both the state of the science and the state of the art of dietetics practice to meet the individualized needs of each patient/client/group (10).

Using the NCP
Even though ADA's Nutrition Care Process will primarily be used to provide nutrition care to individuals in health care settings (inpatient, ambulatory, and extended care), the process also has applicability in a wide variety of community settings. It will be used by dietetics professionals to provide nutrition care to both individuals and groups in community-based agencies and programs for the purpose of health promotion and disease prevention (11,12).

Key Terms
To lay the groundwork and facilitate a clear definition of ADA's Nutrition Care Process, key terms were developed. These definitions provide a frame of reference for the specific components and their functions.

(a) Process is a series of connected steps or actions to achieve an outcome and/or any activity or set of activities that transforms inputs to outputs.

(b) Process Approach is the systematic identification and management of activities and the interactions between activities. A process approach emphasizes the importance of the following:
- understanding and meeting requirements;
- determining if the process adds value;
- determining process performance and effectiveness; and
- using objective measurement for continual improvement of the process (13).

(c) Critical Thinking integrates facts, informed opinions, active listening and observations. It is also a reasoning process in which ideas are produced and evaluated. The Commission on Accreditation of Dietetics Education (CADE) defines critical thinking as "transcending the boundaries of formal education to explore a problem and form a hypothesis and a defensible conclusion" (14). The use of critical thinking provides a unique strength that dietetics professionals bring to the Nutrition Care Process. Further characteristics of critical thinking include the ability to do the following:
- conceptualize;
- think rationally;
- think creatively;
- be inquiring; and
- think autonomously.

Resources

(d) Decision Making is a critical process for choosing the best action to meet a desired goal.

(e) Problem Solving is the process of the following:

- problem identification;
- solution formation;
- implementation; and
- evaluation of the results.

(f) Collaboration is a process by which several individuals or groups with shared concerns are united to address an identified problem or need, leading to the accomplishment of what each could not do separately (15).

DEFINITION OF ADA'S NCP

Using the terms and concepts described above, ADA's Nutrition Care Process is defined as "a systematic problem-solving method that dietetics professionals use to critically think and make decisions to address nutrition related problems and provide safe and effective quality nutrition care."

The Nutrition Care Process consists of four distinct, but interrelated and connected steps: (a) Nutrition Assessment, (b) Nutrition Diagnosis, (c) Nutrition Intervention, and d) Nutrition Monitoring and Evaluation. These four steps were finalized based on extensive review and evaluation of previous works describing nutrition care (16-24). Even though each step builds on the previous one, the process is not linear. Critical thinking and problem solving will frequently require that dietetics professionals revisit previous steps to reassess, add, or revise nutrition diagnoses; modify intervention strategies; and/or evaluate additional outcomes. Figure 2 describes each of these four steps in a similar format consisting of the following:

- definition and purpose;
- key components or substeps with examples as appropriate;
- critical thinking characteristics;
- documentation elements; and
- considerations for continuation, discontinuation, or discharge of care.

Providing nutrition care using ADA's Nutrition Care Process begins when a patient/client/group has been identified at nutrition risk and needs further assistance to achieve or maintain nutrition and health goals. It is also important to recognize that patients/clients who enter the health care system are more likely to have nutrition problems and therefore benefit from receiving nutrition care in this manner. The Nutrition Care Process cycles through the steps of assessment, diagnosis, intervention, and monitoring and evaluation. Nutrition care can involve one or more cycles and ends, ideally, when nutrition goals have been achieved. However, the patient/client/group may choose to end care earlier based on personal or external factors. Using professional judgment, the dietetics professional may discharge the patient/client/group when it is determined that no further progress is likely.

PURPOSE OF NCP

ADA's Nutrition Care Process, as described in Figure 2, gives dietetics professionals a consistent and systematic structure and method by which to think critically and make decisions. It also assists dietetics professionals to scientifically and holistically manage nutrition care, thus helping patients better meet their health and nutrition goals. As dietetics professionals consistently use the Nutrition Care Process, one should expect a higher probability of producing good outcomes. The Nutrition Care Process then begins to establish a link between quality and professional autonomy. Professional autonomy results from being recognized for what we do *well*, not just for who we are. When quality can be demonstrated, as defined previously by the IOM (7,8), then dietetics professionals will stand out as the preferred providers of nutrition services. The Nutrition Care Process, when used consistently, also challenges dietetics professionals to move beyond experience-based practice to reach a higher level of evidence-based practice (9,10).

The Nutrition Care Process does not restrict practice but acknowledges the common dimensions of practice by the following:

- defining a common language that allows nutrition practice to be more measurable;
- creating a format that enables the process to generate quantitative and qualitative data that can then be analyzed and interpreted; and
- serving as the structure to validate nutrition care and showing how the nutrition care that was provided does what it intends to do.

DISTINCTION BETWEEN MNT AND THE NCP

Medical Nutrition Therapy (MNT) was first defined by ADA in the mid-1990s to promote the benefits of managing or treating a disease with nutrition. Its components included an assessment of nutritional status of patients and the provision of either diet modification, counseling, or specialized nutrition therapies. MNT soon became a widely used term to describe a wide variety of nutrition care services provided by dietetics professionals. Since MNT was first introduced, dietetics professionals have gained much credibility among legislators and other health care providers. More recently, MNT has been redefined as part of the 2001 Medicare MNT benefit legislation to be "nutritional diagnostic, therapy, and counseling services for the purpose of disease management, which are furnished by a registered dietitian or nutrition professional" (25).

The intent of the NCP is to describe accurately the spectrum of nutrition care that can be provided by dietetics professionals. Dietetics professionals are uniquely qualified by virtue of academic and supervised practice training and appropriate certification and/or licensure to provide a comprehensive array of professional services relating to the prevention or treatment of nutrition-related illness (14,26). MNT is but one specific type of nutrition care. The NCP articulates the consistent and specific steps a dietetics professional would use when delivering MNT, but it will also be used to guide nutrition education and other preventative nutrition care services. One of the key distinguishing characteristics between MNT and the other nutrition services using the NCP is that MNT always involves an in-depth, comprehensive assessment and individualized care. For example, one individual could receive MNT for diabetes and also nutrition education services or participate in a community-based weight loss program (27). Each service would use the Nutrition Care Process, but the process would be implemented differently; the components of each step of the process would be tailored to the type of service.

By articulating the steps of the Nutrition Care Process, the commonalities (the consistent, standardized, four-step process) of nutrition care are emphasized even though the process is implemented differently for different nutrition services. With a standardized Nutrition Care Process in place, MNT should not be used to describe all of the nutrition services that dietetics professionals provide. As noted above, MNT is the only application of the Nutrition Care Process (28-31). This change in

STEP 1. NUTRITION ASSESSMENT

Basic Definition & Purpose	**"Nutrition Assessment"** is the first step of the Nutrition Care Process. Its purpose is to obtain adequate information in order to identify nutrition-related problems. It is initiated by referral and/or screening of individuals or groups for nutritional risk factors. Nutrition assessment is a systematic process of obtaining, verifying, and interpreting data in order to make decisions about the nature and cause of nutrition-related problems. The specific types of data gathered in the assessment will vary depending on a) practice settings, b) individual/groups' present health status, c) how data are related to outcomes to be measured, d) recommended practices such as ADA's Evidence Based Guides for Practice and e) whether it is an initial assessment or a reassessment. Nutrition assessment requires making comparisons between the information obtained and reliable standards (ideal goals). Nutrition assessment is an on-going, dynamic process that involves not only initial data collection, but also continual reassessment and analysis of patient/client/group needs. Assessment provides the foundation for the nutrition diagnosis at the next step of the Nutrition Care Process.
Data Sources/Tools for Assessment	■ Referral information and/or interdisciplinary records ■ Patient/client interview (across the lifespan) ■ Community-based surveys and focus groups ■ Statistical reports; administrative data ■ Epidemiological studies
Types of Data Collected	■ Nutritional Adequacy (dietary history/detailed nutrient intake) ■ Health Status (anthropometric and biochemical measurements, physical & clinical conditions, physiological and disease status) ■ Functional and Behavioral Status (social and cognitive function, psychological and emotional factors, quality-of-life measures, change readiness)
Nutrition Assessment Components	■ Review dietary intake for factors that affect health conditions and nutrition risk ■ Evaluate health and disease condition for nutrition-related consequences ■ Evaluate psychosocial, functional, and behavioral factors related to food access, selection, preparation, physical activity, and understanding of health condition ■ Evaluate patient/client/group's knowledge, readiness to learn, and potential for changing behaviors ■ Identify standards by which data will be compared ■ Identify possible problem areas for making nutrition diagnoses
Critical Thinking	The following types of critical thinking skills are especially needed in the assessment step: ■ Observing for nonverbal and verbal cues that can guide and prompt effective interviewing methods; ■ Determining appropriate data to collect; ■ Selecting assessment tools and procedures (matching the assessment method to the situation); ■ Applying assessment tools in valid and reliable ways; ■ Distinguishing relevant from irrelevant data; ■ Distinguishing important from unimportant data; ■ Validating the data; ■ Organizing & categorizing the data in a meaningful framework that relates to nutrition problems; and ■ Determining when a problem requires consultation with or referral to another provider.
Documentation of Assessment	Documentation is an on-going process that supports all of the steps in the Nutrition Care Process. Quality documentation of the assessment step should be relevant, accurate, and timely. Inclusion of the following information would further describe quality assessment documentation: ■ Date and time of assessment; ■ Pertinent data collected and comparison with standards; ■ Patient/client/groups' perceptions, values, and motivation related to presenting problems; ■ Changes in patient/client/group's level of understanding, food-related behaviors, and other clinical outcomes for appropriate follow-up; and ■ Reason for discharge/discontinuation if appropriate.
Determination for Continuation of Care	If upon the completion of an initial or reassessment it is determined that the problem cannot be modified by further nutrition care, discharge or discontinuation from this episode of nutrition care may be appropriate.

FIG 2. ADA Nutrition Care Process.

Resources

STEP 2. NUTRITION DIAGNOSIS

Basic Definition & Purpose	**"Nutrition Diagnosis"** is the second step of the Nutrition Care Process, and is the identification and labeling that describes an actual occurrence, risk of, or potential for developing a nutritional problem that dietetics professionals are responsible for treating independently. At the end of the assessment step, data are clustered, analyzed, and synthesized. This will reveal a nutrition diagnostic category from which to formulate a specific nutrition diagnostic statement. Nutrition diagnosis should not be confused with medical diagnosis, which can be defined as a disease or pathology of specific organs or body systems that can be treated or prevented. A nutrition diagnosis changes as the patient/client/group's response changes. A medical diagnosis does not change as long as the disease or condition exists. A patient/client/group may have the medical diagnosis of "Type 2 diabetes mellitus"; however, after performing a nutrition assessment, dietetics professionals may diagnose, for example, "undesirable overweight status" or "excessive carbohydrate intake." Analyzing assessment data and naming the nutrition diagnosis(es) provide a link to setting realistic and measurable expected outcomes, selecting appropriate interventions, and tracking progress in attaining those expected outcomes.
Data Sources/Tools for Diagnosis	■ Organized and clustered assessment data ■ List(s) of nutrition diagnostic categories and nutrition diagnostic labels ■ Currently the profession does not have a standardized list of nutrition diagnoses. However ADA has appointed a Standardized Language Work Group to begin development of standardized language for nutrition diagnoses and intervention. (June 2003)
Nutrition Diagnosis Components (3 distinct parts)	**1. Problem (Diagnostic Label)** The nutrition diagnostic statement describes alterations in the patient/client/group's nutritional status. A diagnostic label (qualifier) is an adjective that describes/qualifies the human response such as: ■ Altered, impaired, ineffective, increased/decreased, risk of, acute or chronic. **2. Etiology (Cause/Contributing Risk Factors)** The related factors (etiologies) are those factors contributing to the existence of, or maintenance of pathophysiological, psychosocial, situational, developmental, cultural, and/or environmental problems. ■ Linked to the problem diagnostic label by words "related to" (RT) ■ It is important not only to state the problem, but to also identify the cause of the problem. □ This helps determine whether or not nutritional intervention will improve the condition or correct the problem. □ It will also identify who is responsible for addressing the problem. Nutrition problems are either caused directly by inadequate intake (primary) or as a result of other medical, genetic, or environmental factors (secondary). □ It is also possible that a nutrition problem can be the cause of another problem. For example, excessive caloric intake may result in unintended weight gain. Understanding the cascade of events helps to determine how to prioritize the interventions. □ It is desirable to target interventions at correcting the cause of the problem whenever possible; however, in some cases treating the signs and symptoms (consequences) of the problem may also be justified. ■ The ranking of nutrition diagnoses permits dietetics professionals to arrange the problems in order of their importance and urgency for the patient/client/group. **3. Signs/Symptoms (Defining Characteristics)** The defining characteristics are a cluster of subjective and objective signs and symptoms established for each nutrition diagnostic category. The defining characteristics, gathered during the assessment phase, provide evidence that a nutrition related problem exists and that the problem identified belongs in the selected diagnostic category. They also quantify the problem and describe its severity: ■ Linked to etiology by words "as evidenced by" (AEB); ■ The symptoms (subjective data) are changes that the patient/client/group feels and expresses verbally to dietetics professionals; and ■ The signs (objective data) are observable changes in the patient/client/group's health status.
Nutrition Diagnostic Statement (PES)	Whenever possible, a nutrition diagnostic statement is written in a PES format that states the Problem (P), the Etiology (E), and the Signs & Symptoms (S). However, if the problem is either a risk (potential) or wellness problem, the nutrition diagnostic statement may have only two elements, Problem (P), and the Etiology (E), since Signs & Symptoms (S) will not yet be exhibited in the patient. A well-written Nutrition Diagnostic Statement should be: 1. Clear and concise 2. Specific: patient/client/group-centered 3. Related to one client problem 4. Accurate: relate to one etiology 5. Based on reliable and accurate assessment data **Examples of Nutrition Diagnosis Statements (PES or PE)** ■ Excessive caloric intake (problem) "related to" frequent consumption of large portions of high fat meals (etiology) "as evidenced by" average daily intake of calories exceeding recommended amount by 500 kcal and 12-pound weight gain during the past 18 months (signs)

FIG 2 cont'd.

- Inappropriate infant feeding practice RT lack of knowledge AEB infant receiving bedtime juice in a bottle
- Unintended weight loss RT inadequate provision of energy by enteral products AEB 6-pound weight loss over past month
- Risk of weight gain RT a recent decrease in daily physical activity following sports injury

Critical Thinking	The following types of critical thinking skills are especially needed in the diagnosis step: ■ Finding patterns and relationships among the data and possible causes; ■ Making inferences ("if this continues to occur, then this is likely to happen"); ■ Stating the problem clearly and singularly; ■ Suspending judgment (be objective and factual); ■ Making interdisciplinary connections; ■ Ruling in/ruling out specific diagnoses; and ■ Prioritizing the relative importance of problems for patient/client/group safety.
Documentation of Diagnosis	Documentation is an on-going process that supports all of the steps in the Nutrition Care Process. Quality documentation of the diagnosis step should be relevant, accurate, and timely. A nutrition diagnosis is the impression of dietetics professionals at a given point in time. Therefore, as more assessment data become available, the documentation of the diagnosis may need to be revised and updated. Inclusion of the following information would further describe quality documentation of this step: ■ Date and time; and ■ Written statement of nutrition diagnosis.
Determination for Continuation of Care	Since the diagnosis step primarily involves naming and describing the problem, the determination for continuation of care seldom occurs at this step. Determination of the continuation of care is more appropriately made at an earlier or later point in the Nutrition Care Process.

STEP 3. NUTRITION INTERVENTION

Basic Definition & Purpose	**"Nutrition Intervention"** is the third step of the Nutrition Care Process. An intervention is a specific set of activities and associated materials used to address the problem. Nutrition interventions are purposefully planned actions designed with the intent of changing a nutrition-related behavior, risk factor, environmental condition, or aspect of health status for an individual, target group, or the community at large. This step involves a) selecting, b) planning, and c) implementing appropriate actions to meet patient/client/groups' nutrition needs. The selection of nutrition interventions is driven by the nutrition diagnosis and provides the basis upon which outcomes are measured and evaluated. Dietetics professionals may actually do the interventions, or may include delegating or coordinating the nutrition care that others provide. All interventions must be based on scientific principles and rationale and, when available, grounded in a high level of quality research (evidence-based interventions). Dietetics professionals work collaboratively with the patient/client/group, family, or caregiver to create a realistic plan that has a good probability of positively influencing the diagnosis/problem. This client-driven process is a key element in the success of this step, distinguishing it from previous planning steps that may or may not have involved the patient/client/group to this degree of participation.
Data Sources/Tools for Interventions	■ Evidence-based nutrition guides for practice and protocols ■ Current research literature ■ Current consensus guidelines and recommendations from other professional organizations ■ Results of outcome management studies or Continuous Quality Index projects. ■ Current patient education materials at appropriate reading level and language ■ Behavior change theories (self-management training, motivational interviewing, behavior modification, modeling)
Nutrition Intervention Components	This step includes two distinct interrelated processes: 1. **Plan the nutrition intervention** (formulate & determine a plan of action) ■ Prioritize the nutrition diagnoses based on severity of problem; safety; patient/client/group's need; likelihood that nutrition intervention will impact problem and patient/client/groups' perception of importance. ■ Consult ADA's *MNT Evidence-Based Guides for Practice* and other practice guides. These resources can assist dietetics professionals in identifying science-based ideal goals and selecting appropriate interventions for MNT. They list appropriate value(s) for control or improvement of the disease or conditions as defined and supported in the literature. ■ Determine patient-focused expected outcomes for each nutrition diagnosis. The expected outcomes are the desired change(s) to be achieved over time as a result of nutrition intervention. They are based on nutrition diagnosis; for example, increasing or decreasing laboratory values, decreasing blood pressure, decreasing weight, increasing use of stanols/sterols, or increasing fiber. Expected outcomes should be written in observable and measurable terms that are clear and concise. They should be patient/client/group-centered and need to be tailored to what is reasonable to the patient's circumstances and appropriate expectations for treatments and outcomes.

FIG 2 cont'd.

Resources

- Confer with patient/client/group, other caregivers or policies and program standards throughout planning step.
- Define intervention plan (for example write a nutrition prescription, provide an education plan or community program, create policies that influence nutrition programs and standards).
- Select specific intervention strategies that are focused on the etiology of the problem and that are known to be effective based on best current knowledge and evidence.
- Define time and frequency of care including intensity, duration, and follow-up.
- Identify resources and/or referrals needed.

2. Implement the nutrition intervention (care is delivered and actions are carried out)
- Implementation is the action phase of the nutrition care process. During implementation, dietetics professionals:
  □ Communicate the plan of nutrition care;
  □ Carry out the plan of nutrition care; and
  □ Continue data collection and modify the plan of care as needed.
- Other characteristics that define quality implementation include:
  □ Individualize the interventions to the setting and client;
  □ Collaborate with other colleagues and health care professionals;
  □ Follow up and verify that implementation is occurring and needs are being met; and
  □ Revise strategies as changes in condition/response occurs.

Critical Thinking	Critical thinking is required to determine which intervention strategies are implemented based on analysis of the assessment data and nutrition diagnosis. The following types of critical thinking skills are especially needed in the intervention step: - Setting goals and prioritizing; - Transferring knowledge from one situation to another; - Defining the nutrition prescription or basic plan; - Making interdisciplinary connections; - Initiating behavioral and other interventions; - Matching intervention strategies with client needs, diagnoses, and values; - Choosing from among alternatives to determine a course of action; and - Specifying the time and frequency of care.
Documentation of Nutrition Interventions	Documentation is an on-going process that supports all of the steps in the Nutrition Care Process. Quality documentation of nutrition interventions should be relevant, accurate, and timely. It should also support further intervention or discharge from care. Changes in patient/client/group's level of understanding and food-related behaviors must be documented along with changes in clinical or functional outcomes to assure appropriate care/case management in the future. Inclusion of the following information would further describe quality documentation of this step: - Date and time; - Specific treatment goals and expected outcomes; - Recommended interventions, individualized for patient; - Any adjustments of plan and justifications; - Patient receptivity; - Referrals made and resources used; - Any other information relevant to providing care and monitoring progress over time; - Plans for follow-up and frequency of care; and - Rationale for discharge if appropriate.
Determination for Continuation of Care	If the patient/client/group has met intervention goals or is not at this time able/ready to make needed changes, the dietetics professional may include discharging the client from this episode of care as part of the planned intervention.

STEP 4. NUTRITION MONITORING AND EVALUATION

Basic Definition & Purpose	"Nutrition Monitoring and Evaluation" is the fourth step of the Nutrition Care Process. *Monitoring* specifically refers to the review and measurement of the patient/client/group's status at a scheduled (preplanned) follow-up point with regard to the nutrition diagnosis, intervention plans/goals, and outcomes, whereas *Evaluation* is the systematic comparison of current findings with previous status, intervention goals, or a reference standard. Monitoring and evaluation use selected outcome indicators (markers) that are relevant to the patient/client/group's defined needs, nutrition diagnosis, nutrition goals, and disease state. Recommended times for follow-up, along with relevant outcomes to be monitored, can be found in ADA's Evidence Based Guides for Practice and other evidence-based sources. The purpose of monitoring and evaluation is to determine the degree to which progress is being made and goals or desired outcomes of nutrition care are being met. It is more than just "watching" what is happening, it requires an active commitment to measuring and recording the appropriate outcome indicators (markers) relevant to the nutrition diagnosis and intervention strategies. Data from this step are used to create an outcomes management system. Refer to Outcomes Management System in text.

FIG 2 cont'd.

	Progress should be monitored, measured, and evaluated on a planned schedule until discharge. Short inpatient stays and lack of return for ambulatory visits do not preclude monitoring, measuring, and evaluation. Innovative methods can be used to contact patients/clients to monitor progress and outcomes. Patient confidential self-report via mailings and telephone follow-up are some possibilities. Patients being followed in disease management programs can also be monitored for changes in nutritional status. Alterations in outcome indicators such as hemoglobin A1C or weight are examples that trigger reactivation of the nutrition care process.
Data Sources/Tools for Monitoring and Evaluation	■ Patient/client/group records ■ Anthropometric measurements, laboratory tests, questionnaires, surveys ■ Patient/client/group (or guardian) interviews/surveys, pretests, and posttests ■ Mail or telephone follow-up ■ ADA's *Evidence Based Guides for Practice* and other evidence-based sources ■ Data collection forms, spreadsheets, and computer programs
Types of Outcomes Collected	The outcome(s) to be measured should be directly related to the nutrition diagnosis and the goals established in the intervention plan. Examples include, but are not limited to: ■ Direct nutrition outcomes (knowledge gained, behavior change, food or nutrient intake changes, improved nutritional status); ■ Clinical and health status outcomes (laboratory values, weight, blood pressure, risk factor profile changes, signs and symptoms, clinical status, infections, complications); ■ Patient/client-centered outcomes (quality of life, satisfaction, self-efficacy, self-management, functional ability); and ■ Health care utilization and cost outcomes (medication changes, special procedures, planned/unplanned clinic visits, preventable hospitalizations, length of hospitalization, prevent or delay nursing home admission).
Nutrition Monitoring and Evaluation Components	This step includes three distinct and interrelated processes: **1. Monitor progress** ■ Check patient/client/group understanding and compliance with plan; ■ Determine if the intervention is being implemented as prescribed; ■ Provide evidence that the plan/intervention strategy is or is not changing patient/client/group behavior or status; ■ Identify other positive or negative outcomes; ■ Gather information indicating reasons for lack of progress; and ■ Support conclusions with evidence. **2. Measure outcomes** ■ Select outcome indicators that are relevant to the nutrition diagnosis or signs or symptoms, nutrition goals, medical diagnosis, and outcomes and quality management goals. ■ Use standardized indicators to: □ Increase the validity and reliability of measurements of change; and □ Facilitate electronic charting, coding, and outcomes measurement. **3. Evaluate outcomes** ■ Compare current findings with previous status, intervention goals, and/or reference standards.
Critical Thinking	The following types of critical thinking skills are especially needed in the monitoring and evaluation step: ■ Selecting appropriate indicators/measures; ■ Using appropriate reference standard for comparison; ■ Defining where patient/client/group is now in terms of expected outcomes; ■ Explaining variance from expected outcomes; ■ Determining factors that help or hinder progress; and ■ Deciding between discharge or continuation of nutrition care.
Documentation of Monitoring and Evaluation	Documentation is an on-going process that supports all of the steps in the Nutrition Care Process and is an integral part of monitoring and evaluation activities. Quality documentation of the monitoring and evaluation step should be relevant, accurate, and timely. It includes a statement of where the patient is now in terms of expected outcomes. Standardized documentation enables pooling of data for outcomes measurement and quality improvement purposes. Quality documentation should also include: ■ Date and time; ■ Specific indicators measured and results; ■ Progress toward goals (incremental small change can be significant therefore use of a Likert type scale may be more descriptive than a "met" or "not met" goal evaluation tool); ■ Factors facilitating or hampering progress; ■ Other positive or negative outcomes; and ■ Future plans for nutrition care, monitoring, and follow up or discharge.
Determination for Continuation of Care	Based on the findings, the dietetics professional makes a decision to actively continue care or discharge the patient/client/group from nutrition care (when necessary and appropriate nutrition care is completed or no further change is expected at this time). If nutrition care is to be continued, the nutrition care process cycles back as necessary to assessment, diagnosis, and/or intervention for additional assessment, refinement of the diagnosis and adjustment and/or reinforcement of the plan. If care does not continue, the patient may still be monitored for a change in status and reentry to nutrition care at a later date.

FIG 2 cont'd.

Resources

describing what dietetics professionals do is truly a paradigm shift. This new paradigm is more complete, takes in more possibilities, and explains observations better. Finally, it allows dietetics professionals to act in ways that are more likely to achieve the results that are desired and expected.

NUTRITION CARE MODEL

The Nutrition Care Model is a visual representation that reflects key concepts of each step of the Nutrition Care Process and illustrates the greater context within which the Nutrition Care Process is conducted. The model also identifies other factors that influence and impact on the quality of nutrition care provided. Refer to Figure 1 for an illustration of the model as described below:

■ Central Core: Relationship between patient/client/group and dietetics professional;
■ Nutrition Care Process: Four steps of the nutrition care process (Figure 2);
■ Outer rings:
■ Middle ring: Strengths and abilities that dietetics professionals bring to the process (dietetics knowledge, skills, and competencies; critical thinking, collaboration, and communication; evidence-based practice, and Code of Ethics) (32);
■ Outer ring: Environmental factors that influence the process (practice settings, health care systems, social systems, and economics);
■ Supporting Systems:
■ Screening and Referral System as access to Nutrition Care; and
■ Outcomes Management System as a means to provide continuous quality improvement to the process.

The model is intended to depict the relationship with which all of these components overlap, interact, and move in a dynamic manner to provide the best quality nutrition care possible.

Central to providing nutrition care is the relationship between the patient/client/group and the dietetics professional. The patient/client/groups' previous educational experiences and readiness to change influence this relationship. The education and training that dietetics professionals receive have very strong components devoted to interpersonal knowledge and skill building such as listening, empathy, coaching, and positive reinforcing.

The middle ring identifies abilities of dietetics professionals that are especially applicable to the Nutrition Care Process. These include the unique dietetics knowledge, skill, and competencies that dietetics professionals bring to the process, in addition to a well-developed capability for critical thinking, collaboration, and communication. Also in this ring is evidence-based practice that emphasizes that nutrition care must incorporate currently available scientific evidence, linking what is done (content) and how it is done (process of care). The Code of Ethics defines the ethical principles by which dietetics professionals should practice (33). Dietetics knowledge and evidence-based practice establish the Nutrition Care Process as unique to dietetics professionals; no other health care professional is qualified to provide nutrition care in this manner. However, the Nutrition Care Process is highly dependent on collaboration and integration within the health care team. As stated above, communication and participation within the health care team are critical for identification of individuals who are appropriate for nutrition care.

The outer ring identifies some of the environmental factors such as practice settings, health care systems, social systems, and economics. These factors impact the ability of the patient/client/group to receive and benefit from the interventions of nutrition care. It is essential that dietetics professionals assess these factors and be able to evaluate the degree to which they may be either a positive or negative influence on the outcomes of care.

Screening and Referral System

Because screening may or may not be accomplished by dietetics professionals, nutrition screening is a supportive system and *not* a step within the Nutrition Care Process. Screening is extremely important; it is an identification step that is outside the actual "care" and provides access to the Nutrition Care Process.

The Nutrition Care Process depends on an effective screening and/or referral process that identifies clients who would benefit from nutrition care or MNT. Screening is defined by the US Preventive Services Task Force as "those preventive services in which a test or standardized examination procedure is used to identify patients requiring special intervention" (34). The major requirements for a screening test to be considered effective are the following:

■ Accuracy as defined by the following three components:
 □ Specificity: Can it identify patients with a condition?
 □ Sensitivity: Can it identify those who do not have the condition?
 □ Positive and negative predictive; and
■ Effectiveness as related to likelihood of positive health outcomes if intervention is provided.

Screening parameters need to be tailored to the population and to the nutrition care services to be provided. For example, the screening parameters identified for a large tertiary acute care institution specializing in oncology would be vastly different than the screening parameters defined for an ambulatory obstetrics clinic. Depending on the setting and institutional policies, the dietetics professional may or may not be directly involved in the screening process. Regardless of whether dietetics professionals are actively involved in conducting the screening process, they are accountable for providing input into the development of appropriate screening parameters to ensure that the screening process asks the right questions. They should also evaluate how effective the screening process is in terms of correctly identifying clients who require nutrition care.

In addition to correctly identifying clients who would benefit from nutrition care, a referral process may be necessary to ensure that the client has an identifiable method of being linked to dietetics professionals who will ultimately provide the nutrition care or medical nutrition therapy. While the nutrition screening and referral is not part of the Nutrition Care Process, it is a critical antecedent step in the overall system (35).

Outcomes Management System

An outcomes management system evaluates the effectiveness and efficiency of the entire process (assessment, diagnosis, interventions, cost, and others), whereas the fourth step of the process "nutrition monitoring and evaluations" refers to the evaluation of the patient/client/group's progress in achieving outcomes.

Because outcomes management is a system's commitment to effective and efficient care, it is depicted outside of the NCP. Outcomes management links care processes and resource uti-

Resources

lization with outcomes. Through outcomes management, relevant data are collected and analyzed in a timely manner so that performance can be adjusted and improved. Findings are compared with such things as past levels of performance; organizational, regional, or national norms; and standards or benchmarks of optimal performance. Generally, this information is reported to providers, administrators, and payors/funders and may be part of administrative databases or required reporting systems.

It requires an infrastructure in which outcomes for the population served are routinely assessed, summarized, and reported. Health care organizations use complex information management systems to manage resources and track performance. Selected information documented throughout the nutrition care process is entered into these central information management systems and structured databases. Examples of centralized data systems in which nutrition care data should be included are the following:

■ basic encounter documentation for billing and cost accounting;

■ tracking of standard indicators for quality assurance and accreditation;

■ pooling data from a large series of patients/clients/groups to determine outcomes; and

■ specially designed studies that link process and outcomes to determine effectiveness and cost effectiveness of diagnostic and intervention approaches.

The major goal of outcomes management is to utilize collected data to improve the quality of care rendered in the future. Monitoring and evaluation data from individuals are pooled/aggregated for the purposes of professional accountability, outcomes management, and systems/processes improvement. Results from a large series of patients/clients can be used to determine the effectiveness of intervention strategies and the impact of nutrition care in improving the overall health of individuals and groups. The effects of well-monitored quality improvement initiatives should be reflected in measurable improvements in outcomes.

Outcomes management comprehensively evaluates the two parts of IOM's definition of quality: outcomes and process. Measuring the relationship between the process and the outcome is essential for quality improvement. To ensure that the quality of patient care is not compromised, the focus of quality improvement efforts should always be directed at the outcome of care (36-43).

FUTURE IMPLICATIONS

Impact on Coverage for Services

Quality-related issues are gaining in importance worldwide. Even though our knowledge base is increasing, the scientific evidence for most clinical practices in all of medicine is modest. So much of what is done in health care does *not* maximize quality or minimize cost (44). A standardized Nutrition Care Process is a necessary foundation tool for gathering valid and reliable data on how quality nutrition care provided by qualified dietetics professionals improves the overall quality of health care provided. Implementing ADA's Nutrition Care Process provides a framework for demonstrating that nutrition care improves outcomes by the following: (a) enhancing the health of individuals, groups, institutions, or health systems; (b) potentially reducing health care costs by decreasing the need for medications, clinic and hospital visits, and preventing or delay-

ing nursing home admissions; and (c) serving as the basis for research, documenting the impact of nutrition care provided by dietetics professionals (45-47).

Developing Scopes and Practice Standards

The work group reviewed the questions raised by delegates regarding the role of the RD and DTR in the Nutrition Care Process. As a result of careful consideration of this important issue, it was concluded that describing the various types of tasks and responsibilities appropriate to each of these credentialed dietetics professionals was yet another professional issue beyond the intent and purpose of developing a standardized Nutrition Care Process.

A scope of practice of a profession is the range of services that the profession is authorized to provide. Scopes of practice, depending on the particular setting in which they are used, can have different applications. They can serve as a legal document for state certification/licensure laws or they might be incorporated into institutional policy and procedure guidelines or job descriptions. Professional scopes of practice should be based on the education, training, skills, and competencies of each profession (48).

As previously noted, a dietetics professional is a person who, by virtue of academic and clinical training and appropriate certification and/or licensure, is uniquely qualified to provide a comprehensive array of professional services relating to prevention and treatment of nutrition-related conditions. A Scope of Practice articulates the roles of the RD, DTR, and advanced-practice RD. Issues to be addressed for the future include the following: (a) the need for a common scope with specialized guidelines and (b) recognition of the rich diversity of practice vs exclusive domains of practice regulation.

Professional standards are "authoritative statements that describe performance common to the profession." As such, standards should encompass the following:

■ articulate the expectations the public can have of a dietetics professional in any practice setting, domain, and/or role;

■ expect and achieve levels of practice against which actual performance can be measured; and

■ serve as a legal reference to describe "reasonable and prudent" dietetics practice.

The Nutrition Care Process effectively reflects the dietetics professional as the unique provider of nutrition care when it is consistently used as a systematic method to think critically and make decisions to provide safe and effective care. ADA's Nutrition Care Process will serve as a guide to develop scopes of practice and standards of practice (49,50). Therefore, the work group recommended that further work be done to use the Nutrition Care Process to describe roles and functions that can be included in scopes of practice. In May 2003, the Board of Directors of ADA established a Practice Definitions Task Force that will identify and differentiate the terms within the profession that need clarification for members, affiliates, and DPGs related to licensure, certification, practice acts, and advanced practice. This task force is also charged to clarify the scope of practice services, clinical privileges, and accountabilities provided by RDs/DTRs based on education, training, and experience.

Education of Dietetics Students

It will be important to review the current CADE Educational Standards to ensure that the language and level of expected competencies are consistent with the entry-level practice of the Nutrition Care Process. Further work by the Commission on Dietetic Registration (CDR) may need to be done to make revisions on the RD and DTR exams to evaluate entry-level competencies needed to practice nutrition care in this way. Revision of texts and other educational materials will also need to incorporate the key principles and steps of this new process (51).

Education and Credentialing of Members

Even though dietetics professionals currently provide nutrition care, this standardized Nutrition Care Process includes some new principles, concepts, and guidelines in each of its steps. This is especially true of steps 2 and 4 (Nutrition Diagnosis and Nutrition Monitoring and Evaluation). Therefore, the implications for education of dietetics professionals and their practice are great. Because a large number of dietetics professionals still are employed in health care systems, a comprehensive educational plan will be essential. A model to be considered when planning education is the one used to educate dietetics professionals on the Professional Development Portfolio (PDP) Process (52). Materials that could be used to provide members with the necessary knowledge and skills in this process could include but not be limited to the following:

■ articles in the *Journal of the American Dietetic Association*;
■ continuing professional education lectures and presentations at affiliate and national meetings;
■ self-study materials; case studies, CD-ROM workbooks, and others;
■ hands-on workshops and training programs;
■ Web-based materials; and
■ inclusion in the learning needs assessment and codes of the Professional Development Portfolio.

Through the development of this educational strategic plan, the benefits to dietetics professionals and other stakeholders will need to be a central theme to promote the change in practice that comes with using this process to provide nutrition care.

Evidence-Based Practice

The pressure to do more with less is dramatically affecting all of health care, including dietetics professionals. This pressure is forcing the health care industry to restructure to be more efficient and cost-effective in delivering care. It will require the use of evidenced-based practice to determine what practices are critical to support outcomes (53,54). The Nutrition Care Process will be invaluable as research is completed to evaluate the services provided by dietetics professionals (55). The Nutrition Care Process will provide the structure for developing the methodology and data collection in individual settings, and the practice-based research networks ADA is in the process of initiating.

Standardized Language

As noted in Step 2 (Nutrition Diagnosis), having a standard taxonomy for nutrition diagnosis would be beneficial. Work in the area of articulating the types of interventions used by dietetics professionals has already begun by the Definitions Work Group under the direction of ADA's Research Committee. Further work to define terms that are part of the Nutrition Care Process will need to continue. Even though the work group provided a list of terms relating to the definition and key concepts of the process, there are opportunities to articulate fur-

ther terms that are consistently used in this process. The Board of Directors of ADA in May 2003 approved continuation and expansion of a task force to address a comprehensive system that includes a process for developing and validating standardized language for nutrition diagnosis, intervention, and outcomes.

SUMMARY

Just as maps are reissued when new roads are built and rivers change course, this Nutrition Care Process and Model reflects recent changes in the nutrition and health care environment. It provides dietetics professionals with the updated "road map" to follow the best path for high-quality patient/client/group-centered nutrition care.

References
1. American Dietetic Association Strategic Plan. Available at: http://eatright.org (member only section). Accessed June 2, 2003.
2. Wheeler D. *Understanding Variation: The Key to Managing Chaos.* 2nd ed. Knoxville, TN: SPC Press; 2000.
3. Shojania KG, Duncan BW, McDonald KM, Wachter RM. Making Health Care Safer: A Critical Analysis of Patient Safety Practices. Evidence Report/Technology Assessment No. 43 (Prepared by the University of California at San Francisco-Stanford Evidence-based Practice Center under Contract No. 290-97-0013). Rockville, MD: Agency for Healthcare Research and Quality; 2001. Report No.: AHRQ Publication No. 01-E058.
4. Potter, Patricia A, Perry, Anne G. *Basic Nursing Theory and Practice.* 4th ed. St Louis: C.V. Mosby; 1998.
5. American Physical Therapy Association. *Guide to Physical Therapist Practice.* 2nd ed. Alexandria, VA; 2001.
6. The Guide to Occupational Therapy Practice. *Am J Occup Ther.* 1999;53:3. Available at http://nweb.pct.edu/homepage/student/NUNJOL02/ot%20process.ppt. Accessed May 30, 2003.
7. Kohn KN, ed. *Medicare: A strategy for Quality Assurance, Volume I.* Committee to Design a Strategy for Quality Review and Assurance in Medicare. Washington, DC: Institute of Medicine. National Academy Press; 1990.
8. Kohn L, Corrigan J, Donaldson M, eds. *To Err Is Human: Building a Safer Health System.* Washington, DC: Committee on Quality of Health Care in America, Institute of Medicine. National Academy Press; 2000.
9. Institute of Medicine. *Crossing the Quality Chasm: A New Health System for the 21st Century.* Committee on Quality in Health Care in America. Rona Briere, ed. Washington, DC: National Academy Press; 2001.
10. Splett P. *Developing and Validating Evidence-Based Guides for Practice: A Tool Kit for Dietetics Professionals.* American Dietetic Association; 1999.
11. Endres JB. *Community Nutrition. Challenges and Opportunities.* Upper Saddle River, NJ: Prentice-Hall, Inc; 1999.
12. Splett P. Planning, Implementation and Evaluation of Nutrition Programs. In: Sharbaugh CO, ed. *Call to Action: Better Nutrition for Mothers, Children, and Families.* Washington, DC: National Center for Education in Maternal and Child Health (NCEMCH); 1990.
13. Batalden PB, Stoltz PA. A framework for the continual improvement of health care: Building and applying professional and improvement knowledge to test changes in daily work. *Jt Comm J Qual Improv.* 1993;19:424-452.
14. CADE Accreditation Handbook. Available at: http://www.eatright.com/cade/standards.html. Accessed March 20, 2003.
15. Alfaro-LeFevre R. Nursing process overview. *Applying Nursing Process. Promoting Collaborative Care.* 5th ed. Lippincott; 2002.
16. Grant A, DeHoog S. *Nutrition Assessment Support and Management.* Northgate Station, WA; 1999.
17. Sandrick, K. Is nutritional diagnosis a critical step in the nutrition care process? *J Am Diet Assoc.* 2002;102:427-431.
18. King LS. What is a diagnosis? *JAMA.* 1967;202:154.
19. Doenges ME. *Application of Nursing Process and Nursing Diagnosis: An Interactive Text for Diagnostic Reasoning,* 3rd ed. Philadelphia, PA: FA Davis Co; 2000.
20. Gallagher-Alred C, Voss AC, Gussler JD. *Nutrition intervention and patient outcomes: a self-study manual.* Columbus, OH: Ross Products Division, Abbott Laboratories; 1995.
21. Splett P, Myers EF. A proposed model for effective nutrition care. *J Am Diet Assoc.* 2001;101:357-363.
22. Lacey K, Cross N. A problem-based nutrition care model that is diagnostic driven and allows for monitoring and managing outcomes. *J Am Diet Assoc.* 2002;102:578-589.
23. Brylinsky C. The Nutrition Care Process. In: Mahan K, Escott-Stump S,

eds. *Krause's Food, Nutrition and Diet Therapy*, 10th ed. Philadelphia, PA: W.B. Saunders Company; 2000:431-451.

24. Hammond MI, Guthrie HA. Nutrition clinic: An integrated component of an undergraduate curriculum. *J Am Diet Assoc.* 1985;85:594.

25. Final MNT Regulations. CMS-1169-FC. Federal Register, November 1, 2001. Department of Health and Human Services. 42 CFR Parts: 405, 410, 411, 414, and 415. Available at: http://cms.hhs.gov/physicians/pfs/cms1169fc.asp. Accessed June 27, 2003.

26. Commission on Dietetic Registration CDR Certifications and State Licensure. Available at: http://www.cdrnet.org/certifications/index.htm. Accessed May 30, 2003.

27. Medicare Coverage Policy Decision: Duration and Frequency of the Medical Nutrition Therapy *(MNT) Benefit* (No. CAG-00097N). Available at: http://cms.hhs.gov/ncdr/memo.asp?id=53. Accessed June 2, 2003.

28. American Dietetic Association Medical Nutrition Therapy Evidence-Based Guides For Practice. Hyperlipidemia Medical Nutrition Therapy Protocol. CD-ROM; 2001.

29. American Dietetic Association. Medical Nutrition Therapy Evidence-Based Guides for Practice. Nutrition Practice Guidelines for Type 1 and 2 Diabetes Mellitus CD-ROM; 2001.

30. American Dietetic Association. Medical Nutrition Therapy Evidence-Based Guides for Practice. Nutrition Practice Guidelines for Gestational Diabetes Mellitus. CD-ROM; 2001.

31. American Dietetic Association Medical Nutrition Therapy Evidence-Based Guides For Practice. Chronic Kidney Disease (non-dialysis) Medical Nutrition Therapy Protocol. CD-ROM; 2002.

32. Gates G. Ethics opinion: Dietetics professionals are ethically obligated to maintain personal competence in practice. *J Am Diet Assoc.* May 2003;103:633-635.

33. Code of Ethics for the Profession of Dietetics. *J Am Diet Assoc.* 1999;99:109-113.

34. US Preventive Services Task Force. Guide to Clinical Preventive Services, 2nd ed. Washington, DC: US Department of Health and Human Services, Office of Disease Prevention and Health Promotion; 1996.

35. Identifying patients at risk: ADA's definitions for nutrition screening and nutrition assessment. *J Am Diet Assoc.* 1994;94:838-839.

36. Donabedian A. *Explorations in Quality Assessment and Monitoring. Volume I: The Definition of Quality and Approaches to Its Assessment.* Ann Arbor, MI: Health Administration Press; 1980.

37. Carey RG, Lloyd RC. *Measuring Quality Improvement in Health Care: A Guide to Statistical Process Control Applications.* New York, Quality Resources; 1995.

38. Eck LH, Slawson DL, Williams R, Smith K, Harmon-Clayton K, Oliver D. A model for making outcomes research standard practice in clinical dietetics. *J Am Diet Assoc.* 1998;98:451-457.

39. Ireton-Jones CS, Gottschlich MM, Bell SJ. *Practice-Oriented Nutrition Research: An Outcomes Measurement Approach.* Gaithersburg, MD: Aspen Publishers, Inc.; 1998.

40. Kaye GL. *Outcomes Management: Linking Research to Practice.* Columbus, OH: Ross Products Division, Abbott Laboratories; 1996.

41. Splett P. *Cost Outcomes of Nutrition Intervention*, a *Three Part Monograph.* Evansville, IN: Mead Johnson & Company; 1996.

42. Plsekk P. 1994. Tutorial: Planning for data collection part I: Asking the right question. *Qual Manage Health Care.* 2:76-81.

43. American Dietetic Association. Israel D, Moore S, eds. *Beyond Nutrition Counseling: Achieving Positive Outcomes Through Nutrition Therapy.* 1996.

44. Stoline AM, Weiner JP. *The New Medical Marketplace: A Physician's Guide to the Health Care System in the 1990s.* Baltimore: Johns Hopkins Press; 1993.

45. Mathematica Policy Research, Inc. Best Practices in Coordinated Care March 22, 2000. Available at: http://www.mathematica-mpr.com/PDFs/bestpractices.pdf. Accessed February 22, 2003.

46. Bisognano MA. New skills needed in medical leadership: The key to achieving business results. *Qual Prog.* 2000;33:32-41.

47. Smith R. Expanding medical nutrition therapy: An argument for evidence-based practices. *J Am Diet Assoc.* 2003;103:313-314.

48. National Council of State Boards of Nursing Model Nursing Practice Act. Available at: http://www.ncsbn.org/public/regulation/nursing_practice_model_practice_act.htm. Accessed June 27, 2003.

49. Professional policies of the American College of Medical Quality (ACMQ). Available at: http://www.acmq.org/profess/list.htm. Accessed June 27, 2003.

50. American Dietetic Association. Standards of professional practice. *J Am Diet Assoc.* 1998;98:83-85.

51. O'Neil EH and the Pew Health Professions Commission. Recreating Health Professional Practice for a New Century. The Fourth Report of the Pew Health Professions Commission. Pew Health Professions Commission; December 1998.

52. Weddle DO. The professional development portfolio process: Setting goals for credentialing. *J Am Diet Assoc.* 2002;102:1439-1444.

53. Sackett DL, Rosenberg WMC, Gray J, Haynes RB, Richardson WS. Evidence based medicine: What it is and what it isn't. *Br Med J.* 1996;312:71-72.

54. Myers EF, Pritchett E, Johnson EQ. Evidence-based practice guides vs. protocols: What's the difference? *J Am Diet Assoc.* 2001;101:1085-1090.

55. Manore MM, Myers EF. Research and the dietetics profession: Making a bigger impact. *J Am Diet Assoc.* 2003;103:108-112.

The Quality Management Committee Work Group developed the Nutrition Care Process and Model with input from the House of Delegates dialog (October 2002 HOD meeting, in Philadelphia, PA). The work group members are the following: Karen Lacey, MS, RD, Chair; Elvira Johnson, MS, RD; Kessey Kieselhorst, MPA, RD; Mary Jane Oakland, PhD, RD, FADA; Carlene Russell, RD, FADA; Patricia Splett, PhD, RD, FADA; Suzanne Bertocchi, DTR, and Tamara Otterstein, DTR; Ellen Pritchett, RD; Esther Myers, PhD, RD, FADA; Harold Holler, RD, and Karri Looby, MS, RD. The work group would like to extend a special thank you to Marion Hammond, MS, and Naoimi Trossler, PhD, RD, for their assistance in development of the Nutrition Care Process and Model.

Resources

Implementing Nutrition Diagnosis, Step Two in the Nutrition Care Process and Model: Challenges and Lessons Learned in Two Health Care Facilities

Jennifer Mathieu; Mandy Foust, RD; Patricia Ouellette, RD

In adherence to the American Dietetic Association's (ADA) Strategic Plan goal of establishing and implementing a standardized Nutrition Care Process (NCP) in the hopes of "increasing demand and utilization of services provided by members" (1), dietetics professionals in two health care facilities established an NCP pilot program in 2005, in collaboration with ADA. The pilot sites were the Virginia Hospital Center in Arlington and the Veterans Affairs Medical Center in San Diego, CA.

This article gives a background on the NCP and Model, the standardized language used in the nutrition diagnosis step, medical record documentation, and an explanation of how the two sites came to participate in the pilot program. It also provides a timeline for each site's implementation of the NCP, including challenges faced and lessons learned. Similarities and differences in approaches will also be discussed. Managers from both facilities will offer advice to facilities who are contemplating implementation of the NCP and nutrition diagnoses in the future.

J. Mathieu is a freelance writer, Houston, TX. M. Foust is clinical nutrition manager, Virginia Hospital Center, Arlington. P. Ouellette is deputy director of nutrition and food services, Veterans Affairs Medical Center, San Diego, CA.

Address correspondence to: Jennifer Mathieu, 5639 Berry Creek Dr, Houston, TX 77017. E-mail: jenmathieu27@yahoo.com

0002-8223/05/10510-0019$30.00/0
doi: 10.1016/j.jada.2005.07.015

BACKGROUND

ADA developed a four-step NCP and Model that appeared in the August 2003 issue of the *Journal*. The NCP consists of four "distinct but interrelated and connected steps"—Nutrition Assessment, Nutrition Diagnosis, Nutrition Intervention, and Nutrition Monitoring and Evaluation (2). The NCP and Model were developed by the Quality Management Committee Work Group with input from the House of Delegates.

This new model calls for dietetics professionals to incorporate a new step—making a nutrition diagnosis—which involves working with defined terminology. It also asks dietetics professionals to chart their diagnosis in the form of a statement that establishes the patient's Problem (diagnostic label), Etiology (cause/contributing risk factors), and Signs and Symptoms (defining characteristics). This is known as a PESS statement, and makes up the heart of the NCP's second step—nutrition diagnosis.

"The second step is the culture shift," says Susan Ramsey, MS, RD, senior manager of medical nutrition services for Sodexho and a member of ADA's Research Committee. "The second step forces us to make a one-line statement. It brings the whole assessment into one clear vision."

According to the article by Lacey and Pritchett, using the new model provides many benefits. The model defines a common language that allows nutrition practice to be more measurable, creates a format that enables the process to generate quantitative and qualitative data that can then be analyzed and interpreted, serves as the structure to validate nutrition care, and shows how the care

that was provided does what it intends to do (2). It also gives the profession a greater sense of autonomy, says Ramsey: "It's given us responsibility for our work instead of looking for permission from others."

The nutrition diagnostic labels and reference sheets were developed by the Standardized Language Task Force, chaired by Sylvia Escott-Stump, MA, RD. It is from this list that dietetics professionals utilizing the NCP list the P (problem) part of the PESS statement. According to Escott-Stump, this Standardized Language will help bring dietetics professionals a new focus and the ability to target their interventions into more effective results that will match the patient nutrition diagnosis (problem).

It is Escott-Stump's belief that documenting nutrition diagnoses, interventions, and outcomes will allow dietetics professionals to better track diagnoses over several clients, allowing the profession to be more likely to track the types of nutrition diagnoses that clients have, and be able to state that the profession affects certain types of acute and chronic diseases more than others.

"For example, now we believe that our impact on cardiovascular, endocrine, and renal diseases is strong, but we may find that our professionals impact gastrointestinal disorders the most," says Escott-Stump. "By having standardized language, we will be able to validate or correct our suspicions."

This pilot implementation of the nutrition care model also tested a new method of charting that differs from the traditional Subjective Objective Assessment Plan format (SOAP). The new ADI template stands for Assessment, Diagnosis, and Intervention (including Monitoring and Evaluation).

According to Dr Esther Myers, PhD, RD, FADA, ADA's Research and Scientific Affairs director, ADA plans to expand these two pilot tests through the Peer Network for Nutrition Diagnosis in the next 2 years. This group of dietetics professionals will receive additional training and networking opportunities to assist them as they implement this new model within their facility and then share their knowledge with other dietetics professionals in their geographical region.

Their experience will be used to determine what additional implementation tools are needed. In addition, a formal research project will be conducted through the Dietetics Practice Based Research Network in early 2006.

IMPLEMENTATION OF THE PROGRAM
Virginia Hospital Center

Mandy Foust, RD and Clinical Nutrition Manager of the Virginia Hospital Center, is contracted through Sodexho to oversee patient services at the 400-bed facility. In December 2004, Foust, who had learned about PESS statements while in school, decided to have her college dietetic intern Anne Avery research current changes and updates in charting for dietetics professionals.

Avery spoke with Dr Myers and discussed the possibility of the Virginia Hospital Center serving as a pilot site for the new model. Foust was excited about the idea for several reasons. "To me, the nutrition care model is a clinically based, concise way of charting that sets goals and is more standardized with other disciplines," she says. Until the implementation of the pilot project, the RDs on staff at the Virginia Hospital Center used the SOAP format of charting.

A conference call took place between Foust, Dr Myers, Avery, and Avery's internship director at Virginia Tech. Foust selected one of her five inpatient registered dietitians (RDs) to serve as the first RD to use the new method. It was decided Avery would present an in-service on the nutrition care model to the dietetics professionals on staff. This in-service provided the RDs with introductory information, the four steps of the NCP, PESS statements, diagnostic labeling, and an explanation of why the changes would be beneficial.

Foust says there were concerns from her staff about the new method. These included that the new ADI charting format would not allow them to be thorough enough and that it seemed "too cookie cutter." Staff also expressed concern that it would be difficult to sum up two or more serious problems in one PESS statement. They also worried that physicians would be wary of the term "nutrition diagnosis."

Over several days in mid-December, Foust arranged meetings with several hospital administrators, including the vice president of the hospital, the chief nursing officer, the medical staff president, and the chief of the nutrition committee to get their feedback on the pilot project. She also kept her supervisor at Sodexho abreast of the situation. "Because I am a contractor, I want to make sure I'm covering my bases," says Foust. She says the Virginia Hospital Center is "very interdisciplinary" and that she wanted there to be an awareness of the upcoming changes.

Administrators initially had questions about how the new method would benefit patients, but Foust says after she met with them and presented them with information on the nutrition care model, they were receptive to the changes. The physician who served as chief of the hospital's nutrition committee had concerns about the idea of a nutrition diagnosis. Foust says she reassured him that the new method did not ask RDs to make a medical diagnosis or interfere with a physician's orders.

After the nutrition committee approved the project in early January 2005, Foust was asked to inform several other hospital staff members about the new format, including the chief of surgery and the chief of surgical education. Because the first RD to participate in the pilot project worked in the intensive care unit (ICU), Foust was also asked to notify the medical director of the ICU, two ICU nurse educators, and the ICU patient care director via formal letters. Responses to these letters encouraged Foust to seek approval for the project from the hospital's patient-monitoring committee.

During the end of January, while waiting for a response from the patient-monitoring committee, Foust met for about an hour each week with the RD who would be the first to use the new method. The RD used actual patients from her daily census to begin practicing PESS statements and ADI charting. Foust shared the results with Dr Myers and the Standardized Language Task Force often. Through early to mid-February, the RD submitted her notes in both the SOAP format and the new format as a way of practicing the new method.

At the end of January, the patient-monitoring committee gave the project its approval. Before implementation officially occurred, Foust requested permission and modified the Hakel-Smith Coding Instrument as an auditing tool to evaluate the charts. She also developed a questionnaire for allied health professionals to give feedback on the new system of charting.

On February 16, 2005, the ICU RD, Korinne Umbaugh, officially began submitting all of her notes using the ADI template. Foust audited two to three charts each day. In late February, a second RD began using the new method of charting. On March 28, a third RD began the process. By the middle of April, all five RDs were using the ADI template, with the fifth RD beginning the process on the second week of the month.

Throughout the entire transition, Foust met formally and informally with staff RDs both individually and in groups. Foust says at least 20 minutes of each weekly hour-long staff meeting continues to be spent discussing the new method of charting and reviewing PESS statements. At this time Foust is editing about 10% of the charts.

Unfortunately, Foust did not receive as many completed questionnaires as she hoped for from allied health professionals. However, her initial chart audits showed that by the end of April the staff had become much more comfortable with the process. Audits revealed notes that steadily became more direct and concise, as well as more outcome-oriented. Extraneous information was not included as often.

Veterans Affairs Medical Center, San Diego

Patricia Ouellette, RD, is the deputy director of nutrition and food services for the Veterans Affairs (VA) Medical

Center in San Diego, CA. The Medical Center is a 238-bed facility. There are three RDs who focus on the inpatient areas of the facility.

In January 2004, the facility's director of nutrition and food service, Ginger Hughes, MS, RD, distributed the August 2003 article by Karen Lacey, MS, RD and Ellen Pritchett, RD, about the NCP that appeared in the *Journal*. The staff was advised to read the article and become familiar with it. In the fall of 2004, internship program director Tere Bush-Zurn and outpatient dietitian Teresa Hilleary received a scholarship to attend the Nutrition Diagnosis Roundtable for Educators workshop at ADA's 2004 Food & Nutrition Conference & Expo. Bush-Zurn and Hilleary relayed what they learned with the rest of their staff when they returned to California.

In November 2004, a staff meeting was held to discuss questions and concerns surrounding the NCP and PESS statements. The staff agreed to start using the PESS statements as soon as possible. After a December 2004 workshop presented by a visiting Lacey, the staff agreed that they wanted to work toward transitioning to the nutrition care model and would serve as a pilot site.

"It evolved after a year of looking at the process and after a lot of discussions with the staff," says Ouellette. "We are a teaching institution and we wanted to challenge ourselves in terms of our practice. We also have a dietetic internship program and feel responsible for providing the interns with the most progressive concepts in our field of practice."

As with the Virginia Hospital Center RDs, the RDs at the VA Medical Center had been using the SOAP format for many years and they had similar concerns over whether the new method would be deemed thorough enough. They were also concerned that one PESS statement would not be enough if the patient had several complicated problems.

Based on staff consensus, in February 2005 the staff started devoting time at the weekly staff meeting to discussing issues related to the new method. The staff practiced writing PESS statements and shared the results with each other during this time. They also discussed questions

and concerns related to the new method.

At the same time, several staff members, including the staff's performance improvement/information technology dietitian, worked separately to develop a point-and-click computer version of the inpatient initial nutrition assessment ADI template that could be used by the inpatient RDs on staff when writing their notes.

During the last week in March, the inpatient RDs spent 1 week writing their notes using both the old SOAP method and the new template. On April 4, the staff officially implemented the new version of charting for the inpatient initial nutrition assessments and stopped using the SOAP method completely. For the first month after the official implementation, Ouellette checked every inpatient initial nutrition assessment chart note and provided weekly feedback to the staff.

In May, the auditing components were incorporated into the NFS Periodic Performance Review plan implemented as part of the Joint Commission on Accreditation of Healthcare Organizations' continuous readiness philosophy. Although not required, they believed this was a good way to continue to audit and document the process.

Ouellette continued to meet with RDs individually as problems and questions developed about the change. Her initial audits revealed that the majority of the staff used the same five to six diagnostic labels. She also assessed that after 2 weeks of using the new ADI template exclusively, PESS statements markedly improved and chart notes became more focused and concise. After 3 weeks, the amount of time spent on the notes shortened, suggesting that the staff was becoming more comfortable with the process.

In regard to diagnostic labels, Ouellette's staff began the practice of utilizing two diagnostic labels and combining them into one PESS statement if the two conditions were closely related (eg, difficulty swallowing and chewing difficulty).

The monitoring component of the process still needs to be observed carefully, as many of Ouellette's staff members are not yet in the habit of stating which specific laboratory tests need to be performed.

SIMILARITIES AND DIFFERENCES

The biggest difference between the two sites was the time spent seeking approval for the project before proceeding. As a contractor, Foust believed she needed to secure approval from several different administrators before beginning implementation. Ouellette's approval process occurred much more informally. Ouellette says this is because the VA allows flexibility in how Nutrition and Food Service processes are carried out.

Another difference centered on the way staff RDs began participating in the implementation. Ouellette's staff discussed the process for about a year before they all began the new method of charting at the same time. Ouellette and her staff wanted to work with only one inpatient charting template at a time, and this allowed them to do so. Also, Ouellette believed that if the SOAP method template was available, RDs might be tempted to go back to the old format that they felt most comfortable using.

After the staff in-service, Foust started one of her RDs on the new method and others followed over a period of months. As the implementation was occurring, the staff had several meetings to discuss the new changes. Foust believed this gradual method of implementation allowed time for RDs who were having trouble with the new method to learn from RDs who were actively working with it.

The similarities between both sites included the increased amount of administrative time spent on the change (especially at the manager level) as well as the decision to focus the change on inpatient areas only. Foust and Ouellette both said this decision was made because inpatient cases tend to be more complex, and if these cases could be dealt with successfully it would be even easier to make the transition with outpatient cases. The sites shared another similarity in that the types of concerns held by the staffs were nearly identical, as were the challenges they faced and the lessons they learned.

CHALLENGES AND LESSONS LEARNED

According to Foust and Ouellette, the biggest challenge for both sites was assisting their RDs in completely changing the way they think about their chart notes. "It's a brand new language," says Foust. "My RDs are already seeing 14, 16 patients a day, and it's a long process when you're starting something new."

Both managers say their RDs had a hard time excluding extraneous language. In the SOAP format, for example, RDs were used to including information about everything from decades-old surgeries, the patient's general mood, and other aspects of the patient's condition that are not relevant to a nutrition diagnosis. With the nutrition care model, the charting must be much more exact. "This new method requires us to focus on establishing a nutrition label and forces us to restrict our charting to what is relevant to that nutritional diagnosis," says Ouellette.

Also challenging for the RDs was the creation of the PESS statements. "They initially roadblock with the PESS," says Foust. "It is a completely different way of formatting your thoughts. It's moving from a very conversational way of charting to a more clinical-sounding, concise note. This results in a struggle when first charting."

Staff members at both sites had concerns over what to do when there seemed to be two separate but equally important problems. After discussions with Dr Myers, it was decided that, on occasion, two PESS statements can be used.

Ouellette adds that another challenge comes from the fact that the nutrition care model means a different way of approaching formatting the chart note. "The chart note really has to be decided after determining the PESS statement," says Ouellette. "The statement can only be determined after a thorough nutritional assessment. The chart review and patient consultation method are the same, but the structuring of the chart note is quite different. We no longer do this in a linear fashion. We start from the middle with the PESS statement and complete both ends—assessment and goals—from there."

RDs also struggled with how to write PESS statements for patients that simply had no nutrition risk. Foust says she urged her staff to recognize that if they were experts in making a nutrition diagnosis, they could say that at certain times there is no nutrition diagnosis. Ouellette adds that it might be a good idea to create a category of "potential" diagnostic labels that could be used for patients who are basically stable with tube feedings or dialysis, but who still need to be monitored.

While the PESS statement proved to be the most difficult hurdle, RDs also had to learn to be more specific when it came time to express how they would monitor and evaluate their patients. It wasn't enough to write "monitor labs," says Foust. "You need to give specific labs and then follow with an explanation and expected outcomes."

For managers, keeping morale of staff up was a challenge. This was especially true for RDs who spoke of feeling stifled by the new method and who constantly feared they were making a mistake. Managers learned they needed to spend extra time encouraging their RDs and reminding them that they were working on a cutting-edge project.

"All of my RDs are competent and brilliant," says Foust. "Changing the way they chart and implementing new techniques can cause doubt. This can potentially alter their clinical self-confidence, and you want to maintain a positive outlook to avoid this."

Both Foust and Ouellette say it was beneficial to work in groups on PESS statements and learn from each other, being sure to highlight well-written charts as well as the ones that that needed attention. Foust and Ouellette also learned that not every RD would learn at the same pace. While RDs who had been in the profession for a shorter amount of time were often able to grasp the concept faster, Ouellette adds that, in general, the RDs who had the easiest time were the ones with personality types that adjusted well to change, regardless of experience level.

ADVICE TO SITES READY FOR IMPLEMENTATION

Both Foust and Ouellette offer similar advice to sites seeking to implement the NCP and model. Both suggest an in-service for the staff and the distribution of materials well ahead of implementation. Ouellette also suggests providing training from a knowledgeable source, as was the case with Karen Lacey speaking to her staff using ADA slides describing the NCP.

Both managers suggest setting aside a generous portion of the weekly staff meeting time to discuss the model, review PESS statements, answer questions, and motivate the staff with positive feedback.

While Foust and Ouellette had different experiences in terms of seeking approval from the administration to implement the program, both suggest allowing time to meet with the necessary people in the facility, as the approval needed will differ from facility to facility.

Most of all, Ouellette and Foust suggest that future managers and staffs remind themselves that transitioning to the nutrition care model is a beneficial but time-consuming process that requires patience. Both say they have seen marked improvements among their staff over time, and many of the initial challenges have been overcome with patience and practice.

"You're changing the way you're thinking, you're changing the way you're charting—it's a huge change," says Ouellette. "There are no short-cuts you can take, but my staff is excited about being on the forefront. It's certainly a worthwhile thing."

Adds Foust, "This continues to be an excellent, groundbreaking experience."

The authors would like to acknowledge the contributions of the following people in the preparation of this article: Susan Ramsey, MS, RD, senior manager of medical nutrition services for Sodexho who also serves on ADA's Research Committee; Sylvia Escott-Stump, MA, RD, Standardized Language Task Force Chair; and Esther Myers, PhD, RD, FADA, ADA's Research and Scientific Affairs director.

References

1. American Dietetic Association Strategic Plan. Available at: http://www.eatright.org (member-only section). Accessed April 17, 2005.
2. Lacey K, Pritchett E. Nutrition Care Process and Model: ADA adopts road map to quality care and outcomes management. *J Am Diet Assoc.* 2003;103:1061-1072.

Resources

OF PROFESSIONAL INTEREST

TIMELINES OF IMPLEMENTATION

Virginia Hospital Center

December 2004
- Idea of participating in pilot project presented to facility.
- Staff in-service held to educate staff about the NCP, ADI charting, and PESS statements.
- Meetings between clinical nutrition manager and hospital administrators to discuss the NCP and seek approval for participation in the pilot project.

January 2005
- Hospital nutrition committee approves the pilot project.
- Other hospital administrators, including those on the unit where the first RD to participate in the project works, are informed of the pilot project.
- The hospital's patient-monitoring committee approves the pilot project.
- Throughout the month of January, the first RD to take part in the project meets regularly with clinical nutrition manager to practice ADI charting and PESS statements.
- Clinical nutrition manager obtains permission and modifies the Hakel-Smith Coding Instrument as a way of auditing charts.

February 2005
- From early to mid-February, the first RD to participate in the project charts using both the ADI and SOAP formats before formally transitioning to the ADI method alone on February 16.
- In late February, a second RD begins to exclusively use the ADI method of charting.

March 2005
- By the end of March, a third RD has transitioned to the ADI method of charting.
- Throughout the entire process, the clinical nutrition manager meets formally and informally with RDs both individually and in groups to discuss concerns and monitor progress.
- Throughout the process, at least 20 minutes of each weekly staff meeting are devoted to reviewing the ADI method of charting, PESS statements, questions, and concerns.

April 2005
- By the start of April, a fourth RD is exclusively using the ADI method of charting, with the fifth and final RD making the transition by mid-April.
- The clinical nutrition manager audits 10% of charts.

Veterans Affairs Medical Center, San Diego

January 2004
- Director of nutrition and food services distributes journal articles about the NCP to staff.

October 2004
- Two staff members attend the Nutrition Diagnosis Roundtable for Educators workshop at ADA's Food & Nutrition Conference & Expo and share what they learn with the rest of the staff upon their return.

November 2004
- A staff meeting is held to discuss questions and concerns surrounding the NCP and PESS statements.

December 2004
- ADA's Karen Lacey, Chair of ADA's Quality Management Working Group on the NCP, provides the staff with a workshop on the NCP.

February 2005
- The staff begins to devote time during each weekly staff meeting to practice using the new method and to share PESS statements.
- Several staff members, including the staff's performance improvement/information technology dietitian, develop a point-and-click computer version of the ADI template for the staff to use.

March 2005
- Toward the end of March, the staff spends 1 week using both the SOAP format and the new ADI template to chart notes.

April 2005
- On April 4, the staff officially implements the new method of charting exclusively.
- The deputy director of nutrition and food service checks each inpatient initial nutrition assessment chart note and provides feedback to individuals.

May 2005
- Ongoing auditing was accomplished by incorporating the auditing elements into the periodic performance review plan implemented to ensure continuous readiness for the Joint Commission on Accreditation of Healthcare Organization's review.

NUTRITION CARE PROCESS AND MODEL WORK GROUP

Karen Lacey, MS, RD, Chair
Elvira Johnson, MS, RD
Kessey Kieselhorst, MPA, RD
Mary Jane Oakland, PhD, RD, FADA
Carlene Russell, RD, FADA
Patricia Splett, PhD, RD, FADA
Staff Liaisons:
Harold Holler, RD
Esther Myers, PhD, RD, FADA
Ellen Pritchett, RD
Karri Looby, MS, RD

The work group would like to extend a special thank you to Marion Hammond, MS, and Naomi Trostler, PhD, RD, for their assistance in development of the NCP and Model.

STANDARDIZED LANGUAGE TASK FORCE

Sylvia Escott-Stump, MA, RD, Chair
Peter Beyer, MS, RD
Christina Biesemeier, MS, RD, FADA
Pam Charney, MS, RD
Marion Franz, MS, RD
Karen Lacey, MS, RD
Carrie LePeyre, RD
Kathleen Niedert, MBA, RD, FADA
Mary Jane Oakland, PhD, RD, FADA
Patricia Splett, PhD, MPH, RD
Frances Tyus, MS, RD

The task force would like to extend a special thank you to Naomi Trostler, PhD, RD, FADA.

Resources

SUBJECT: NUTRITION CONTROLLED VOCABULARY/TERMINOLOGY MAINTENANCE/REVIEW	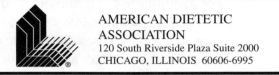 AMERICAN DIETETIC ASSOCIATION 120 South Riverside Plaza Suite 2000 CHICAGO, ILLINOIS 60606-6995

Effective Date: April 2005
Revision Date: December 2006
Review Date: December 2006

PURPOSE:

This policy establishes the process followed by the Nutrition Care Process/Standardized Language (NCP/SL) Committee to maintain a current Nutrition Care Process and list of nutrition controlled vocabulary terminology that document the Nutrition Care Process.

STRUCTURE:

The NCP/SL Committee is a joint House of Delegates and Board of Directors Committee and provides semi-annual reports to both bodies.

PROCEDURES:

The NCP/SL Committee accepts proposals for additions or modifications to the Nutrition Diagnosis, Intervention, and/or Monitoring and Evaluation terminology as follows:

1. Any individual ADA member or Dietetic Practice Group can submit proposals for modification or additions by submitting the following:
    a. Proposed terminology addition or modification letter
    b. Reference worksheet for proposed addition or modification
    c. Case example of when the additional or modified term will be used
2. For modifications or additions to the terminology, the NCP/SL will designate two committee members to review the submission to establish:
    a. Is the term already represented by an existing term?
        i. If yes, the new term can be added as a synonym for the existing term or replace the existing term.
        ii. If no, then the term can be considered for addition to the list of terms as long as it meets the need for describing elements of dietetics practice in the context of the nutrition care process.
    b. Does the term overlap with an existing term, but add new elements?
        i. If yes, then the existing term can be modified to include the new elements or the proposed term can be clarified to be distinctly different from the existing term through a dialogue with the proposal submitter.
        ii. If no, then consider adding new term
    c. Is the term distinct and separate from all existing terms?
        i. If yes, then ensure that the term is in the context of dietetics practice within the Nutrition Care Process and consider adding to list of terms.
        ii. If no, then work with proposal submitter to discuss how to integrate into existing terms or create a separate term.

Edition: 2008

3. For additions to the terminology, the NCP/SL will also ask the Research Committee to recommend a research expert to review the submission. Furthermore, a practitioner content expert can be added at the discretion of the NCP/SL Chair to review the submissions for either additions or modifications and establish the items noted above and:
   a. Is the content of the submission consistent with current practice and/or research in this practice area?
      i. If yes, then ensure that the term is in the context of dietetics practice within the Nutrition Care Process and consider adding to list of terms.
      ii. If no, then work with proposal submitter to discuss how to integrate into existing terms or create a separate term.
4. The reviewers will provide a recommendation for accepting (adding or modifying the terminology) or denying the submission to the NCP/SL committee at the routine face-to-face meetings or teleconferences.
5. The NCP/SL will prepare a summary of comments and one representative of the NCP/SL will confer with the proposal submitter after the initial discussion to answer questions and discuss the initial input from the NCP/SL Committee. If the proposal submitter is not satisfied with the direction proposed by the NCP/SL, then they will be invited to submit additional documentation and have time on the next teleconference/meeting agenda to personally present their concerns.
6. It is anticipated that an uncontested review will take approximately 6 months.
7. Changes or modifications accepted by the NCP/SL will be integrated into the Nutrition Diagnosis, Intervention, and/or Monitoring and Evaluation terminology that is published on an annual basis.

STAFFING:
Governance and Scientific Affairs and Research provide staff support for Research Committee functions.

ATTACHMENTS:
1. Letter template for proposing a **New Term** for Nutrition Diagnostic terminology
2. Letter template for proposing a **New Term** for Nutrition Intervention terminology
3. Letter template for proposing a **New Term** for Nutrition Monitoring and Evaluation terminology
4. Letter template for proposing **Modifications** to the Nutrition Diagnosis, Intervention, and/or Monitoring and Evaluation terminology
5. Template for reference sheet to support **additions/modifications** to Nutrition Diagnosis terminology
6. Template for reference sheet to support **additions/modifications** to Nutrition Intervention terminology
7. Template for reference sheet to support **additions/modifications** to the Nutrition Monitoring and Evaluation terminology

SUBJECT: NUTRITION CONTROLLED VOCABULARY/TERMINOLOGY MAINTENANCE/REVIEW

Attachment 1: Letter Template for Proposing **New Term** for **Nutrition Diagnostic Terminology**

Date: _____

To:　　NCP/SL Committee
　　　　Scientific Affairs and Research
　　　　American Dietetic Association
　　　　120 South Riverside Plaza, Suite 2000
　　　　Chicago, IL 60606-6995
　　　　emyers@eatright.org; lornstein@eatright.org

Subject:　Proposed **Addition** to **Nutrition Diagnostic Terminology**

(I/We) would like to propose a new term, _____ (Proposed term to add to the Nutrition Diagnostic Terminology list). The reason I/we believe that this term should be added is as follows: (insert concise rationale for change and may include brief example of when the situation arose that the current term was inadequately defined)

1. (Insert first statement of rationale.)
2. (Insert second statement of rationale, if applicable.)
3. (Insert example of situation where this modification was needed.)

Other terms that are similar with explanations of why they do not exactly match our new proposed term are as follows:

1. (Insert term.) – (Insert 2-3 sentences to illustrate why the existing term does not meet your need.)
2. (Insert term.) – (Insert 2-3 sentences to illustrate why the existing term does not meet your need)
3. (Add as many as applicable.)

Attached is the a reference sheet that includes the label name, proposed domain and category, definition, examples of etiologies and signs and symptoms, references, and a case that illustrates when this term would be used and the corresponding PES statement that would be used in medical record documentation.

The point of contact for this proposal is _____ (insert name), who can be reached at _____ (best contact telephone number) and _____ (e-mail address).

Thank you for considering our request.

Signature block

(Organizational unit if applicable)

Attachments: (1) Completed Reference Sheet, (2) Case

Edition: 2008

**SUBJECT: NUTRITION CONTROLLED VOCABULARY/TERMINOLOGY
MAINTENANCE/REVIEW**

Attachment 2: Letter Template for Proposing **New Term** for **Nutrition Intervention Terminology**

Date: _____

To: NCP/SL Committee
        Scientific Affairs and Research
        American Dietetic Association
        120 South Riverside Plaza, Suite 2000
        Chicago, IL 60606-6995
        emyers@eatright.org; lornstein@eatright.org

Subject: Proposed **Addition** to **Nutrition Intervention Terminology**

(I/We) would like to propose a new term, _____ (Proposed term to add
to the Nutrition Intervention Terminology list). The reason I/we believe that this term should
be added is as follows: (insert concise rationale for change and may include brief example of
when the situation arose that the current term was inadequately defined)
   1. (Insert first statement of rationale.)
   2. (Insert second statement of rationale, if applicable.)
   3. (Insert example of situation where this modification was needed.)

Other terms that are similar with explanations of why they do not exactly match our new
proposed term are as follows:
   1. (Insert term.) – (Insert 2-3 sentences to illustrate why the existing term does not meet
       your need.)
   2. (Insert term.) – (Insert 2-3 sentences to illustrate why the existing term does not meet
       your need)
   3. (Add as many as applicable.)

Attached is the a reference sheet that includes the label name, proposed domain, definition,
details of the nutrition intervention, nutrition diagnostic terminology with which it is
typically used, other considerations, and references, <u>and</u> a case that illustrates when this term
would be used.

The point of contact for this proposal is _____ (insert
name), who can be reached at _____ (best contact telephone number) and
_____ (e-mail address).

Thank you for considering our request.

Signature block
(Organizational unit if applicable)

Attachments: (1) Completed Reference Sheet, (2) Case

SUBJECT: NUTRITION CONTROLLED VOCABULARY/TERMINOLOGY MAINTENANCE/REVIEW

Attachment 3: Letter Template for Proposing **New Term for Nutrition Monitoring and Evaluation Terminology**

Date: _____

To: NCP/SL Committee
        Scientific Affairs and Research
        American Dietetic Association
        120 South Riverside Plaza, Suite 2000
        Chicago, IL 60606-6995
        emyers@eatright.org; lornstein@eatright.org

Subject: Proposed **Addition** to **Nutrition Monitoring and Evaluation Terminology**

(I/We) would like to propose a new term, _____ (Proposed term to add to the Nutrition Monitoring and Evaluation Terminology list). The reason I/we believe that this term should be added is as follows: (insert concise rationale for change and may include brief example of when the situation arose that the current term was inadequately defined)
  4. (Insert first statement of rationale.)
  5. (Insert second statement of rationale, if applicable.)
  6. (Insert example of situation where this addition was needed.)

Other terms that are similar with explanations of why they do not exactly match our new proposed term are as follows:
  4. (Insert term) – (Insert 2-3 sentences to illustrate why the existing term does not meet your need.)
  5. (Insert term) – (Insert 2-3 sentences to illustrate why the existing term does not meet your need)
  6. (Add as many as applicable.)

Attached is a reference sheet that includes the outcome label, domain, label definition, potential indicators, data sources, nutrition interventions and diagnoses with which it is typically used, evaluation criteria (goal/reference standard), patient/client example, and a case that illustrates when this term would be used.

The point of contact for this proposal is _____ (insert name), who can be reached at _____ (best contact telephone number) and _____ (e-mail address).

Thank you for considering our request.

Signature block
(Organizational unit if applicable)

Attachments: (1) Completed Reference Sheet, (2) Case

Edition: 2008

Attachment 4: Letter Template for Proposing **Modifications** to the Nutrition Diagnosis, Intervention, or Monitoring and Evaluation Terminology

Date: _____

To: NCP/SL Committee
        Scientific Affairs and Research
        American Dietetic Association
        120 South Riverside Plaza, Suite 2000
        Chicago, IL 60606-6995
        emyers@eatright.org; lornstein@eatright.org

Subject: Proposed **Modification** to an existing term in Nutrition Diagnosis, Intervention, or Monitoring and Evaluation Terminology

(I/We) would like to propose a modification of the term, _____ (insert Number and Name from current Nutrition Diagnosis, Intervention, or Monitoring and Evaluation Terminology lists). The reason I/we believe that this term should be modified is as follows (insert concise rationale for change and may include brief example of when the situation arose that the current term was inadequately defined):
    1. (Insert first statement of rationale.)
    2. (Insert second statement of rationale, if applicable.)
    3. (Insert example of situation where this modification was needed.)

Attached is the revised Nutrition Diagnosis, Intervention, or Monitoring and Evaluation Terminology reference sheet that shows the changes highlighted or bolded for your consideration. Attached is also a case that illustrates when the modified term would be used.

The point of contact for this proposal is _____ (insert name), who can be reached at _____ (best contact telephone number) and _____ (e-mail address).

Thank you for considering our request.

Signature block
(Organizational unit if applicable)

Attachments: (1) Modified Reference Sheet, (2) Case

SUBJECT: NUTRITION CONTROLLED VOCABULARY/TERMINOLOGY MAINTENANCE/REVIEW

Attachment 5: Template for Reference Sheet to support **additions/modifications** to Nutrition Diagnostic Terminology

DOMAIN
(Intake, Clinical or Behavioral-Environmental)

Category
(e.g., Functional Balance)

Nutrition Diagnostic Label (Leave number blank)
(Insert 1- to 4-word label)

Definition
(Insert 1 sentence that describes the intent of the label)

Etiology (Cause/Contributing Risk Factors)
Factors gathered during the nutrition assessment process that contribute to the existence of or the maintenance of pathophysiological, psychosocial, situational, developmental, cultural, and/or environmental problems.

- (Insert common etiologies for Nutrition Diagnostic Label)

Signs/Symptoms (Defining Characteristics)
A typical cluster of subjective and objective signs and symptoms gathered during the nutrition assessment process that provide evidence that a problem exists; quantify the problem and describe its severity.

Nutrition Assessment Category	Potential Indicators of this Nutrition Diagnosis (one or more must be present)
Biochemical Data, Medical Tests and Procedures	• (Insert as appropriate)
Anthropometric Measurements	• (Insert as appropriate)
Physical Exam Findings	• (Insert as appropriate)
Food/Nutrition History	• (Insert as appropriate)
Client History	• (Insert as appropriate)

References
(Cite references)

Edition: 2008

SUBJECT: NUTRITION CONTROLLED VOCABULARY/TERMINOLOGY MAINTENANCE/REVIEW

Attachment 6: Template for Reference Sheet to support **additions/modifications** to Nutrition Intervention Terminology

---

Nutrition Intervention Label (Leave number blank)

(Insert 1- to 4-word label)

DOMAIN

(Food and/or Nutrient Delivery, Nutrition Education, Nutrition Counseling, or Coordination of Nutrition Care)

Definition

(Insert 1 sentence that describes the intent of the label)

Details of Intervention

A typical intervention might be further described related the following details.

- Insert as appropriate

Typically used with the following

Nutrition Diagnostic Terminology Used in PES Statements	Common Examples (Not intended to be inclusive)
Nutrition Diagnoses	• (Insert as appropriate)
Etiology	• (Insert as appropriate)
Signs and Symptoms	• (Insert as appropriate)

Other considerations (*e.g., patient/client negotiation, patient/client needs and desires, readiness to change*)

List other considerations

References

(Cite references)

Attachment 7: Template for Reference Sheet to support **additions/modifications** to Nutrition Monitoring and Evaluation Terminology

Nutrition Monitoring and Intervention Outcome Label (Leave number blank)
(Insert 1- to 4-word label)

DOMAIN
(Nutrition-Related Behavioral and Environmental Outcomes, Food and Nutrient Intake Outcomes, Nutrition-Related Physical Sign and Symptom Outcomes, Nutrition-Related Patient/Client-Centered Outcomes)

Definition: (Insert 1 sentence that describes the intent of the outcome label)
Monitoring:

Potential Indicators

(Insert as appropriate)
(Insert as appropriate)
(Insert as appropriate)
(Insert as appropriate)

Examples of the measurement methods or data sources for these outcome indicators: (Insert)

Typically used to measure the outcomes for the following domains of nutrition interventions: (Insert)

Typically used to monitor and evaluate change in the following nutrition diagnoses: (Insert)

Evaluation:

Criteria for evaluation:

Comparison to Goal or Reference Standard:

1) Goal (tailored to patient/client needs)
OR
2) Reference standard

(Continued on next page)

Edition: 2008

Attachment 7: Template for Reference Sheet to support **additions/modifications** to Nutrition Monitoring and Evaluation Terminology

Patient/Client Example:

Indicator(s) selected:
> (Insert as appropriate)
> (Insert as appropriate)

Criteria for evaluation:

Comparison to Goal or Reference Standard:
> 1) Goal: (Insert)
>
> OR
>
> 2) Reference standard: (Insert)

Sample monitoring and evaluation documentation for this outcome:

Initial encounter with patient/client	(Insert)
Re-assessment after nutrition intervention	(Insert)

References
(Cite references)

Standardized Language Task Force and Terminology Expert Reviewers

Standardized Language Task Force

Chair
Annalynn Skipper, PhD, RD, FADA
Task Force Member 2005-2007

Vice Chair
Nancy Lewis, PhD, RD, FADA
Task Force Member 2005-2007

Judy Beto, PhD, RD, LD, FADA
Task Force Member 2006-2007

Pam Charney, PhD, RD, CNSD
Task Force Member 2003-2007

Claudia A. Conkin, MS RD LD
Task Force Member 2006-2007

Susan Cowen, MS, RD, CSP
Task Force Member 2006

Mary Russell, MS, RD, LDN, CNSD
Task Force Member 2005-2007

Patricia Splett, PhD, MPH, RD
Task Force Past Chair and Member 2003-2007

Donna A Israel, PhD, RD, LD, LPC, FADA
Task Force Member 2005-2007

Elise Smith, MA, RD, LD
Task Force Member 2006-2007

Joanne Shearer, MS, RD, CDE, LN
Ex-Officio/QM Committee
Task Force Member 2005-2007

Kristy Hendricks, DSc, RD
Ex-Officio/Research Committee
Task Force Member 2005-2007

Kathleen Rourke, PhD, RD, RN, CHES
Ex-Officio/BOD
Task Force Member 2006-2007

Standardized Language Task Force Past Members and Contributors

Peter Beyer, MS, RD, LD
Task Force Member 2003-2006

Christina Biesemeier, MS, RD, LDN, FADA
Task Force Member 2003-2005

Sylvia Escott-Stump, MA, RD, LDN
Task Force Past Chair and Member 2003-2006

Marion Franz, MS, RD, CDE
Task Force Member 2003-2005

Trisha Fuhrman, MS, RD, LD, FADA, CNSD
Task Force Member 2005-2006

Karen Lacey, MS, RD, CD
Task Force Member 2003-2005

Robin Leonhardt, RD
Attended Face-to-Face Meeting in Summer 2003

Kathleen Niedert, MBA, RD, LD, FADA
Task Force Member 2003-2005

Mary Jane Oakland, PhD, RD, LD, FADA
Task Force Member 2003-2006

Frances Tyus, MS, RD, LD
Task Force Member 2003-2005

Naomi Trostler, PhD, RD
Task Force Member 2004-2005

Staff Liaisons
Esther Myers, PhD, RD, FADA
Director of Scientific Affairs and Research
American Dietetic Association
E-mail: emyers@eatright.org

Kay B. Howarter, MS, RD, LD
Senior Research Manager, Evidence Analysis Library
American Dietetic Association
E-mail: khowarter@eatright.org

Pam Michael, MBA, RD
Director, Nutrition Services Coverage Team
American Dietetic Association
E-Mail: pmichael@eatright.org

Lt Col Vivian Hutson, MA, MHA, RD, LD, FACHE
Staff Liaison 2003-2004

Ellen Pritchett, RD, CPHQ
Staff Liaison 2003-2005

Major Kim Thomsen, MA, MHA, RD, LD, CHE
Staff Liaison 2005-2006

Consultants
Melinda L. Jenkins, PhD, FNP
Donna G. Pertel, MEd, RD
Annalynn Skipper, PhD, RD, FADA
Joanne M. Spahn, MS, RD, FADA

Edition: 2008

Standardized Language Task Force and Terminology Expert Reviewers

Expert Reviewers

Nutrition Diagnosis Terminology

Keith-Thomas Ayoob, PhD, RD (Albert Einstein)	Kenneth Kudsk, MD (University of Wisconsin)
Charlette R. Gallagher Allred, PhD, RD (Retired-Ross Labs)	Johanna Lappe, PhD, RN (Creighton University)
Katherine Beals, PhD, RD (Industry, formerly Ball State)	Don Layman, PhD (University of Illinois-Champaign)
Jeannmarie Beiseigel, PhD, RD (USDA)	Edith Lerner, PhD (Case Western Reserve University)
Carol Braunschweig, PhD, RD (University of Illinois, Chicago)	Nancy Lewis, PhD, RD (University of Nebraska-Lincoln)
Larry Cheskin, MD (Johns Hopkins)	Alice Lichtenstein, DSc (Tufts)
Mary Cluskey, PhD, RD (Oregon State)	Melinda Manore, PhD, RD (Oregon State)
Kathy Cobb, MS, RD (Centers for Disease Control)	Judith Marlett, PhD, RD (University of Wisconsin)
Wendy Mueller Cunnigham, PhD, RD (Cal State)	Joel Mason, MD (Tufts)
Anne Daly, MS, RD, BC-ADM, CDE (Springfield, IL)	Laura Matarese, MS, RD, CNSD (Cleveland Clinic)
Linda Delahanty, MS, RD (Harvard)	Rebecca Mullis, PhD, RD (Georgia)
Johanna Dwyer, DSc, RD (Tufts)	Maureen A. Murtaugh, PhD, RD (University of Utah)
Joan Fischer, PhD, RD (University of Georgia)	Eileen Stellefson Myers, PhD, RD (Private practice)
Trisha Fuhrman, MS, RD (Coram Healthcare)	Ellen Parham, PhD, RD (Northern Illinois University)
Emily Gier, MS, RD (Cornell)	Kristina Penniston, PhD, RD (University of Wisconsin)
Leah Graves, MS, RD (Saint Francis Hospital, Tulsa, OK)	Maggie Powers, MS, RD, CDE (International Diabetes Center)
Geoffrey Greene, PhD, RD (University of Rhode Island)	Marla Reicks, PhD, RD (University of MN)
Ann Grandjean, EdD, RD (International Center for Sports Nutrition)	Denise Baird Schwartz, MS, RD, CNSD (Clinical practice)
Janice Harris, PhD, RD (University of Kansas)	Moshe Shike, MD (Memorial Sloan Kettering)
Celia Hayes, MS, RD (HRSA)	Annalynn Skipper, PhD, RD, FADA (Nutrition Consultant)
Bob Heaney, MD (Creighton University)	Joanne Slavin, PhD, RD (University of Minnesota)
Jim Hill, MD (University of Colorado)	Helen Smiciklas-Wright, PhD, RD (Penn State)
Andrea Hutchins, PhD, RD (Arizona State University East, Mesa, AZ)	Bonnie Spear, PhD, RD (University of Alabama, Birmingham
Elizabeth Jeffery, PhD (University of Illinois, Champaign)	Riva Touger-Decker, PhD, RD (UMDNJ)
Elvira Johnson, MS, RD (Private practice)	Linda A. Vaughan, PhD, RD (Arizona State University)
Sondra King, PhD, RD (Northern Illinois University)	Jody Vogelzang, MS, RD, LD, CD, FADA (Texas Women's University)
Joel Kopple, MD (UCLA)	Anne Voss, PhD, RD (Ross Labs)
Jessica Krenkel, MS, RD (University of Nevada)	Jonathan Waitman, MD (Cornell)
Molly Kretsch, PhD, RD (USDA)	Lyn Wheeler, MS, RD, CD, FADA, CDE (Indiana University School of Medicine)
Penny Kris-Etherton, PhD, RD (Penn State)	Robert Wolfe, PhD (University of Texas)
Laurie A. Kruzich, MS, RD (Iowa State)	Allison Yates, PhD, RD (Industry, formerly Director of the IOM Food and Nutrition Board)

Standardized Language Task Force and Terminology Expert Reviewers

Expert Reviewers

Nutrition Intervention Terminology

Rene Brand, RD, LN (Rapid City Regional Hospital)	Tay Kennedy, PhD, RD (Oklahoma State University)
Nicole Clark, MS, RD, CDE, LDN (University of Indiana of Pennsylvania)	Kathy Keim, PhD, RD, LDN (Rush University Medical Center)
Marion J Franz, MS, RD, CDE (International Diabetes Center)	Molly Kellogg, RD, LCSW (Psychotherapist, Nutrition Therapist & Writer)
Shirley Gerrior, PhD, RD, LD (USDA)	Ida Laquatra, PhD, RD (H.J. Heinz Company)
Laura Graney, MS, RD, CD (Sheboygan County WI, Health. and Human Services)	Kathleen C. Niedert, MBA, CSG, RD, LD, FADA (Principal, Omega Health Associates Iowa)
Joanne Guthrie, PhD, RD (USDA)	Mary Ellen E. Posthauer, RD, CD, LD (Supreme Care West, Inc.)
Mary Hise, PhD, RD (University of Kansas Medical Center)	Rebecca S. Reeves, D.Ph., R.D., FADA (Baylor College of Medicine, Houston)
Carol Ireton-Jones, PhD, RD, LD, CNSD (Coram, Inc)	Linda G. Snetselaar, PhD, RD (University of Iowa)

Expert Reviewers

Nutrition Monitoring and Evaluation Terminology

Barbara Ainsworth, PhD, MPH (Arizona State University)	David Holben, PhD, RD (Ohio University)
Judith Barr, MEd, ScD (Northeastern University)	Maddy Houghton, PhD, RD (University of Idaho)
Janet Beary, PhD, RD (Washington State University)	Wanda Howell PhD,RD (University of Arizona)
Jackie Boucher, MS, RD, CDE (Health Partners, Minneapolis, MN)	Ashima Kant, PhD, RD (SUNY Queens)
Catherine Christie, PhD, RD, LD/N, FADA (University of North Florida)	Kendra Kattelmann, PhD, RD (South Dakota State)
Mary Cluskey, PhD, RD, LD (Oregon State University)	Kathy Keim, PhD, RD, LDN (Rush University Medical Center)
Charlene Compher, PhD, RD, FADA, CNSD (University of Pennsylvania, Philadelphia)	Jana Kicklighter, PhD, RD (University of Georgia)
Martha Sue Dale, MAg, RD/LDN (University of Florida, Gainesville)	Penny M. Kris-Etherton, PhD, RD (The Pennsylvania State University)
Judy Driskell, PhD, RD (University of Nebraska)	Laurie Kruzich, MS, RD (Iowa State)
David Frankenfield, MS, RD, CNSD (The Pennsyvania State University)	Susan Kynast-Gales, PhD, RD (Washington State)
Marion J. Franz, MS, RD, CDE (Nutrition Concepts by Franz, Inc., Minneapolis, MN)	Tami J. Mackle, MS, RD (UMDNJ)
Susan Fullmer, PhD, RD (Brigham Young)	Mary Marian, MS,RD (University of Arizona)
Karen Glanz, PhD, MPH (Emory University)	Melinda Maryniuk, MEd, RD (Harvard University)
Mary Gregoire, PhD, RD (Rush University Medical Center)	Linda Massey PhD, RD (Washington State)
Amy E. Griel, PhD (The Pennsylvania State University)	Nancy Nevin-Folino, MEd, RD, CSP, FADA (Children's Medical Center Dayton)
Linda Griffith, PhD, RD (University of Kansas)	Kathleen C. Niedert, MBA, CSG, RD, LD, FADA (Principal, Omega Health Associates Iowa)
Kathy Hammond, MS, RN, RD, LD, CNSD (Chartwell, Inc., Sharpsburg, GA)	Sandy Procter, PhD, RD (Kansas State University)
Joan Heins, MA, RD, CDE (Washington University, St Louis, MO)	Michelle Rockwell, MS, RD (Sports Nutrition Consultant)

Edition: 2008

Standardized Language Task Force and Terminology Expert Reviewers

Expert Reviewers

Nutrition Monitoring and Evaluation Terminology, continued

Nancy Rodriguez, PhD, RD (University of Connecticut)	Mary Story PhD, RD (University of Minnesota)
Carlene Russell, MS, RD, LD (Iowa Department of Elder Affairs)	Diane Sowa, MS, RD (Rush University Medical Center)
Linda Snetselaar, PhD, RD (University of Iowa)	Joy Winzerling PhD, RD (University of Arizona)
Bonnie Spear, PhD, RD (University of Alabama Birmingham)	Judith Wylie–Rosett, EdD, RD (Albert Einstein College of Medicine)
Jamie Stang, PhD, RD (University of Minnesota)	

Additional Reviewers

Linda Roberts and Associates, Wheaton IL
Registered Dietitians at Malcolm Grow USAF Medical Center, Washington, DC
Registered Dietitians at Rush Medical Center, Chicago, IL
Registered Dietitians at US Dewitt Army Hospital, Fort Belvoir, VA
Registered Dietitians at USDA Women's Infants and Children, Washington DC
Registered Dietitians at Walter Reed Medical Center, Washington, DC

FEEDBACK FORM

Name: _____

Book: _____

Publication year: _____

Please provide feedback on the revisions you would suggest to the next edition of the *International Dietetics and Nutrition Terminology (IDNT) Reference Manual: Standardized Language for the Nutrition Care Process, First Edition*. Please indicate whether each section should be included and identify what questions you would like answered in the next edition as well as additional materials that you would find helpful.

The following items should be included in the next edition:

Please Check

	YES	NO

Nutrition Care Process Summary

	YES	NO

Step 1: Nutrition Assessment *SNAPshot*
Introduction
Matrix

Step 2: Nutrition Diagnosis *SNAPshot*
Introduction
Terminology
Terms and Definitions
Reference Sheets

Step 3: Nutrition Intervention *SNAPshot*
Introduction
Terminology
Terms and Definitions
Reference Sheets

Step 4: Nutrition Monitoring and Evaluation *SNAPshot*
Introduction
Terminology
Terms and Definitions
Reference Sheets

Bibliography
Other _____

What questions would you like answered in the next edition?

What additional materials would be helpful in the next edition?

Please mail form or e-mail information to: Scientific Affairs and Research, American Dietetic Association, Nutrition Care Process/Standardized Language Committee, 120 South Riverside Plaza, Suite 2000, Chicago, IL 60606-6995. emyers@eatright.org; lornstein@eatright.org

Edition: 2008

INTAKE NI

Defined as "actual problems related to intake of energy, nutrients, fluids, bioactive substances through oral diet or nutrition support"

Energy Balance (1)

Defined as "actual or estimated changes in energy (kcal)" balance

❏ Unused	NI-1.1
❏ Increased energy expenditure	NI-1.2
❏ Unused	NI-1.3
❏ Inadequate energy intake	NI-1.4
❏ Excessive energy intake	NI-1.5

Oral or Nutrition Support Intake (2)

Defined as "actual or estimated food and beverage intake from oral diet or nutrition support compared with patient goal"

❏ Inadequate oral food/beverage intake	NI-2.1
❏ Excessive oral food/beverage intake	NI-2.2
❏ Inadequate intake from enteral/parenteral nutrition	NI-2.3
❏ Excessive intake from enteral/parenteral nutrition	NI-2.4
❏ Inappropriate infusion of enteral/parenteral nutrition (use with caution)	NI-2.5

Fluid Intake (3)

Defined as "actual or estimated fluid intake compared with patient goal"

❏ Inadequate fluid intake	NI-3.1
❏ Excessive fluid intake	NI-3.2

Bioactive Substances (4)

Defined as "actual or observed intake of bioactive substances, including single or multiple functional food components, ingredients, dietary supplements, alcohol"

❏ Inadequate bioactive substance intake	NI-4.1
❏ Excessive bioactive substance intake	NI-4.2
❏ Excessive alcohol intake	NI-4.3

Nutrient (5)

Defined as "actual or estimated intake of specific nutrient groups or single nutrients as compared with desired levels"

❏ Increased nutrient needs (specify)	NI-5.1
❏ Evident protein-energy malnutrition	NI-5.2
❏ Inadequate protein-energy intake	NI-5.3
❏ Decreased nutrient needs (specify)	NI-5.4
❏ Imbalance of nutrients	NI-5.5

Fat and Cholesterol (5.6)

❏ Inadequate fat intake	NI-5.6.1
❏ Excessive fat intake	NI-5.6.2
❏ Inappropriate intake of food fats (specify)	NI-5.6.3

Protein (5.7)

❏ Inadequate protein intake	NI-5.7.1
❏ Excessive protein intake	NI-5.7.2
❏ Inappropriate intake of amino acids (specify)	NI-5.7.3

Carbohydrate and Fiber (5.8)

❏ Inadequate carbohydrate intake	NI-5.8.1
❏ Excessive carbohydrate intake	NI-5.8.2
❏ Inappropriate intake of types of carbohydrate (specify)	NI-5.8.3
❏ Inconsistent carbohydrate intake	NI-5.8.4
❏ Inadequate fiber intake	NI-5.8.5
❏ Excessive fiber intake	NI-5.8.6

Vitamin (5.9)

❏ Inadequate vitamin intake	NI-5.9.1
❏ Excessive vitamin intake	NI-5.9.2

(specify)
❏ A   ❏ C
❏ Thiamin   ❏ D
❏ Riboflavin ❏ E
❏ Niacin   ❏ K
❏ Folate   ❏ Other

Mineral (5.10)

❏ Inadequate mineral intake (specify)	NI-5.10.1

❏ Calcium   ❏ Iron
❏ Potassium ❏ Zinc
❏ Other

❏ Excessive mineral intake (specify)	NI-5.10.2

❏ Calcium   ❏ Iron
❏ Potassium ❏ Zinc
❏ Other

CLINICAL NC

Defined as "nutritional findings/problems identified that relate to medical or physical conditions."

Functional (1)

Defined as "change in physical or mechanical functioning that interferes with or prevents desired nutritional consequences."

❏ Swallowing difficulty	NC-1.1
❏ Chewing (masticatory) difficulty	NC-1.2
❏ Breastfeeding difficulty	NC-1.3
❏ Altered GI function	NC-1.4

Biochemical (2)

Defined as "change in capacity to metabolize nutrients as a result of medications, surgery, or as indicated by altered lab values."

❏ Impaired nutrient utilization	NC-2.1
❏ Altered nutrition-related laboratory values	NC-2.2
❏ Food-medication interaction (specify)	NC-2.3

Weight (3)

Defined as "chronic weight or changed weight status when compared with usual or desired body weight."

❏ Underweight	NC-3.1
❏ Involuntary weight loss	NC-3.2
❏ Overweight/obesity	NC-3.3
❏ Involuntary weight gain	NC-3.4

BEHAVIORAL-ENVIRONMENTAL NB

Defined as "nutritional findings/problems identified that relate to knowledge, attitudes/beliefs, physical environment, access to food, or food safety."

Knowledge and Beliefs (1)

Defined as "actual knowledge and beliefs as observed or documented"

❏ Food- and nutrition-related knowledge deficit	NB-1.1
❏ Harmful beliefs/attitudes about food- or nutrition-related topics (use with caution)	NB-1.2
❏ Not ready for diet/lifestyle change	NB-1.3
❏ Self-monitoring deficit	NB-1.4
❏ Disordered eating pattern	NB-1.5
❏ Limited adherence to nutrition-related recommendations	NB-1.6
❏ Undesirable food choices	NB-1.7

Physical Activity and Function (2)

Defined as "actual physical activity, self-care, and quality-of-life problems as reported, observed, or documented."

❏ Physical inactivity	NB-2.1
❏ Excessive exercise	NB-2.2
❏ Inability or lack of desire to manage self-care	NB-2.3
❏ Impaired ability to prepare foods/meals	NB-2.4
❏ Poor nutrition quality of life	NB-2.5
❏ Self-feeding difficulty	NB-2.6

Food Safety and Access (3)

Defined as "actual problems with food access or food safety"

❏ Intake of unsafe food	NB-3.1
❏ Limited access to food	NB-3.2

Edition: 2008

NUTRITION COUNSELING C

Theoretical Basis/Approach (1)

The theories or models used to design and implement an intervention.

- □ Cognitive-Behavioral Theory — C-1.2
- □ Health Belief Model — C-1.3
- □ Social Learning Theory — C-1.4
- □ Transtheoretical Model/Stages of Change — C-1.5
- □ Other — C-1.6
  (specify) _____

Strategies (2)

Selectively applied evidence-based methods or plans of action designed to achieve a particular goal.

- □ Motivational interviewing — C-2.1
- □ Goal setting — C-2.2
- □ Self-monitoring — C-2.3
- □ Problem solving — C-2.4
- □ Social support — C-2.5
- □ Stress management — C-2.6
- □ Stimulus control — C-2.7
- □ Cognitive restructuring — C-2.8
- □ Relapse prevention — C-2.9
- □ Rewards/contingency management — C-2.10
- □ Other — (specify) _____

COORDINATION OF NUTRITION CARE RC

Coordination of Other Care During Nutrition Care (1)

Facilitating services with other professionals, institutions, or agencies during nutrition care.

- □ Team meeting — RC-1.1
- □ Referral to RD with different expertise — RC-1.2
- □ Collaboration/referral to other providers — RC-1.3
- □ Referral to community agencies/programs — RC-1.4
  (specify) _____

Discharge and Transfer of Nutrition Care to New Setting or Provider (2)

Discharge planning and transfer of nutrition care from one level or location of care to another.

- □ Collaboration/referral to otherProviders — RC-2.1
- □ Referral to community agencies/programs — RC-2.2
  (specify) _____

Feeding Environment (5)

Adjustment of the factors where food is served that impact food consumption.

- □ Lighting — ND-5.1
- □ Odors — ND-5.2
- □ Distractions — ND-5.3
- □ Table height — ND-5.4
- □ Table service/set up — ND-5.5
- □ Room temperature — ND-5.6
- □ Other — ND-5.7
  (specify) _____

Nutrition-Related Medication Management (6)

Modification of a drug or herbal to optimize patient/client nutritional or health status.

- □ Initiate — ND-6.1
- □ Dose change — ND-6.2
- □ Form change — ND-6.3
- □ Route change — ND-6.4
- □ Administration schedule — ND-6.5
- □ Discontinue — ND-6.6
  (specify) _____

NUTRITION EDUCATION E

Initial/Brief Nutrition Education (1)

Build or reinforce basic or essential nutrition-related knowledge.

- □ Purpose of the nutrition education — E-1.1
- □ Priority modifications — E-1.2
- □ Survival information — E-1.3
- □ Other — E-1.4
  (specify) _____

Comprehensive Nutrition Education (2)

Instruction or training leading to in-depth nutrition-related knowledge or skills.

- □ Purpose of the nutrition education — E-2.1
- □ Recommended modifications — E-2.2
- □ Advanced or related topics — E-2.3
- □ Result interpretation — E-2.4
- □ Skill development — E-2.5
- □ Other — E-2.6
  (specify) _____

FOOD AND/OR NUTRIENT DELIVERY ND

Meal and Snacks (1)

Regular eating event (meal); food served between regular meals (snack).

- □ General/healthful diet — ND-1.1
- □ Modify distribution, type, or amount of food and nutrients within meals or at specified time — ND-1.2
- □ Specific foods/beverages or groups — ND-1.3
- □ Other — ND-1.4
  (specify) _____

Enteral and Parenteral Nutrition (2)

Nutrition provided through the GI tract via tube, catheter, or stoma (enteral) or intravenously (centrally or peripherally) (parenteral).

- □ Initiate EN or PN — ND-2.1
- □ Modify rate, concentration, composition or schedule — ND-2.2
- □ Discontinue EN or PN — ND-2.3
- □ Insert enteral feeding tube — ND-2.4
- □ Site care — ND-2.5
- □ Other — ND-2.6
  (specify) _____

Supplements (3)

Medical Food Supplements (3.1)

Commercial or prepared foods or beverages that supplement energy, protein, carbohydrate, fiber, fat intake.

Type
- □ Commercial beverage — ND-3.1.1
- □ Commercial food — ND-3.1.2
- □ Modified beverage — ND-3.1.3
- □ Modified food — ND-3.1.4
- □ Purpose — ND-3.1.5
  (specify) _____

Vitamin and Mineral Supplements (3.2)

Supplemental vitamins or minerals.

- □ Multivitamin/mineral — ND-3.2.1
- □ Multi-trace elements — ND-3.2.2
- □ Vitamin — ND-3.2.3
  - □ A   □ Riboflavin
  - □ C   □ Niacin
  - □ D   □ Folate
  - □ E   □ B6
  - □ K   □ B12
  - □ Thiamin
  - □ Other (specify) _____
- □ Mineral — ND-3.2.4
  - □ Calcium   □ Phosphorus
  - □ Iron   □ Potassium
  - □ Magnesium   □ Zinc
  - □ Other (specify) _____

Bioactive Substance Supplement (3.3)

Supplemental bioactive substances.

- □ Initiate — ND-3.3.1
- □ Dose change — ND-3.3.2
- □ Form change — ND-3.3.3
- □ Route change — ND-3.3.4
- □ Administration schedule — ND-3.3.5
- □ Discontinue — ND-3.3.6
  (specify) _____

Feeding Assistance (4)

Accommodation or assistance in eating.

- □ Adaptive equipment — ND-4.1
- □ Feeding position — ND-4.2
- □ Meal set-up — ND-4.3
- □ Mouth care — ND-4.4
- □ Other (specify) — ND-4.5
  (specify) _____

Edition: 2008

Food and Beverage (2)
Foods and food groups and fluids from all sources, e.g., food, beverages, supplements.

Fluid/Beverage intake (2.1)
❑ Oral Fluids Amounts (*water, coffee/tea, juice, milk, soda*)   FI-2.1.1
❑ Food derived fluids   FI-2.1.2
❑ IV Fluids   FI-2.1.3
❑ Liquid meal replacement   FI-2.1.4

Food intake (2.2)
❑ Food variety   FI-2.2.1
❑ Number of food group servings   FI-2.2.2
  (*grains, fruits, vegetables, milk/dairy, meat/protein substitutes*)
❑ Healthy Eating Index   FI-2.2.3
❑ Children's Diet Quality Index   FI-2.2.4
❑ Revised Children's Diet Quality Index   FI-2.2.5

Enteral and Parenteral (3)
Specialized nutrition support intake from all sources, e.g., enteral and parenteral routes.

Enteral/parenteral nutrition intake (3.1)
❑ Access   FI-3.1.1
❑ Formula/solution   FI-3.1.2
❑ Discontinuation   FI-3.1.3
❑ Initiation   FI-3.1.4
❑ Rate/schedule   FI-3.1.5

Bioactive Substances (4)
Alcohol, plant stanol and sterol esters, soy protein, psyllium and β-glucan, and caffeine intake from all sources, e.g., food, beverages, supplements, and via enteral and parenteral routes.

Alcohol intake (4.1)
❑ Drink size/volume   FI-4.1.1
❑ Frequency   FI-4.1.2

Bioactive substance intake (4.2)
❑ Plant sterol and stanol esters   FI-4.2.1
❑ Soy protein   FI-4.2.2
❑ Psyllium and β-glucan   FI-4.2.3

Caffeine intake (4.3)
❑ Total caffeine   FI-4.3.1

Macronutrients (5)
Carbohydrate, fiber, protein, and fat and cholesterol intake from all sources, e.g., food, beverages, supplements, and via enteral and parenteral routes.

Fat and cholesterol intake (5.1)
❑ Total fat   FI-5.1.1
❑ Saturated fat   FI-5.1.2
❑ Trans fatty acids   FI-5.1.3

❑ Polyunsaturated fat   FI-5.1.4
❑ Monounsaturated fat   FI-5.1.5
❑ Omega-3 fatty acids   FI-5.1.6
  (*marine/plant derived, alpha-linolenic acid*)
❑ Dietary cholesterol   FI-5.1.7

Protein intake (5.2)
❑ Total protein   FI-5.2.1
❑ High biological value protein   FI-5.2.2
❑ Casein   FI-5.2.3
❑ Whey   FI-5.2.4
❑ Soy protein   FI-5.2.5
❑ Amino acids   FI-5.2.6
❑ Essential amino acids   FI-5.2.7

Carbohydrate intake (5.3)
❑ Total carbohydrate   FI-5.3.1
❑ Sugar   FI-5.3.2
❑ Starch   FI-5.3.3
❑ Glycemic index   FI-5.3.4
❑ Glycemic load   FI-5.3.5

Fiber intake (5.4)
❑ Total fiber   FI-5.4.1
❑ Soluble fiber   FI-5.4.2
❑ Insoluble fiber (*fructo-oligosaccharides*)   FI-5.4.3

Micronutrients (6)
Vitamins and mineral intake from all sources, e.g., food, beverages, supplements, and via enteral and parenteral routes.

Vitamin intake (6.1)
❑ A   ❑ Riboflavin
❑ C   ❑ Niacin
❑ D   ❑ Folate
❑ E   ❑ B6
❑ K   ❑ B12
❑ Thiamin
❑ Other (specify) _____

Mineral/element intake (6.2)
❑ Calcium   ❑ Potassium
❑ Iron   ❑ Sodium
❑ Magnesium   ❑ Zinc
❑ Phosphorus
❑ Other (specify) _____

**NUTRITION-RELATED
BEHAVIORAL-ENVIRONMENTAL OUTCOMES**   BE

Knowledge/Beliefs (1)
Improved understanding of nutrition concepts and change in beliefs and attitudes that increase the probability that the patient/client will successfully implement nutrition prescription/goal.

Beliefs and attitudes (1.1)
❑ Readiness to change   BE-1.1.1
❑ Perceived consequence of change   BE-1.1.2
❑ Perceived costs versus benefits of change   BE-1.1.3
❑ Perceived risk   BE-1.1.4
❑ Outcome expectancy   BE-1.1.5
❑ Conflict with personal/family value system   BE-1.1.6
❑ Self-efficacy (*breastfeeding, eating, weight loss*)   BE-1.1.7

Food and nutrition knowledge (1.2)
❑ Level of knowledge   BE-1.2.1
  (*e.g., none, limited, minimal, substantial, and extensive*)
❑ Areas of knowledge   BE-1.2.2
  (*food/nutrient requirements, physiological functions, disease/condition, nutrition recommendations, food products, consequences of food behavior, food label understanding, self-management parameters*)

Behavior (2)
Patient/client activities and actions necessary to achieve nutrition-related goals.

Ability to plan meals/snacks (2.1)
❑ Meal/snack planning ability   BE-2.1.1

Ability to select healthful food/meals (2.2)
❑ Food/meal selection   BE-2.2.1

Ability to prepare food/meals (2.3)
❑ Food/meal preparation ability   BE-2.3.1

Adherence (2.4)
❑ Self-reported adherence   BE-2.4.1

Goal setting (2.5)
❑ Goal setting ability   BE-2.5.1

Portion control (2.6)
❑ Portion size eaten   BE-2.6.1

Self-care management (2.7)
❑ Self-care management ability   BE-2.7.1

Self-monitoring (2.8)
❑ Self-monitoring ability   BE-2.8.1

Social support (2.9)
❑ Ability to build and utilize social support   BE-2.9.1

Stimulus control (2.10)
❑ Ability to manage behavior in response to stimuli   BE-2.10.1

Access (3)
Availability of a sufficient quantity of safe, healthful food.

Access to food (3.1)
❑ Access to a sufficient quantity of healthful food   BE-3.1.1
❑ Access to safe food   BE-3.1.2

Physical Activity and Function (4)
Improved physical activity and ability to engage in specific tasks (e.g., breastfeeding).

Breastfeeding success (4.1)
❑ Initiation of breastfeeding   BE-4.1.1
❑ Duration of breastfeeding   BE-4.1.2
❑ Exclusive breastfeeding   BE-4.1.3
❑ Breastfeeding problems   BE-4.1.4

Nutrition-related ADLs and IADLs (4.2)
❑ Acceptance of assistance with eating   BE-4.2.1
❑ Ability to use adaptive eating devices   BE-4.2.2
❑ Time taken to eat and consume meals   BE-4.2.3
❑ Ability to shop for food   BE-4.2.4
❑ Nutrition-related ADL   BE-4.2.5
❑ Nutrition-related IADL   BE-4.2.6

Physical activity (4.3)
❑ Consistency/frequency   BE-4.3.1
❑ Duration   BE-4.3.2
❑ Intensity   BE-4.3.3
❑ Strength   BE-4.3.4

FOOD AND NUTRIENT INTAKE OUTCOMES   FI
Energy intake (1)
Total energy intake from all sources, e.g., food, beverages, supplements, and via enteral and parenteral routes.

Energy intake (1.1)
❑ Total energy intake   FI 1.1.1

NUTRITION-RELATED PHYSICAL SIGN/SYMPTOM OUTCOMES — S

Anthropometric (1)
Measures such as weight, body mass index (BMI) percentile/age, waist circumference, and length.

Body composition/Growth (1.1)

❑ Body mass index (kg/m2)	S-1.1.1
❑ IBW or UBW percentage	S-1.1.2
❑ Growth pattern *(head circumference, length/height, weight for length/stature, BMI percentile/age, also see Weight change)*	S-1.1.3
❑ Weight/weight change *(e.g. % change , weight gain /day)*	S-1.1.4
❑ Lean body mass, fat free mass	S-1.1.5
❑ Mid-arm muscle circumference	S-1.1.6
❑ Body fat percentage	S-1.1.7
❑ Triceps skin fold	S-1.1.8
❑ Waist circumference	S-1.1.9
❑ Waist-hip ratio	S-1.1.10
❑ Bone age	S-1.1.11
❑ Bone mineral density	S-1.1.12

Biochemical and Medical Tests (2)
Lab values or medical tests such as glucose, lipids, electrolytes, and fecal fat test.

Acid-base balance (2.1)

❑ pH, serum	S-2.1.1
❑ Bicarbonate	S-2.1.2
❑ Partial pressure of carbondioxide in arterial blood	S-2.1.3

Electrolyte and renal profile (2.2)

❑ BUN	S-2.2.1
❑ Creatinine	S-2.2.2
❑ BUN:creatinine ratio	S-2.2.3
❑ Glomerular filtration rate	S-2.2.4
❑ Sodium	S-2.2.5
❑ Chloride	S-2.2.6
❑ Potassium	S-2.2.7
❑ Magnesium	S-2.2.8

Electrolyte and renal profile (2.2) (cont'd)

❑ Calcium	S-2.2.9
❑ Calcium, ionized	S-2.2.10
❑ Phosphorus	S-2.2.11
❑ Serum osmolality	S-2.2.12
❑ Parathyroid hormone	S-2.2.13

Essential fatty acid profile (2.3)

❑ Triene:Tetraene ratio	S-2.3.1

Gastrointestinal profile (2.4)

❑ Amylase	S-2.4.1
❑ Alkaline phophatase	S-2.4.2
❑ Alanine aminotransferase	S-2.4.3
❑ Aspartate aminotransferase	S-2.4.4
❑ Gamma glutamyl transferase	S-2.4.5
❑ Bilirubin, total	S-2.4.6
❑ Ammonia, serum	S-2.4.7
❑ Prothrombin time	S-2.4.8
❑ Partial thromboplastin time	S-2.4.9
❑ INR (ratio)	S-2.4.10
❑ Fecal fat	S-2.4.11

Glucose profile (2.5)

❑ Glucose, fasting	S-2.5.1
❑ Glucose, casual	S-2.5.2
❑ HgbA1c	S-2.5.3
❑ Pre-prandial capillary plasma glucose	S-2.5.4
❑ Peak postprandial capillary plasma glucose	S-2.5.5

Lipid profile (2.6)

❑ Cholesterol, serum	S-2.6.1
❑ Cholesterol, HDL	S-2.6.2
❑ Cholesterol, LDL	S-2.6.3
❑ Triglycerides, serum	S-2.6.4

Mineral profile (2.7)

❑ Copper, serum	S-2.7.1
❑ Iodine, urinary excretion	S-2.7.2
❑ Thyroid stimulating hormone	S-2.7.3
❑ Zinc, plasma	S-2.7.4

Nutritional anemia profile (2.8)

❑ Hemoglobin	S-2.8.1
❑ Hematocrit	S-2.8.2
❑ Mean corpuscular volume	S-2.8.3
❑ Red blood cell folate	S-2.8.5
❑ Red cell distribution width	S-2.8.6
❑ Serum B12	S-2.8.7
❑ Serum methylmalonic acid	S-2.8.8
❑ Serum folate	S-2.8.9
❑ Serum homocysteine	S-2.8.10
❑ Serum ferritin	S-2.8.11
❑ Serum iron	S-2.8.12
❑ Total iron-binding capacity	S-2.8.13
❑ Transferrin saturation	S-2.8.14

Protein profile (2.9)

❑ Albumin	S-2.9.1
❑ Prealbumin	S-2.9.2
❑ Transferrin	S-2.9.3
❑ Phenylalanine, plasma	S-2.9.4
❑ Tyrosine, plasma	S-2.9.5

Respiratory quotient (2.10)

❑ RQ	S-2.10.1

Urine profile (2.11)

❑ Urine color	S-2.11.1
❑ Urine osmolality	S-2.11.2
❑ Urine specific gravity	S-2.11.3
❑ Urine tests *(e.g., ketones, sugar, protein)*	S-2.11.4
❑ Urine volume	S-2.11.5

Vitamin profile (2.12)

❑ Vitamin A *(serum or plasma retinol)*	S-2.12.1
❑ Vitamin C *(plasma or serum)*	S-2.12.2
❑ Vitamin D *(25-hydroxy)*	S-2.12.3
❑ Vitamin E *(plasma alpha-tocopherol)*	S-2.12.4
❑ Thiamin *(activity coefficient for erythrocyte transketolase activity)*	S-2.12.5
❑ Riboflavin *(activity coefficient for erythrocyte glutathione reductase activity)*	S-2.12.6
❑ Niacin *(urinary N'methyl-nicotinamide concentration)*	S-2.12.7
❑ Vitamin B6 *(plasma or serum pyridoxal 5'phosphate concentration)*	S-2.12.8

Physical Examination (3)
Physical exam parameters such as such as edema, nausea, vomiting, bowel function, skin integrity, and blood pressure.

Nutrition physical exam findings (3.1)

❑ Cardiovascular-pulmonary *(pulmonary edema)*	S-3.1.1
❑ Extremities, musculo-skeletal *(e.g., nails, subcutaneous fat, muscle)*	S-3.1.2
❑ Gastrointestinal *(e.g., nausea, vomiting, bowel function)*	S-3.1.3
❑ Head and neck *(e.g., tongue, mouth, and hair changes)*	S-3.1.4
❑ Neurological *(e.g., confusion, fine/gross motor)*	S-3.1.5
❑ Skin *(e.g., appearance, turgor, integrity)*	S-3.1.6
❑ Vital signs *(blood pressure, respiratory rate)*	S-3.1.7

NUTRITION-RELATED PATIENT/CLIENT-CENTERED OUTCOMES — PC

Nutrition Quality of Life (1)
Patient/client's perception of his/her nutrition intervention and its impact on life.

Nutrition quality of life (1.1)

❑ Food impact	PC-1.1.1
❑ Physical state	PC-1.1.2
❑ Psychological factors	PC-1.1.3
❑ Self-image	PC-1.1.4
❑ Self-efficacy	PC-1.1.5
❑ Social/interpersonal factors	PC-1.1.6
❑ Nutrition quality of life score	PC-1.1.7

Satisfaction (2)
To be added